TREATING TROUBLED CHILDREN
AND THEIR FAMILIES

TREATING TROUBLED CHILDREN AND THEIR FAMILIES

Ellen F. Wachtel

THE GUILFORD PRESS
New York London

*This book is dedicated to my brother, Joel,
to my children, Kenneth and Karen,
and to my husband, Paul;
each in his or her own way has taught me
about the multiple dimensions of love.*

©1994; Preface: A Decade Later ©2004 Ellen F. Wachtel
Published by The Guilford Press
A Division of Guilford Publications, Inc.
72 Spring Street, New York, NY 10012
www.guilford.com

Paperback edition 2004

Printed in the United States of America

This book is printed on acid-free paper.

Last digit is print number: 9   8   7

Library of Congress Cataloging-in-Publication Data

Wachtel, Ellen F.
    Treating troubled children and their families / Ellen F. Wachtel
      p.   cm.
    Includes bibliographical references and index.
    ISBN 0-89862-007-4 (hc.)—ISBN 1-59385-072-7 (pbk.)
    1. Child psychotherapy.   2. Family psychotherapy.   I. Title.
RJ504.W23   1994
618.92′8914—dc20
                                                      94-8553
                                                        CIP

Preface: A Decade Later

In the decade since *Treating Troubled Children and Their Families* was first published, I have given dozens of workshops to mental health professionals both in the United States and abroad on the approach to working with children and families described in this book. And although over the years I have added a variety of clinical interventions to my work, it has been gratifying to see how the basic approach spelled out in the book has remained helpful to both parents and professionals. Many of the participants in my workshops have told me that they first read the book as students in graduate school but keep the book handy because they refer to it again and again when they are feeling "stuck."

It also has been rewarding to see that the central tenets of the approach—integrating an in-depth understanding of the individual issues of the child into work with the family; translating complex understandings into active and concrete interventions; utilizing the adults in the child's life as the agents of change; integrating systemic, psychodynamic, behavioral, and cognitive perspectives; emphasizing positives; working collaboratively with teachers, parents, foster parents, and other significant adults in the child's life—have been applicable to work with ethnically and economically diverse populations.

Over the years I have found that the ideas in this book lend themselves not only to therapy with emotionally troubled children and their families, but to consultations with parents around developmental challenges and crises that are part of the normal stresses and strains of parenting. Parents have been grateful for the very specific suggestions that emerge when one combines in-depth understanding of the child's concerns with systemic, behavioral, and cognitive approaches. As can be seen in the dozens of case examples throughout this book, small changes can have profound effects.

Among the new ideas introduced subsequent to the original publication of the book, perhaps the most important is what I have called the "language of becoming." I have found that by noticing and reflecting back the specific ways in which the child is *becoming* more able to calm himself, more self-confident, more affectionate to his brother, etc., the parent gives a meta-message that one's personality is not set in stone but rather is something that evolves and changes over time. I have found that parents, children, and therapists have all eagerly embraced this new intervention, which helps children change how they think about themselves. As a supplement to this book, I strongly suggest that readers look at an article I wrote on this topic, "The Language of Becoming: Helping Children Change How They Think about Themselves" (*Family Process,* Vol. 40, No. 4, 2001).

The "language of becoming" can only be used effectively, however, when some noticeable change, albeit small, has actually occurred, and the work described in this book is the meat and potatoes of helping children and families to make those changes. The publication of a paperback edition will make the book available to students in psychiatric and pediatric residencies, clinical and school psychology, counseling, social work, psychiatric nursing, and other professions concerned with mental health and the well-being of children. My thanks to all the readers and workshop participants whose feedback has enlivened my practice and furthered my thinking on these issues. I look forward to yet more lively exchanges. Please feel free to contact me at *efwachtel@yahoo.com.*

ELLEN F. WACHTEL

Acknowledgments

The seeds from which the ideas in this book germinated were planted in the rich intellectual soil of the Ackerman Institute for Family Therapy, where in 1974 and then from 1976 until 1978 I received intensive training in family therapy. Under the directorship of Donald Bloch, the Ackerman Institute was, and still is today (now under the directorship of Peter Steinglass), a true intellectual mecca where diverse ideas can be explored, argued, tested, elaborated on, and sometimes retired. It was there that I was exposed to the brilliant systemic understandings and reframings of Olga Silverstein, with whom I trained, as well as to stimulating presentations of psychodynamic perspectives on family interactions. My thanks go to the faculty at Ackerman as well as to my fellow students, who now, as Ackerman faculty, continue the tradition of intellectual openness and commitment to finding the best ways of helping families.

My thanks too go to my colleagues in the Society for the Exploration of Psychotherapy Integration (SEPI). My work with both families and individuals has been greatly influenced by the stimulation of formal presentations and informal conversations at SEPI meetings and by articles in its journal, the *Journal of Psychotherapy Integration*. One of the cases discussed in the last chapter was first written up for that journal (1992; copyright 1992 by Plenum Press, reprinted by permission) and was greatly enhanced by the probing comments and questions of the journal's editor, Hal Arkowitz.

Another of the cases discussed in Chapter 9 first appeared in the *Journal of Marital and Family Therapy* (1987; copyright 1987 by the American Association for Marriage and Family Therapy, reprinted by permission). I am grateful to Alan Gurman, who was then editor (and is also a member of SEPI), for offering extremely useful feedback which helped me clarify and sharpen the ideas that are the foundations for this book.

Still another of the cases presented here originally appeared in the *Journal of Strategic and Systemic Therapies* (1990; copyright 1990 by Donald Efron, reprinted by permission). I wish to thank the editor for permission to reprint parts of that article here.

The excellent students from the New York University Clinical Psychology Ph.D. program whom I have supervised over the years have contributed much to the ideas in this book. Their highly intelligent questions challenged me to carefully think through my approach and I have learned a great deal by helping them integrate the various perspectives to which they have been exposed in their training.

I want also to thank Marsha Shelov, a dear friend and colleague from my student days at Ackerman, for her excitement, encouragement, and help in getting my first article on integration published ("Learning Family Therapy: The Dilemmas of an Individual Therapist," 1979). Over the years we have had many valuable exchanges about ways to better help children and families and she and her colleagues at the Taconic Counseling Group have done very innovative work which they have shared with me.

Special thanks too goes to Zina Steinberg for the time and care she gave to reading several chapters. Her experience as an educator, researcher, child therapist, and family therapist made her comments particularly useful.

Maria Alba Fisch, as usual, gave of herself with great generosity. Her fine mind, sensitivity, and expertise on working with children made her feedback on several chapters a precious gift.

And last, a word about the thanks I owe to my husband, Paul Wachtel. We did not know it at the time, but when we first met nearly 30 years ago the quest for integration had begun. Although I was then in law school, my undergraduate education had been strongly Adlerian in orientation, and I was at that point rather fiercely opposed to psychoanalysis. Much to my chagrin, Paul, fresh out of graduate school, had psychoanalytic leanings! Laughter, friendship, passion, and most of all love overcame our incompatibilities, and together we have lived a life in which the dynamic tension between individually evolving viewpoints has been constantly stimulating and enriching. To thank my husband for his help on this book seems almost besides the point. Yes, his editorial assistance was invaluable. He went over every word with a fine-toothed comb and his opinion on substantive points as well were of tremendous importance to me. Yet, in keeping with the theme of this book, I cannot really separate out the part from the whole. He has been my supporter, fan, friend, lover, intellectual mate, and father to our children, and though we are very much separate individuals we have also shaped and created one another. My gratitude to him is for his very being and our whole life together.

Preface

This book is not a finished product. For many years I have been search-
ing for ways to better help young children who are having a difficult time
of it, and even as the fruits of this quest appear in print the approach
continues to evolve. Each case seems to require at least some variation
in what I have done before, and questions and challenges remain. I am
more and more impressed, for instance, with the power of siblings to
affect each other's core sense of self and hope in the future to better understand and influence this process. And I wonder too about how to better help youngsters who are sorely deficient in empathy or who just do
not seem to be attuned to social cues or even to their physical environment. My goal here, therefore, is not to present a neatly packaged therapeutic program but rather to describe a general point of view which I
hope will stimulate readers to explore and experiment on their own. I
would like very much to hear from readers and find out where the recommendations in this book have and have not proved helpful. I would like
as well to learn about new applications and variations that readers develop.

    Despite the numerous variations in the work presented here, several
features are constants. To begin with, this is primarily a short-term approach. There are, to be sure, children who require long-term intensive
psychotherapy. Occasionally, I refer a child with whom I am working
for such work, and on other occasions I take on a family in which the
child is or has been in a more long-term individual treatment. But whenever
possible, I try to make use of the resiliency and growth potential of both
children and parents and intervene actively to mobilize for change more
rapidly than is sometimes thought possible. To be sure, there are
conflicts—in both parents and children—that are deep and protracted
and require much work. It is an error to assume, for example, that just
because parents *want* to change they will be able to do so quickly and

consistently. It is equally an error to ground one's approach on theories that, in stressing "deep" pathology, inevitably reach the conclusion in case after case that only long term intensive therapy will overcome inevitable and entrenched resistances. A distinguishing feature of the approach described here is an abiding—if also skeptical—faith in the capacity of people to change and a persistent emphasis on making contact with, and enhancing, their adaptive resources and simple goodwill. Often the crucial difference in whether a parent, for example, seems malevolent or simply someone not doing well with his or her child at a particular point is whether the therapist *sees* the parent as malevolent. One's eyes must be open, to be sure, but so must one's heart.

It will be apparent to the reader that my role as therapist is in a large measure as coach and catalyst. It is the parent with whom the child spends the greatest amount of time and who is usually the most powerful emotional force in the child's life. My aim as a therapist is, one might say, to "give away" my skills, to enable the *parent* to become the key therapeutic agent in the child's life. My role is certainly an active one—this kind of work, indeed, can be exhausting—but it is in the empowerment and enlightenment of the parent that it bears fruit.

Although I received my doctorate from a program that at the time was almost exclusively psychoanalytically oriented, and do work with individuals in a modified form of psychodynamic therapy (see Wachtel & Wachtel [1986], *Family Dynamics and Individual Psychotherapy*), the work I am about to describe derives largely from my training as a family therapist. Yet, the avoidance of strict categorizations of this sort is largely what this book is about. All too often too neatly defined professional identities limit our therapeutic options. Although child therapists may occasionally have a family session or family therapists may sometimes see a child alone, there is often a sense that one is breaking a rule and working outside the paradigm to which one subscribes. Identification with a particular school of therapy limits not only *who* we see but *what* we see as well. Like the blind men of the famous Sufi fable who each describe only a part of the elephant, we may end up with an image of the problem which though partially correct is not the whole truth.

This book is part of a larger integrative project in which I and many others share. Increasingly therapists from a variety of persuasions have been finding that the orientation in which they were trained provides them not only with a lens to focus but with blinders as well. Through my participation in the Society for the Exploration of Psychotherapy Integration I have seen the excitement and the increase in understanding that come when therapists of a variety of orientations talk to each other rather than just debate. In this book I am attempting to continue that dialogue, but I am also to some degree talking to myself. I continually ask myself how psychodynamic and behavioral perspectives can enhance the family systems orientations that was my first language, so to speak, for thinking about children and their difficulties.

The majority of integrative efforts thus far have been directed toward work with adults. It is my hope in this book to make a contribution to the application of integrative thinking toward work with young children and their families. The particular form of integration I am describing is intended primarily for work with families where the child manifesting difficulties is a preadolescent or younger. Although the use of multiple perspectives to understand the various facets of a child's difficulties would, of course, be applicable to adolescents as well as to young children, the methods and interventions that are described are not necessarily transferable to work with teens. Many adolescents require privacy and the promise of confidentiality if they are going to feel comfortable talking about their difficulties, and the free flow of information which is part of the work with parents and young children is often not appropriate with adolescents.

I have randomly throughout this book referred to the therapist, the parent, and the child (when either is being referred to in the abstract rather than as a particular actual individual) sometimes as he and sometimes as she. This accomplishes the purpose of correcting the bias inherent in the traditional use of he as the abstract pronoun while avoiding the awkwardness of sentences strewn with "he and she" or "him and her."

Needless to say, the details of the identities of the families discussed have been altered. I have made a variety of changes in the identifying features of the children and the parents in order to protect their privacy. In all instances the essence of the children's characteristics and difficulties and of the therapeutic challenge they presented has been retained.

Contents

1

The Child as an Individual: An Introduction to Child-in-Family Therapy

F amily systems thinking offers a unique and major advance in our understanding of children's difficulties. Viewing children's problems as a product of ongoing interactions, rather than simply a reflection of something coming from within, provides a crucial perspective that we forget at our peril. Today, almost 40 years since its inception, the systemic model has gained wide acceptance not only within the profession but among the general public as well.

Yet despite the general recognition of the importance of the systemic dimension in children's difficulties, family therapists tend not to be regarded as experts on children's problems. Schools and mental health professionals still tend to refer troubled children to therapists identified as child therapists. They regard family therapy as a possible adjunct to the child's individual treatment rather than as an appropriate therapeutic modality in itself.

Systems approaches and individually oriented approaches to psychotherapy have been seen as contradictory orientations about which the clinician must make a choice. Although there have been many attempts to explore the interface between the two perspectives when working with adults, the literature on integrating systemic and individual perspectives with young children is quite sparse. With few exceptions (e.g., Duhl & Duhl, 1981; Feldman, 1985, 1988, 1992; Gold, 1988; Pinsof, 1983), clinicians working with young children line up in camps; family therapists see child therapists as "pathologizing" children (Combrinck-Graham,

1989; Haley, 1976; Kaslow & Racusin, 1990), while child therapists see family therapists as oversimplifying and ignoring the child's intrapsychic life (McDermott & Char, 1974).

This book argues that the reason family therapy has not fully taken hold in the treatment of problems centered on children's difficulties is that in their efforts to develop strictly systemic perspectives, family therapists have tended to act as if the decades of child therapy that preceded the systemic perspective simply had no relevance. Ironically, an approach developed to broaden our perspective and rescue the child from being labeled as the "patient" has unwittingly led to the *neglect* of the child by many family therapists. In a fashion uncomfortably (and almost literally) replicating the proverbial saying, family therapists have "thrown out the baby with the bath water."

When parents consult a family therapist because of a troubled child, they are likely to detect in the therapist's questions the verbal equivalent of a raised eyebrow. Trained to be alert to covert alliances between a symptomatic child and a parent or to the role a child having difficulties plays in a troubled marriage, family therapists aim in the first few sessions to redefine the problem as systemic rather than that of the individual child. From its inception, family therapy looked at the child's difficulties with a wide-angle lens. Instead of seeing the family *of* the patient, the family was regarded *as* the patient (Bloch & LaPerriere, 1973).

One needs only to read the child therapy literature to realize what a dramatic and profound paradigm shift the systemic perspective entailed. No longer was the child's problem regarded as something that resided *within* him, with the implication that the *child* needed to or could be "fixed," but rather a youngster's emotional difficulties were understood both as a symptom of family dysfunction and as serving a role in the family's life. Anyone who has ever watched videotapes or studied the theories of Salvador Minuchin, for instance, can have no doubt of the validity and power of this point of view.

This book's starting point lies in this extraordinarily valuable work. Its intention is not to challenge or disregard the advances in understanding that family systems thinking has brought, but rather to modify what I believe is an imbalance that has developed. Specifically, I wish to call attention to what I would call top-down systemic thinking — systemic thinking that focuses too much on the influence of the system on the child and insufficiently on the reverse.

Now that it is a mature discipline, family therapy no longer needs to stake out its claim against any and all contenders. Instead, family therapy must find a way to use and creatively integrate into family work with children that which is valuable in other approaches. In so doing, it will also make it possible for therapists who primarily identify themselves as child therapists — whether psychoanalytic, behavioral, or any other persuasion — to incorporate a systemic perspective into their work. This, I believe, will be a gain for both points of view.

THE EXCLUSION OF CHILDREN
FROM FAMILY THERAPY

Although many of the most influential clinicians and theoreticians in the field of family therapy have advocated the inclusion of children in sessions (Ackerman, 1970; Minuchin, 1974; Satir, 1964; Keith & Whitaker, 1981), it is nonetheless common for family therapist to dismiss children from the work after just a few sessions. Notwithstanding the commitment in principle to circular notions of causality, in practice, systemic thinking can lead to an almost exclusive concentration on the adult side of interactions. As Korner and Brown (1990) note on the basis of a survey about the beliefs and practices of familiy therapists, "The exclusion of children from family psychotherapy appears to be a fairly common and widespread practice" (p. 427). As Chasin and White (1989) put it:

> Children are excluded as a matter of course by therapists whose theoretical persuasions justify their working principally or entirely with adults and their families of origin (Bowen, 1978). Yet many who espouse approaches that call for direct observations and intervention with members of all generations omit children from most sessions in practice. Perhaps the most popular explanation they give for this omission is that the heart of the problem and the ultimate key to the solution lie in the parental subsystem: therefore, seeing the parents alone is the most efficient way to help the family. (p. 6)

Unfortunately, many family therapists feel ill-equipped to work with young children even when they do recognize the importance of doing so. The exclusion of children from meetings seems to reflect discomfort with having children in the sessions at least as much as it does an overreliance on theoretical perspectives linking children's symptoms to marital dysfunction (Bloch, 1976; Chasin & White, 1989; Combrinck-Graham, 1986, 1991; Keith, 1986, Korner, 1988; Zilbach, 1986). Zilbach (1986), who examined attitudes of family therapists toward the inclusion of children through both a review of the literature and direct interviews, concludes that "many family therapists only minimally recognize when, how, or why they exclude children. . . . Exclusion is often based on inner reluctance or even strong aversion to playing with children" (p. 20). Combrinck-Graham (1986) similarly notes that in addition to excluding children because the child's dysfunction is seen as resulting from a problem in the marriage, family therapists "have little training in working with children; therefore, they tend to avoid it, if possible" (p. x).[1]

Keith (1986) has suggested that family therapists may exclude children because "the spontaneity that children add may cause confusion so that the therapist feels incompetent" (p. 2). Diller (1991) quotes Chasin, president of the American Family Therapy Association and director of the Cambridge Family Institute, as saying:

> It's a long-standing embarrassment in the field, that people expect family therapists to be good at working with children, but often they have no training or information to do this work, as well as no experience, no interest and no energy. As a result they find very ingenious ways of doing good work . . . while managing to avoid dealing directly with kids. (p. 18)

Recently, there has been some increased attention in the literature to the question of how to incorporate young children in family sessions and use their presence for therapeutic purposes (Benson, Schindler-Zimmerman, & Martin, 1991; Chasin & White, 1989; Zilbach, 1986). Nonetheless, as Combrinck-Graham (1991) puts it, "[There is] a dearth of literature about children in family therapy, and there is a general impression that children, especially the very young, are either excluded from treatment altogether or treated by specially trained therapists in individual sessions" (p. 373).

This volume aims to contribute to filling this gap. Its intent is to give therapists not only a theoretical framework that incorporates individual and systemic perspectives but also specific recommendations regarding ways to engage youngsters meaningfully in family therapy.

THE CHILD AND THE SYSTEM:
A REVIEW OF SYSTEMIC HYPOTHESES

I wish to begin with a brief review of what the systemic perspective offers and what has been left out. Family therapy provided an invaluable corrective to the individualistic assumptions that long dominated work with children. However, in most cases an exclusively systemic perspective is not enough. To be maximally effective, clinicians need also to utilize in their work with families both psychodynamic and behavioral understandings of the child as an individual. This book presents the ideas and methods of a fully integrative approach, and it is my hope that it will prove useful to a wide range of therapists.

The Triangulation of Children

Perhaps the most uniformly accepted idea in family therapy is that a child's difficulties are usually linked to some conflict between adults in the family. When one looks at a child's problems through a systemic lens, one frequently sees that the child is part of a triangular interaction in which stress between adults is either deflected or expressed through the child's difficulties. Minuchin (1974) calls these types of interactions "rigid triads."

Various types of triadic systems are possible. For instance, there may be constantly shifting coalitions in the family in which adults who are in covert conflict with one another subtly attempt to enlist the child's support. The child's symptoms may be an expression of the stress he feels about having to make loyalty-laden choices. When there is open conflict between adults, a stable, rather than shifting, coalition may be formed in which a child identifies with one parent only, at the price of becoming alienated from the other parent, who is regarded as the outsider if not the enemy.

A couple may also use their child to aid in the *denial* of conflict between themselves. Minuchin calls this kind of triad "detouring." The "detouring–attacking" mode is one in which the parents unite in their assessment of their child as "bad" and in need of parental control. Similarly, parents can mask their differences by the "detouring–supportive" mode in which they jointly focus on a child who is considered "sick."

The Child as Self-Sacrificing

From a variety of family systems perspectives (E. Wachtel & P. Wachtel, 1986), children are regarded as sacrificing themselves in order to prevent the disintegration of the parents' marriage. Whereas the concept of "triangulation" tends to see the child as being assigned a role and sucked up by the system, the self-sacrifing view regards the youngster as rather actively engaged in maintaining a "troubled" role for the sake of the family. Self-sacrifice on the part of symptomatic family members (children as well as adults) is regarded as a regular concomitant of attachment and family ties. Over and over again this theme is discussed in the literature. Haley (1979) and Boszormenyi-Nagy and Ulrich (1981), for example, whose theories have little else in common, agree in seeing the child's difficulties as arising out of loyalty to parents and a wish to save the parents' marriage from destruction. The psychoanalytically oriented family therapist Robin Skynner (1981) observes that "the 'sick' member . . . colludes in the process out of a deep, if unconscious, recognition that he is preserving the parent, the marriage or the family as a whole from disintegrating, out of a motive of attachment as well as guilt" (pp. 46–47). Similarly, the decidedly unpsychoanalytic view of Madanes (1984), which regards interactions around children's symptoms as metaphors for other problematic interactions in the family, approaches symptomatic behavior in children by asking, "In what way is the child's plan helpful and what is unfortunate about this mode of helpfulness? The child's plan to help the parents often creates a problem worse than the one he is intending to solve" (Madanes, 1986, p. 185). Still another distinctive approach to symptomatic family members, the Milan school, with its emphasis on paradox and prescriptions, assumes that the symptomatic individual is in some way being helpful to the family and reframes the problem as the apparently ill child's really being the one who is taking responsibility for the family (Hoffman, 1981).

The Child as Receptacle for Projections

A related commonly held systemic understanding of children's symptoms is that the child has become the receptacle for projections and distortions on the part of the parents.[2] Disowned aspects of the self are embodied in the child, and the parents, through identification with the child, can both reject and gratify conflictual aspects of the self. Projective identification may be thought of as something like "having your cake and eating it too." Ackerman (1966), one of the earliest writers to apply the psychodynamic idea of projection, to families describes a case in which the nonconforming, difficult child "was not really the outsider, different and alien . . . [but] was their spokesman in an important but neglected area of life" (p. 236). Similarly, Stierlin (1977) regards the symptomatic child as the "delegate" of the family, who is perceived by the family as the cause of its misery but who in actuality represents "their disowned badness or madness" (p. 203). Framo (1980) too points out that "intimates collusively carry psychic functions for each other" (p. viii).

In practical terms, this perspective means that when a family therapist sees an angry, acting-out child, not only does the therapist ask himself what function this behavior serves in the family system, but also how anger and aggression are dealt with by other family members. For example, a parent who is defending against his own anger at authority figures may give messages to the child regarding the child's hostile behavior to teachers who say "don't" and "do" at one and the same time. The concept of projective identification suggests that the parent can reinforce his defenses against anger by expressing disapproval, and at the same time can vicariously gratify the forbidden wish through identification with the child.

It is important to note that the parent does not merely "see" in the child traits that are not there but, rather, often stimulates and induces concerns and anxieties which then *do* become the child's. Laing (1965), calling this process mystification, describes the parents as actively but covertly molding the child's feelings while disqualifying or invalidating the child's self-determined and differentiated point of view It is the nature of collusive defense mechanisms that this process is going on unconsciously.

Children as Embodying Ghosts from the Past

A similar process occurs when a child, rather than being induced to embody significant but conflictual aspects of the self, is instead led to play out roles of significant others in one's past with whom there is unfinished business. Thus, a child who has unconscious conflicts around dependency may be confused because she is picking up a *parent's* wish to be parented. Or, conversely, a child may be plagued by monstrously angry feelings because a parent is working through some issues around a tyrannical parent. The child is not simply *seen* as "tyrannical" but is actually induced to behave that way. In other instances parents look to their children for the closeness and nurturance that was missing in their childhood. Many family therapists believe that children who are having difficulty with separation are staying home in order to look after a parent whose needs for nurturing have not been satisfied.

GOING BEYOND SYMPTOM RELIEF

Armed with these three concepts — (1) that there is a structural problem in the family in which the symptomatic child is part of a dysfunctional triangle, (2) that the child is sacrificing himself in order to hold the family together, and (3) that the child is induced into acting out disowned aspects of self or is playing the role of family members with whom there is unfinished business — family therapists have succeeded impressively in looking at the child's problem with a wide-angle lens. The literature is replete with reports of the rapid alleviation of symptoms in children when these kinds of systemic analyses are used.

Generally, symptom alleviation is the primary or even exclusive goal in a family therapist's work with children. This is because it is commonly believed that once the child is relieved of her role as symptom bearer for the family, she will get back on the normal developmental path and no special interventions will be necessary (Keith, 1986). Although this certainly may be the case in some instances, rapid and dramatic symptom relief may distract therapists from working with the child on issues that are not so obvious or as easily resolved. Family therapists often put unnecessary limitations on what they can offer children. For instance, the rapid response of a suicidal adolescent to interventions based on an understanding of her behavior as a reaction to her parent's imminent separation (Madanes, 1986) could be thought of as the *beginning* of the work with the child rather than the end. Unless we address individual issues such as the child's difficulty in knowing and expressing her feelings, or the child's inability to calm herself down, her feeling of being overwhelmed and having no options, or her sense of despair—we do the child a serious disservice. Although the child might do "fine" in the sense of getting back on track (going to school, relating to peers), without a more in-depth approach one wonders how she will handle future stress. Fear of pathologizing children has led to an excessive "normalizing" of children who could really benefit from further psychotherapeutic work.

McDermott and Char (1974) have argued that "specialized attention and skill need to be paid to the disturbed child in order to understand and to treat him and his problems. He has a right to be a patient, and understood and treated as a patient, just as much as his parents" (p. 428). Though many family therapists still feel that as "the health of the family expands so does the children's health" (Keith, 1986, p. 2), there has been increasing concern on the part of family therapists that the children's dysfunction is being treated solely as a marital issue (Combrinck-Graham, 1986). Papp (1986) has described as a "common myth" of family therapy that if you relieve children of their role as mediator they will be symptom free and well adjusted. Similarly, Rosman (1986) points out that "releasing the child from his role as savior doesn't automatically enable him to develop normally. Children may be left after their 'cure' with enormous social–emotional handicaps" (p. 229).

Our assessment of the "success" of family treatment depends on what we are looking at. Sider (1984) has pointed out the following:

> The choice of therapeutic modality involves a decision about a specific outcome as well as the means of achieving that end. Psychoanalysts may aim for structural character change, family therapists for improved family dynamics, behaviorists for anxiety reduction and psychopharmacologists for relief of psychotic symptoms. (p. 390)

Most family therapists do seem to exclude from their work with young children and their families consideration of the child's internal psychic reality. Little attention is given to such questions as the following: What is the child's self-image? Does the child experience the world as a hostile or dangerous place? Is he frightened of his own anger? Does the child have the ego capacities that one would expect at this age? Can she modulate anxiety? Has there been a failure to differentiate from a parent? Is there difficulty in accepting good and bad aspects of self and others so that "splitting" occurs? What are the kind and extent of the child's defense mechanisms? We do a disservice to children and families if we fail to address these questions. By meeting with children alone and integrating an in-depth understanding of the symptomatic child into the family work, therapists can address such concerns without pathologizing children or engaging them and their families in long-term therapy. Chapter 4 gives specific guidelines for using individual meetings with the child to assess these broader issues and Chapters 7 and 8 describe ways to work with families and children to resolve unconscious conflicts and to modify maladaptive defense mechanisms.

Some Unfortunate Consequences of Top-Down Systemic Thinking

As discussed earlier in this chapter, the systemic perspective ironically can result in a failure to really get to know the children in the family. When family therapists see marital problems and troubled children, they tend to assume that the marital difficulties came *first* and in that sense caused the child to have problems. Often insufficient attention is given to the possibility that the marital problems may have partly arisen out of the stress of attempting to deal with a difficult and troubled child.

Bogdan (1986), in an article titled "Do Families Really Need Problems?," pointed out:

> When a child acts up, it might indeed happen that his parents' attention gets focused on him, and therefore, the parents have fewer opportunities to argue between themselves. *At issue is not the existence of such patterns, but their appropriate interpretation. Are these consequences accidental or are they, for lack of a better word, meaningful?* (p. 30, italics added)

In "The Undeclared War between Child and Family Therapy," McDermott and Char (1974) point out the obvious fact that marital problems do not always create disturbed children. They criticize family therapists for not giving sufficient attention to the child "who has his own changing characteristics, perceptions, needs distortions and capacities which make him different from the adults in the system. . . . The child is not simply a pawn in the game-playing between adults" (p. 425). There is much truth in this characterization of family therapy, although the solution is not to abandon a systemic approach but rather to find ways to be more responsive to the children.

An exclusively systemic theoretical perspective leads not only to the dismissal of children from sessions, as discussed earlier in the chapter, but also to children's often remaining essentially *unknown* even when they *are* included in sessions. Children (even outgoing ones) are generally harder to get to know than adults. Unlike adults, who—at least in comparison to children—tend to be adept at talking descriptively about themselves, and who thus become known to us as individuals, children are often known only in terms of their role in the family system. When we perceive children exclusively through systemic lenses, it is easy for us to overlook children's idiosyncratic characteristics and regard them in such noncomplex categorical terms as "parentified child," "triangulated child," "mother's ally" and "father's spokesman." With children, much more than with adults, special efforts must be made to get to know them more fully.

With some modifications in traditional ways of working, family therapists can readily get a more in depth sense of the child's individual strengths and difficulties. It is important to know, for example, how a child's temperaments and anxieties contribute to family dysfunction or how the child's efforts to deal with his or her anxieties affect the system. Without this sort of information we are essentially working with one hand tied behind our back. Children have a life that exists separate and apart from their families', and some of their concerns are best understood from an individual rather than a systemic perspective. Top-down systemic approaches do not leave room to incorporate into the work such questions as the following: What are the child's unconscious conflicts that might be contributing to his or her difficulties? What is the child's coping style? Does the child withdraw from difficult tasks or does he or she persist even when frustrated? Does the child have poor social skills? Is she excessively cautious? reckless? obsessive? Much of this book elaborates on how this type of information might be obtained and then worked with in the context of family therapy.

Another unfortunate consequence of top-down systemic thinking is that often we do not make sufficient use of the child's capacity to alter problematic interactions and consequently to alter the family system. With few exceptions (e.g., Combrinck-Graham, 1986; Guerin & Gordon, 1986; Stierlin, 1977), family therapists do not focus on the child's role in maintaining problematic patterns of interaction. A number of years ago, Montalvo and Haley (1973) published a fascinating article on child therapy titled "In Defense of Child Therapy," in which they point out that many family therapists disregard therapeutic approaches that have a long and respected history and thus overlook the valuable contributions made by earlier therapeutic modes. Detailing the many ways that individual work with a child leads to structural change in the family, they conclude that it is the inadvertent but inevitable *systemic* effects that lead to change. They argue, for instance, that the child who regresses as a result of individual therapy influences the therapist to influence the parents, or that when the child therapist's permissiveness in the session leads to an exaggeration of out-of-control behavior at home, this in turn provokes the parents to set limits.

Although there seems to be a great deal of truth to Montalvo and

Haley's analysis, the one aspect of child therapy that is not addressed is the direct help the child gets in resolving intrapsychic as well as interpersonal difficulties and in changing his or her side of problematic interactions. The fact that changes in the child brought about *directly* by the child therapy might in turn initiate further changes in the family is a phenomenon that is completely ignored. The assumption is that only systemic interventions really help, and embedded in their ironic "praise" of individual therapy is the same top-down assumption that still dominates the family therapy literature: When parents change, the child gets better.

Although they may come to therapy reluctantly, children generally feel quite miserable about the difficulties they are having with parents and teachers. Even if they are in fact playing a "saving, self-sacrificing" role in the family, they are usually not at all happy with the state of affairs generated by their being the "identified patient." Most children are highly motivated to solve their problems and feel upset about the negative interactions they are having with parents, teachers, or peers. Often they feel stuck and simply do not know what to do to make things better. The eagerness with which many young children take in suggestions on ways to interact differently is underutilized by therapists who believe that the child needs to hold on to his symptom because it is serving a function in the family. Concentration on the adult side of interactions leads to neglect of a powerful force for change, the child's wish for harmonious relationships. Chapter 8 details ways to help children change their side of problematic systemic interactions.

Perhaps the most important unfortunate limitation of top-down thinking is that children are not being offered the direct and specific help they need in overcoming their difficulties. Thus, when family therapists do include in the systemic work a focus on the child's role in interactions, they generally do not provide direct assistance to the child in resolving individual issues. Like the trickle-down theory of conservative economists, who believe that those at the bottom of our society will be best aided by attending to the circumstance of those on top, skewed or top-down systemic thinking regards direct attention to the individuals most in trouble as somehow counterproductive. A broader view of family therapy would incorporate an understanding of the child's individual issues into the systemic work. Active interventions designed to address such individual issues as the child's oversensitivity to criticism, low self-esteem, poor relationships with peers, and conflicts around aggression, to name but a few, would be incorporated into the work. Chapters 7 and 8 elaborate on how sessions with the whole family, various subsystems, and the child alone can incorporate and directly address these individual issues of the child.

AN INTEGRATIVE APPROACH

The work with families described in this book is "integrative" in two senses of the word. First, it integrates individual and systemic theoretical perspectives on emotional distress and psychopathology. Second, it is integrative in that it borrows and modifies interventions developed in a variety of therapeutic orientations, such as behavior therapy, cognitive therapy, and psychoanalytically oriented therapy. An underlying assumption is that one can utilize some of the therapeutic interventions of a variety of approaches without fully subscribing to any particular school's conceptualization of the problem. Nor is it necessary to adopt *in toto* the clinical practices generally associated with that particular approach. Thus, as described in an earlier work (E. Wachtel & P. Wachtel, 1986), individual therapy based on psychodynamic understanding can fruitfully incorporate active interventions derived from behavioral and systemic approaches (methods generally eschewed by traditional psychodynamic therapists on the grounds that they obscure the development of the transference). Similarly, family therapy can incorporate some behavioral or psychodynamic interventions without losing the centrality of a systemic perspective.

SYSTEMS AND THE PARTIAL
AUTONOMY OF INDIVIDUALS

Family therapy was founded on the notion that focusing on the individual who is manifesting a problem is misguided. The basic epistemologic premise of family therapy is that causality is circular, not linear. Family therapists felt uncomfortable emphasizing any one individual's difficulties because to do so seemed to violate the basic tenet of systemic work—that what seems like an individual problem is actually part and parcel of dysfunctional interactions among a number of people all of whom contribute equally to the troubled state of affairs. Recently, systemic notions of circular causality have come under close scrutiny as family therapists confront the reality of family violence and sexual abuse. It is beyond the scope of this book to go into detail about the extremely important attempts to reconcile feminist and systemic perspectives (Bogard, 1986; Cottone & Greenwell, 1992; Fish, 1990; Goldner, 1985; Goldner, Penn, Sheinberg, & Walker, 1990; Luepnitz, 1988; Sheinberg, 1992) except to say that these challenges to traditional systemic thinking make clear that adherence to strict notions of mutual causality and the idea that the symptom bearer is equally responsible for what happens in the family is untenable in certain situations. Crucial to the approach described in this book is the idea that one does not have to abandon notions of circular causality (in the sense of recursive interpersonal patterns) to accept and work with such observations as the following: (1) One family member may be suffering more than others, (2) one family member may be contributing more to a problem than others, (3) one family member may have more "baggage" from the past than others, (4) some problems of individuals may be more internalized than others and therefore not as responsive to changes in the family's system of interaction.

Often we stretch too hard to find mutuality, complementarity, and collusion in symptoms and thereby overlook what any experienced family therapist knows—that all family members are not equally troubled. Imber-Black (1986) points out that although the various parts of a system interact, in reality some parts are "more equal" than others and do not fit neatly into a pure systemic epistemology. Her point is succinctly made when she says, "Some circles are more oval than round" (p. 524).

In a written debate on this issue, Dell acknowledges that the epistemological concept of circular causality might be of limited relevance in actual therapeutic work (Dell, 1986). He resolves the conflict between clinician's experience and Batesonian epistemology by concluding that the concept of causality has different meaning to the clinician and to the theoretician. Whereas epistemologists speak of causality at the level of explanation, the clinician uses causality as a description of experience. Wynne (1986), also addressing the problem from the point of view of a clinician, goes even further in stating that "at the pragmatic level of therapeutic effectiveness, nonlineality equals therapeutic ineffectiveness" (p. 255) and that almost all therapeutic interventions are in fact linear.

Although there is some risk of masking the family issues by paying too much attention to the troubled child, not to focus on the child is often to deprive the child of the assistance he or she needs and deserves.

THE IDEA OF THE "INDIVIDUAL"

A related yet separate concept that has inhibited family therapists from working on individual issues is the notion that it does not make sense to consider the individual as an entity that in some way exists apart from the context in which he or she lives. The "classical" systemic view is perhaps best expressed by Haley. In a recent debate on the issue of whether it is necessary or useful to include an individual perspective in systemic work, Haley (1987) states that "[for] a theory of therapy it is best not to assume that motivation comes from within the individual" (p. 39). He believes that "the idea that a person's emotions and ideas are a product of his social situation, not that the social situation is a product of a person's ideas and feelings" (p. 39) is central to family therapy and states that "when you focus on the individual I don't think you can see simultaneously what is happening in the system" (p. 39).

Recently, there has been increasing recognition of the need to include individual perspectives in family work. A number of authors have attempted to make a bridge between the two perspectives. Nichols (1987) points out, for example:

> In families almost no interaction is simply the result of group processes. Even when the process of interaction seems to take a life of its own, it is the product of personalities. . . . We need this dual vision to see family processes as both shaped by the emergent properties of the system itself and also as originating in the individual needs and actions of family members. (p. 32)

Nichols's work with families includes attending to the subjective experience and private motivations of family members.

Attempts to integrate individual and systemic dimensions cover a wide range of perspectives (Carter, 1987; Kramer, 1980; Lebow, 1984, 1987; Moultrup, 1981, 1986; Sander, 1979). Schwartz (1987), for instance, focuses on the "multiple selves" we all have. He believes that "the power that human systems—especially families—exert upon us comes from their ability to evoke particular sub-selves within us" (p. 30). A number of theorists have utilized object relations theory (Friedman, 1978; Scharff & Scharff, 1987; Slipp, 1984) as well as self psychology (Kirschner & Kirschner, 1986) to bridge the gap between individual and systemic perspectives. Others have attempted to integrate behavioral and systemic perspectives (e.g., Barton & Alexander, 1981; Duncan & Parks, 1988). And still others attempt to include in their integration systemic, behavioral, and psychodynamic considerations (Feldman, 1985, 1992; Gold, 1988; Gurman, 1981; Pinsof, 1983).

Despite the fact that the individual development of the child is inextricably linked to interactions in the family (P. Minuchin, 1985, 1988), I find it helpful, in terms of the actual clinical work with children and their families, to keep the concepts of individual and system somewhat separate. Though holistic approaches have much to be said for them, dualistic conceptualizations may lend themselves more readily to intervening on the individual level. One can think of individual concerns and difficulties as *influencing* and being *influenced by* the system yet having a separate and distinct existence. Symptoms in both adults and children are therefore partially autonomous from the system in which they flourish and which, in fact, they may play a role in maintaining. Like the ocean and the bay, the tides and currents in the larger system influence those of the smaller, but the smaller nonetheless has its own identity: the composition, direction, and force of its waters cannot be fully understood just by knowing the characteristics of the larger body or system.

Just as individual developmental orientations too often ignore the system in which the child lives (P. Minuchin, 1985), family therapists are not sufficiently attentive to what the child as an *individual* is bringing to the system and how he or she helps shape family interactions. By working to understand and help the child more fully as an individual as well as offering direct assistance in changing his role in the system, the family therapist tremendously enhances his own effectiveness.

CYCLICAL PSYCHODYNAMICS

Formulating hypotheses that integrate psychodynamic notions of intrapsychic conflict with behavioral and systemic perspectives is facilitated by a theoretical orientation, cyclical psychodynamics (P. Wachtel, 1977, 1987, 1993), which highlights the complex bidirectional interplay between internal psychological structures and the person's ongoing transactions with other people. On the one hand, unconscious wishes, fears, and conflicts continuously shape current interactions and sometimes lead to behavior and affects that seem out of keeping with current realities. On the other hand, unconscious wishes, fears, and conflicts are *themselves* shaped by ongoing events. Their frequent resemblance to the psychic structures of early childhood is due not to a direct preservation of early experiences through fixation or arrest but to a dynamic process of reciprocal influence and evolution. As a consequence of the existing psychological structures and their power to shape how we experience events, a new situation is likely to take on the characteristics of earlier ones in significant ways. In turn, the new (yet similar) experiences brought about in this way feed back to maintain the earlier internal structures in roughly the same general outlines.

Of course, in many aspects of personality and development change does occur both in overt behavior and in internal structures. That is the essence of growth and change. But when significant conflict and repression are at play, a variety of forces makes it likely that there will be a reciprocal maintenance of the same old pattern, both internally and in manifest transactions with others. Thus, interventions designed to address the individual's daily actions and interactions bear on his deeper psychological structures as well as the manifest interpersonal behavior that is their target.

It should be evident that the cyclical psychodynamic perspective provides a bridge as well between psychodynamic concepts and systemic notions of circular causality (see also E. Wachtel & P. Wachtel, 1986). Both the child's individual attempts (conscious and unconscious) to deal with problematic wishes and fears and the family's attempted "solutions" to problems may inadvertently hinder the successful resolution of conflict and lead to the development of symptoms. Thus, the individual psychodynamic component of this proposed integration, though focusing in one sense on the *internal* life of the child, is, in another sense, interpersonal by nature.

As in other psychodynamic perspectives, the cyclical psychodynamic understanding of a child's difficulties highlights the ways that the child's behavior is a product of unconscious motivations, fantasies, impulses, and conflicts and stresses that these unconscious concerns are being kept out of awareness by various defense mechanisms. But the cyclical psychodynamic view, rather than seeing the individual's impulses, fantasies, object representations, self-representations, and images of internal and manifest transactions as directly preserved remnants of early life, focuses instead on how the child's needs and defense mechanisms of his inner world intersect with the family system in ways that keep alive the very same anxieties, conflicts, and relational images. Whatever the original source of the child's unconscious anxieties (temperament, traumatic experiences, or family interactions), it is *current* interactions that maintain (and are maintained by) unconscious concerns and it is in large measure *modifications* of current interactions that will ultimately resolve the difficulties.

Another reason for the emphasis on current interactions is that the ways children — or adults for that matter — go about either defending against or expressing their unconscious concerns often have the unfortunate ironic consequence of making the problem worse. For example, a child who fears abandonment may respond to this unarticulated anxiety by crying so much that her parents no longer leave her with sitters. But this attempted solution leads to a set of ironic consequences. The parents, for example, begin to resent the child, because they no longer have a life of their own. The child, in turn, sensing the parents' resentment about the imposition on their life, may become even more afraid of abandonment. Moreover, because the child is not left even with a responsible sitter or relative, the parents have inadvertently prevented her from learning gradually to cope with separation and from having experiences that would disconfirm her fears.

Just as current interactions can exacerbate the child's unconscious concerns, so too can new experiences alleviate them. Helping the family behave in ways that have a positive impact on the child's unconscious wishes and conflicts is an important element of the approach being described in this book. Chapter 7 elaborates on the many ways in which a psychodynamic understanding of a child's difficulties can be addressed by carefully planned changes in current interactions. With guidance from the therapist, parents can have a positive influence on what psychoanalysts have traditionally regarded as "deeply buried" and "inaccessible" unconscious material. Thus, the task is not only to help families break the cycles that have inadvertently kept the unconscious worries alive, but also to utilize the child's environment as a powerful force for change.

BORROWING FROM OTHER MODALITIES

The family therapy literature is filled with a wide range of creative interventions that aim at altering dysfunctional family patterns and extricating the child from problematic roles. Much of the integrative work described in this book borrows from this rich literature, and many standard family therapy techniques are employed to alter covert alliances and facilitate structural changes in how the family operates. When it comes, however, to integrating behavioral methods into systemic work with young children or to finding active ways to address a child's unconscious conflicts, the clinician has little accumulated knowledge to fall back on.[3] Even rarer still is the integration of psychodynamic and systemic formulations to design active interventions that focus on the child's unconscious anxieties.

A search of the literature does, however, reveal *some* interesting clinical examples of family work where the child's difficulties are addressed through multiple perspectives. For example, Duhl and Duhl (1981), in their chapter on integrative family therapy, describe their work with a not quite 5-year-old child who had been having continuous nightmares since the age of 3. One of her current symptoms, besides severe social problems, was that she would not let her mother pick her up and comfort her. The article describes the use of puppet play to help the child express unconscious feelings. Conversing with the child through puppets, the Duhls enabled the little girl to express unarticulated feelings of anger and sadness regarding a 6-week separation from the mother which had occurred 2 years earlier, following the birth of a sibling.

Lindblad-Goldberg (1986), in "Elective Mutism in Families with Young Children," demonstrates a different kind of integration than Duhl and Duhl's. She designs a behavioral intervention that involves the gradual desensitization of the child to the stepfather with rewards of M&M candies every time the child moves closer to the feared stepparent. In addition to this direct intervention designed to deal with the child's anxiety, Lindblad-Goldberg helps the family make structural changes and addresses the child's mutism as an expression of the mother's difficulty with anger.

Waters and Lawrence (1993) playfully and ingeniously convert an understanding of what a child is feeling (often obtained by meeting with the youngster alone) into "projects" that enable the child to find more adaptive solutions to what is bothering him.

Still another type of integration incorporates some of the ideas and techniques of cognitive psychotherapy (Feldman, 1992; Gold, 1988).

Though much of this work is interesting and seems potentially quite useful, a more systematic attention to the incorporation of other modalities in work with young children is needed. Clearly, there are a variety of ways to address more directly the individual issues of the child and to integrate the understanding of the individual with systemic interventions. It is important for family therapists to have a better grasp of alternative ways to think about children's difficulties as well as a wider repertoire of interventions directed at alleviating the child's distress.

A PRELIMINARY LOOK AT THE INTEGRATIVE MODEL

The work with families and symptomatic young children described in this book is founded on the assumption that both the individual and systemic meaning of the symptom must be addressed. Problematic behavior in children expresses individual concerns and defense mechanisms on the one hand and family systems issues and family defense operations on the other. It is important for the family therapist to get to know young children better and to learn how to formulate psychodynamic hypotheses about unconscious conflict. The cyclical psychodynamic perspective utilized here readily lends itself to a combining of individual and interpersonal perspectives. It views what conventional psychodynamic thinkers regard as "deep" issues rooted in one's earliest experiences as stemming not solely from past events but rather as kept alive by current interactions. Because current interactions feed the intrapsychic issues, interventions designed to alter interactions have a wide-reaching effect. Psychodynamic formulations are used to create interventions that both alter the family system and address directly the child's unconscious concerns. Behavioral and cognitive interventions are used to address directly the symptomatic behavior.

The therapeutic work described in this book proceeds on several levels at once. It can be thought of as a three-pronged approach in which (1) the symptomatic behavior is blocked, (2) the unconscious concerns that made the symptom necessary are addressed, and (3) the systemic issues surrounding the child's difficulties are explored and worked with. In this approach, psychodynamic understanding of the problem and behavioral methods targeted at the symptom go hand and hand. The therapist *simultaneously* helps the parents to understand the child's concerns and encourages them to make clear to the child that the "symptomatic" behavior will not be allowed to prevail. Often when the parents no longer allow the child to act out his concerns in self-defeating ways, the child becomes motivated to get help for his difficulties. Thus, for example, with an overly aggressive youngster parents are helped to set limits even before the child's aggression is understood. The child, feeling more pressure from the parents to behave better, tends to be more receptive to interventions that will help him understand and control his feelings. Thus, the second prong of this approach addresses the unconscious concerns that made this form of behavior seem necessary to the child: Is the aggression a defense against feelings of vulnerability? How can the child be helped by the family, and possibly the therapist directly, to feel less vulnerable so that she can give up the aggression? Third, the therapist works with the systemic issues surrounding the child's difficulties. Is there a taboo in the family about showing vulnerability? Is the child expressing hostility for someone else? What is the family's role in maintaining the child's difficulties?

The reader will soon see that the relative balance of systemic, psychodynamic, behavioral, and cognitive interventions varies greatly from case to case. There is no formula one can apply. Sometimes straight systemic interventions seem to be enough. At other times psychodynamic formulations seem to be at the heart of the issue. Though it is, of course, difficult to live with ambiguity, it is simply not the case that all problems of young children and families are caused by the same set of influences or will be helped by the same set of interventions. Therapists working with families and young children need to be "inclusive" rather than "exclusive" in their point of view. They need to pick and choose, borrow, and reshape from all those who have something to offer distressed and troubled children. Most important of all is that therapists learn to think about children's difficulties from a variety of perspectives and that they have in their repertoire a wide range of interventions.

To address this complex reality is the task of this book.

2

Meeting with Parents Alone:
Understanding Their Concerns

F amily therapy literature is replete with references to overcoming
the resistance of families. Images of "doing battle" and outman-
euvering intransigent systems abound. There are showdowns, confrontations, and strategies for dealing with the toughest of cases, which
were called by some "high rollers" or "barracudas" (Bergman, 1985). Hoffman (1981) pointed out that "implicit in most therapies is an adversary
position, usually covert, sometimes overt. . . . An ineffective therapist
is like a fisherman whose line hangs limp in the water; at times there is
a tug—the fish nibbles, then gets away" (p. 328). Often, it seems that
the first few sessions with families require the therapist to "outwit" or
outwait the family. Many therapists refuse to see a family when one of
the members requested does not arrive for a first session. Napier and
Whitaker (1978), for instance, talk about the battle for structure which
the therapist must win at the outset. They feel that the family, in not
making sure all members have arrived, is testing what they, the therapists,
can handle and finding out "one way or another . . . how much power
we had" (p. 10).

There is increasing consensus that perhaps we have overrated
resistance and the homeostatic tendencies of systems (Dell, 1982; Hoffman, 1981). Anderson and Stewart (1983) point out that not all families
display equal degrees of resistance, and although they see it as inevitable
to some degree, resistance is almost always accompanied by a wish for
relief from distress. I believe that much of the resistance encountered in
conventional family therapy is the result of the "hierarchical, acting upon"
stance that many therapists take with families. As Hoffman (1988) puts

it, "So many models of family therapy have kept therapists standing on a mountaintop or hidden behind a screen" (p. 56). When therapy is something done *to* families rather than a collaborative effort *with* them, families are not likely to be fully cooperative (deShazer, 1985).

Recently, ideas from theories of social constructivism have begun to influence clinical work (Goolishian & Anderson, 1992; Hoffman, 1990, 1991; Sheinberg, 1992). Sheinberg (1992) notes the following:

> Currently, "conversation" and "reflection" have replaced the more instrumental language of "strategy" and "intervention." As our theoretical metaphors have moved away from physics and biology toward social and cultural descriptions, clinical practice has moved away from the hierarchical and "definitive" toward the collaborative and the hypothetical. (p. 201)

Instead of looking for a particular systemic meaning of a problem, therapists working within a constructivist model think of their work in terms of helping the family find new narratives or explanatory stories which, in turn, enable family members to act differently. The role of the therapist is not to help restructure the family but to ask questions and to converse with the family in a way that helps the family to alter pre-existing belief systems about the family's past as well as its future (Penn, 1985; Tomm, 1987, 1988). Of course, everything a therapist says during an interview is itself an intervention (E. Wachtel, 1993), but the collaborative attitude implied in a conversational mode of therapy is much less likely to generate resistance.

Regardless of how one approaches the work, however, it will still be the case that some families will be reluctant to change familiar, entrenched patterns that have proven to be destructive. Yet, even these families are generally *ambivalent,* not just *negative,* toward the prospect of change. Often, family members, adults as well as children, readily accept and even embrace suggestions for changed ways of interacting. It is clinically nonproductive to assume that families necessarily *need* the identified patient to remain in her position. Moreover, even if there is *some* "benefit" to the couple or family in having a "troubled" child, clinical experience suggests that resistance to change can be substantially reduced by a respectful attitude toward the parents' concerns.

A first principle of the approach described in this book is that it is better to start out with the assumption that most parents consulting us (even those who are *sent* by schools) truly want help for their child. Although they may regard the difficulties as the child's and not the family's, they are usually at least somewhat amenable to making changes in the family system that will help the child. Capitalizing on this wish, and nurturing the desire for change which coexists with "resistance," is the goal of the first meeting.

BUILDING TRUST:
ESTABLISHING A COLLABORATIVE RELATIONSHIP

Many family therapists feel that it is important to start the process of family therapy by meeting with the family as a whole. Challenging the family's notion that it is the *child's* problem rather than a *family* problem is regarded by some as step one in the process of change (Kirschner & Kirschner, 1886; Pinsof, 1981). The approach described in this book starts with a wholly opposite stance. The parents are allowed, and even encouraged, to focus on the child and his or her difficulties as they are perceived by the parent. Paradoxically, by so doing, the parents ultimately are less resistant to systemic interventions. Parents are asked *not* to bring their children to the first meeting. Instead, they are told that the therapist would like to hear from them about their concerns and what thoughts they might have as to the child's difficulties. When parents are divorced it is generally best initially to meet with each parent separately. Since one aim of the first meeting with parents is to help them feel free to express any and every concern they have, this is best achieved in private meetings with the therapist. Even in the unfortunately far too rare case of amiable divorces, couples generally are somewhat guarded with one another and will open up more fully in an individual meeting.

Meetings alone with parents are held regularly. It is important, therefore, to keep in mind that the initial meeting is not an intake interview after which the real work will begin. Rather, it is the first of many interviews held with the parents and, therefore, the therapist should not feel pressured to get all the information described here in one meeting. Throughout the work we continually engage the parents as collaborators in devising a plan for helping the child. As we get to know the child better we give the parents feedback about what we see and ask for continual updates on their perceptions of things at home.

Fundamental to establishing rapport with parents is an attitude of respect for their concerns and what they know about their children. Too often, therapists (family therapists as well as child therapists) convey, instead of respect, skepticism and superior knowledge. Parents may distort, project, and use their children in systemic warfare, yet, unless the parent is suffering from severe psychological difficulties in which reality testing is impaired, they know a great deal that is true about their children. If the therapist believes as I do, that she really *can* learn a lot about the child from the parents, the parents will feel valued and in turn will value the advice of the "expert." In the first session, as in subsequent sessions with the parents, the tone and stance the therapist takes are collaborative. Together, the parents and therapist will try to figure out what is wrong and what can be done to help the troubled child. After the parents have had an opportunity to detail their concerns (this is described later), the therapist explains in the first session that almost always the best way to help young children is to work with both the child and the family. Although the child will be seen for individual sessions from time to time, most of the therapeutic work will be done by the parents at home. The role of the therapist is to help them help their child. Family meetings, individual sessions with the child, and meetings alone with parents will be intermingled. Most parents feel quite comfortable with this approach. Though they sometimes do have the wish to send their child off to be fixed up by a child therapist, they are generally relieved by an approach that builds on the wish to parent. Even parents who are terribly worn out and frustrated seem to respond somewhat positively (though often hesitantly) to the idea that the therapist will help them help their child. Relinquishing parental roles to a child therapist can feel like a failure, and most parents are happy to have one more opportunity, with some coaching by the family therapist, to turn things around themselves.

The fact that this approach is fairly short term is another important consideration for most parents. It is a financial burden as well as a logistical one to have a young child in long-term individual treatment. Many parents feel a good deal of resentment at having to spend so much money on a troubled child. Though they may recognize the need for help, their frustration and anger at the child may manifest itself in irritation at having to spend time and money because the child is "difficult." Giving parents an opportunity to express these feelings, as well as assuring them that with their participation the work will be as brief as possible, further minimizes resistance.

PARENTAL GUILT

Many parents who consult therapists about their children feel extremely guilty. They worry that they have done something to create these problems. Parents may feel depressed by the tension surrounding family life. Not infrequently the weekends are the hardest time and they look forward to going back to work on Monday. Some parents have a hidden worry that they no longer love their child. Life with a difficult child can feel miserable. Overwhelmed and angry, parents sometimes feel that this particular child is ruining their life and is negatively affecting their marriage as well as the lives of other children in the family. "Confessing" these feelings to the therapist can be a great relief: If these confessions are met with empathy and some reassurance, a powerful therapeutic alliance is formed.

One way to help parents feel comfortable enough to express such "dark" feelings in a first session is to allow them to ventilate, complain, criticize, and worry about their child *without* the therapist's interjecting questions and comments that underscore that the problem is a systemic one. We must be careful not to rescue the child from the role of identified patient too soon, for to do so is to weaken the alliance with the parents which gives us leverage for systemic change. It is because it is important to allow the parents freedom to "let it all out" so to speak that I do not include the children in these meetings. Parents naturally and appropriately hold back when speaking in the child's presence and will not only withhold important information about the child but will be careful not to reveal their disturbingly negative emotions in regard to the youngster. In the session alone with the parents I encourage them to feel free to talk about these negative feelings by stating something like, "Many parents who are having a very rough time with a child are disturbed by how negatively they are feeling. Often children are being so difficult that they are literally turning the parents off. Has it gotten that bad for you?" Couched in this way (the child is turning the parent off) the parent feels understood and is relieved to reveal the dreaded feeling—that he no longer likes the child. Knowing that it is not uncommon to feel this way is a great relief. Reassurance that in the therapist's experience as the negative interactions with the child change the positive feelings will return is important to impart. The therapist holds out the hope that working with the child and the family will lead to the return of warmth and love for the child.

It is often helpful to ask the parents to reflect on whether there are *any* moments when the child is acting in a way that makes it possible to enjoy time together. By asking this question in a way that does not *yet* challenge the idea that the child is the problem, the therapist enables the parents to not feel criticized and to become less defensive. Thus, they are often able to say that there are times when they *do* enjoy the child and to recognize that sometimes it is *they* not the child who may be acting differently. If parents leave a first meeting with the sense that they have been heard, understood, not judged, respected, and even helped to focus on times they feel positive about the youngster, a big step has been taken toward successful systemic interventions.

ASSESSING THE ATTITUDE TOWARD THE SYMPTOM AND ITS PLACE IN THE SYSTEM

Of course, not all parents feel as negatively about their difficult children as described previously. Part of the assessment in the first interview is to learn what the parents' idiosyncratic attitudes are toward their child and his or her difficulties. The therapist must listen carefully for the metaphors and adjectives used to describe the child. Thus we are not simply gathering information about the child but also information about the projections, fantasies, and anxieties of the parent. This in turn gives us a piece of the systemic information we ultimately need to work effectively with the family.

For example, two sets of parents came in the same week describing a difficult youngster (one child was 5 and the other 7) who in each case was referred by the child's school because of behavior problems in the classroom. Interestingly, in both instances the parents reported mild difficulties at home but did not regard these as major problems and would not have sought help but for the acting out in school. Neither set of parents was at their wit's end or harboring extremely negative feelings toward their child. Both sets could express a good deal of warmth and saw many positives in their child despite the fact that their child had always been difficult. Yet despite these important similarities there were some subtle differences in attitude which are important to know in designing "good fit" family interventions.

Thus, one set of parents, whom I will call the Smiths, described their son's aggressive behavior with other children as reflecting his "headstrong" nature and his determination to "stand his ground." Mother said with humor and admiration in her voice that "he's a real New Yorker." Father joined in with reminiscences of the days in the sandbox when his son did not play quietly like some children but instead was always defending his turf. Both recalled that the child's teacher, though concerned about the excessively aggressive response to minor provocations, did say that the child was always reacting to *something* and never hit when completely unprovoked. They emphasized that despite his apparent overreactions he was very well liked and sought out by many children.

These parents felt a good deal of pride in their child and when asked could enumerate many wonderful traits the child possessed. Even his "negatives" were perceived to a large degree as positive. Their main concern was that his defiance and strong will would interfere with learning in that he often got into power struggles with teachers. Both parents highly valued academic success and it was the child's failure to learn as much as he could that worried them. In working with these parents it would be extremely important to work within their rubric—concern for a cooperative attitude with teachers. Clearly, it was important to the parents that the child be tough and not let others push him around. The therapist must begin the work with an acceptance of this value and design interventions that would build on or at least do not tread on this concern.

Contrast the report of the Walker family (described more fully in Chapter 9). Like the child just described, this boy too was well liked by children and adults. He was described by both parents as having a serious problem with overreacting and they were concerned that he could do something that would be seriously harmful to another child. They supervised him as much as possible and went on class trips to ensure that the stress of dealing with an unfamiliar situation did not lead to a rageful episode. Both parents agreed that he seemed like a volcano which could erupt at any time with no notice whatsoever. He had trouble distinguishing intentional assaults by other children from accidents and responded with extreme aggression (punching, pushing) to the accidental pushing and shoving that can happen in crowded situations. Both parents felt that the child's hair-trigger temper was the result of a constant frustration he lived with because of a mild learning disability which made reading a difficult undertaking. Like the Smiths, the Walkers had no trouble elaborating on many of the wonderful qualities the child possessed. Like the Smiths, they felt both proud and protective of their son. However, there is a clear difference in the way they experienced the child's aggressiveness. A good deal of anxiety surrounded their description of his behavior and they seemed to regard his responses as somewhat "paranoid." Though in fact there were some differences in the aggressive behavior of these two boys (there were many nuances to the behavior that needed further clarification), nonetheless, the differences in the attitudes of the parents were very striking and important to consider in the systemic work that followed.

THE PARENTS' EXPLANATIONS OF THE PROBLEM

As seen in the previous examples, parental explanations for children's difficulties are often embedded in the descriptions of the child's problems. It is helpful to listen for and to encourage elaboration of these explanations since the "stories" one constructs about a problem determine the types of solutions attempted. By giving the parents the privacy and encouragement to express their belief systems, the therapist gains important information about where to intervene systemically. Furthermore, knowing parental explanations as early as possible helps us avoid direct clashes in perspective until a good working alliance is established. It is not that we never confront and challenge the parents' theory, but rather that we wait until trust has developed. Many parents welcome hearing an expert disconfirm their explanation, as frequently the parents' view of the child is a much more pessimistic one than the therapist's. In order to take in the therapist's more positive view of the situation they need to feel that a real assessment of the child has taken place. Challenging ideas of pathology too soon may seem to families to be insincere or glib in that the therapist does not appear to have sufficient information to make the alternative views believable.

For example, one mother described with horror that her 6-year-old daughter was simply mean. She reportedly "tortured" her friends psychologically, made "stabbing" comments to them, and seldom showed warmth to either parent. The child's father noticed the same behavior, was upset by it, but did not impute the same meaning to this profile that his wife did. The father felt that the child was a highly intense, intelligent child who got frustrated easily. Mother, on the other hand, saw a close resemblance between the child and the maternal grandmother, who had a history of psychiatric hospitalizations and who, when home, had tormented her family with her nastiness. This woman's reactions to her daughter were based in part on anger at her own mother but also on fear of serious psychiatric problems in the future.

In this case, mother was not reassured until the therapist met with the child alone and witnessed the child's "nastiness" first hand. Giving the parents feedback in regard to what had been discovered in the individual session was an essential component of making alternative explanations credible.[1] Only then could the mother accept with relief the therapist's assertion that this child was not as seriously disturbed as she might appear. Systemic explanations were more readily accepted once mother's concerns as to the child's psychopathology were put to rest.

Not infrequently, single parents view the child's problems as stemming from a similarity to the divorced spouse. It is important to note that it is not just that the child is being used as a pawn in a power struggle between warring parents but rather that one parent is truly concerned and dismayed by the child's identification with and modeling of the other parent. Often parents feel quite guilty as well as hopeless about this explanation of the child's difficulties. Again, the parent's explanation should not be immediately challenged. While carefully avoiding tilting toward an alliance with one of the parents, as both parents need to be worked with if at all possible, the therapist must convey to each parent that his or her concerns will be taken seriously and not merely dismissed as vindictiveness toward the ex-spouse. Many, though not all, parents want to rise above their own hurts and frustrations to protect the child from undue psychological harm from the divorce and will eventually accept a more complex explanation for the problem than the one that locks the child into an unwelcome identification.

Sometimes parents have psychoanalytic explanations of their child's difficulties that derive from their own experience with psychoanalysis or from having first tried individual therapy for the child with a psychoanalytically oriented practitioner. For instance, a parent may see the child's behavior as a reflection of repressed anger, sibling rivalry, or never having resolved separation problems or as an "oedipal" issue. Although there is often some truth to these explanations, the parents' "understanding" attitude may in fact be part of the problem. Parents may not be helping the child develop healthy defense mechanisms (see Chapter 5) or may fail to set appropriate limits out of a misguided notion that a child should not "repress" his feelings no matter what form the expression of emotion takes.

Noticing Differences in Parental Attitudes and Belief Systems

An important clue to understanding the systemic contribution to the child's difficulties is the differences in parental attitudes toward the child. One parent may express much more empathy for the child than the other does. Not infrequently, one parent is concerned that the school is being too hard on the child and making a big fuss about nothing. Or, one parent may talk about the child quite negatively while the other corrects, qualifies, and generally takes the role of providing a larger perspective. It is more common that parents will not be in agreement on the causes, seriousness, or strategies regarding the symptomatic child. Generally the differences reflect differences in *degree* of upset about a problem rather than extreme divergences of opinion. The fact of parental disagreement per se is usually not enough to warrant a systemic hypothesis regarding the role of the symptom in marital discord. More important than the disagreement is the emotional climate in which these differences exist. Sometimes, for instance, one parent will volunteer that the other parent does not see it the same way or that the child behaves very differently with the spouse. This can be a source of relief for a parent. Parents who feel guilty about their own negative feelings may *want* the other parent to feel differently about the child. The opposite may also be true—that a parent who feels guilt ridden may want the other parent to confirm that the child is, in fact, quite difficult, unpleasant, and hard to love.

It is helpful to try to assess whether the disagreements the parents have about the child reflect *other* marital difficulties or whether the differences—even when intense—derive *from* the stress and guilt evoked by having a troubled child. Though many parents are hesitant in a first meeting to discuss marital difficulties, they are generally quite responsive to questions regarding their differences in attitude toward the child and the effect of these differences on their marriage. Questions about whether the child is always on their mind or whether they can sometimes go out together and not talk about the child are helpful in assessing whether the child is the cement holding the relationship together.

When meeting with the therapist alone, parents often reveal cross-generational alliances which, because of their wish to present a united front to their children, are less apparent in family meetings. In discussing a child's behavior and feelings, a parent may make it clear that he or she identifies with what the youngster is feeling. Thus, for instance, one woman said she understood her young son's obstinacy as deriving from the fact that his father (her husband) was a perfectionist who constantly corrected the child as well as her. In another case the mother saw the clinginess of a 4-year-old as stemming from the fact that she was starving for her father whose busy career involved late meetings at the office and foreign travel. Although she minimized the degree to which she too felt deprived when her husband worked late and traveled, it was clear that she supported her daughter's protests. Similarly, one man said that he felt his wife nagged their 8-year-old son too much in regard to household chores but described his own reaction to her nagging as "I'm used to it so it doesn't bother me."

Differing attitudes toward a child's behavior and difficulties are generally most apparent when parents are separated or divorced. It is important to assess whether the parents simply experience the child differently, whether the child, in fact, *acts* differently with the two parents, or whether it is some combination of the two factors. In separate meetings with each parent (and with stepparent if applicable) the therapist explores this issue. When parents trust that the therapist is not allied with the other parent (even if only one parent initiated treatment) they are often less defensive and more willing to confirm the other parent's perceptions and concerns. Even when parents are in agreement as to the existence of a problem, rarely is there a consistent approach in the two homes. Even in the most cooperative of divorces, ex-spouses often disapprove of some aspects of one another's parenting. For instance, one parent may feel that the best way to treat an anxious child is to offer a good deal of comforting and reassurance while the other parent may feel that this is totally wrong and is instead "tough" with a fearful child.

Perhaps one of the most difficult aspects of being divorced is coming to terms with the reality that one has little or no influence on the experiences that one's children have with their other parent. Often, a hidden agenda of one parent is that the therapist will influence the other parent to behave differently with the child. Although in ongoing meetings with each parent the therapist does try to coordinate an approach to the child's difficulties and will, of course, discuss ways that changed behavior could be helpful to the child, no amount of therapeutic rapport will change the fact that the parents may have different values and tolerances. In individual sessions with each parent the therapist tries to help them accept that it is simply a fact of life that expectations and tolerances in each home are different and that it can even be beneficial to a child to have a varied experience.

GATHERING INFORMATION FOR SYSTEMIC, PSYCHODYNAMIC, AND BEHAVIORAL HYPOTHESES

Sessions alone with parents give us an opportunity to ask questions that we would not want to ask in the child's presence.[2] What we observe about the child in our office, either alone or with the family, often does not tell us much about how the child acts at home or in school. I have seen children behave in a perfectly calm, self-assured manner in the family sessions when in "real life" they are often tense and irritable. Even without observing the worrisome behavior we can get a fairly good sense of the child by encouraging the parents to relate recent problems as well as what they can recollect from the past.

One can begin by asking each parent (in separate sessions if they are divorced) to say *everything* they are concerned about. After a list of all their "worries" is generated, the parents are asked to elaborate on each problem with details and examples. Thus, for example, one mother said, "Susie gets overexcited; her exuberance goes too far." In this and other instances, it can be misleading to assume based on our experiences with other children that we know what the parent means. A concrete (and preferably recent) example can give us the type of information we need to be sure we understand. Susie, it turned out, "was so involved in singing" that she could not or would not stop even when her mother asked her to come to the table and her younger brother started screaming over the song in order to be heard. Exuberance? Perhaps. But more likely this description tells us more about systemic dynamics and anger than it does about enthusiasm.

MAJOR OMISSIONS

Most therapists have had the disturbing experience of realizing that they have been working without some very basic information. Parents often do not think to tell us about major events that may have affected the child. Generally they are not consciously withholding information but may simply have not stored the information under the category of "important event." However, although minimizing significant events may simply be due to a lack of psychological sophistication, it can also reflect parental discomfort in thinking about the event from the child's perspective. Identifying with the feelings of one's child can be quite painful and thus many parents tend to minimize the impact of difficult experiences on the child. Often it is not until well into the work that some new and important information is spontaneously discussed. Unless we make a concerted effort to get this information at the outset, we may discover for instance, months into the work, that a single parent had a live-in lover for several years who was not mentioned because he or she had not been part of their lives for quite some time, or that a parent had been at home and out of work for a year, putting the whole family under financial and emotional strain.

For this reason it is important to jog the parents' memory with specific questions.

Have there been any deaths in the family? Any deaths of close friends? Have any close family members been seriously ill emotionally or physically? Have any family members been hospitalized? Have they moved? Changed babysitters? Has there been serious marital strife leading to a separation? Have there been lengthy separations for any other reason? Have any teachers with whom the child was particularly close left abruptly? At what age did the mother (or father) return to work? If the parents are separated or divorced, what was the emotional climate in the house during and after the separation. Was there any period when the child did not see a parent. Have any pets died?

Have any close family members been the victim of crime? Has the house been robbed?

Has the child known any children who suffered the loss of a parent? Has the child known any children who died or were seriously injured in an accident?

What is the child's health history? Has the child had any serious illnesses? Has the child had any unusually unpleasant medical procedures? Did the child achieve developmental milestones at a normal age? Was there delayed speech? Was the child precociously verbal? Have there been any worries in regard to the child's health or mental and physical development?

Have there been fertility problems? Have there been miscarriages? How late in pregnancy?

What is the employment history of each parent? Has the family been under financial stress?

I also inquire about incidents with other children or siblings that might have left emotional scars. One 8-year-old, for instance, had, years earlier, thrown a truck at a younger brother causing serious injury. Children growing up in urban areas have sometimes witnessed crimes or been frightened by the mentally disturbed homeless. I inquire as to whether there have ever been any intense family scenes that the child may have witnesses or experienced in some way.

INFORMATION ABOUT INTERACTIONS WITH TEACHERS, BABYSITTERS, AND OTHER SIGNIFICANT ADULTS

The women's movement, the high rate of divorce, and economic pressures to make ends meet make working mothers the rule rather than the exception these days. Many children, at a very young age, are entrusted to the care of babysitters or day-care staff. Many start nursery school by 2½ and by first grade spend 6 to 8 hours a day in school and after-school programs. The adults with whom children interact in these settings play a significant role in the development of their sense of self and should not be ignored. Parents and therapists too, who are often working parents themselves—frequently tend to minimize the impact of these relationships (both negative and positive) on a child's image of himself. Not infrequently, difficult children are disliked by their teachers and caretakers who do not have the bonds of love as a countervailing force to the negative feelings engendered by interactions with a resistant and negativistic child. On the other hand, some teachers and caretakers are exceptionally warm and sympathetic and despite the problem behavior, genuinely like the child. It is important to inquire about the parents' impression of these relationships. Who were the teachers toward whom the child felt most warmly? How did the child react when he or she changed teachers—relieved or with feelings of loss? What is the current teacher's attitude toward the child's difficulties as far as the parents can tell? Do the parents regard the teacher as too lenient or too demanding? Were there any teachers with whom the child had a particularly close bond? Has the child ever been regarded by the teacher and parents of other children as the class troublemaker who was an undesirable companion to the "good" kids? The parent's impressions may, of course, not be correct, and later more information about this will be obtained by speaking directly with the child's current teacher, but getting the parents' views on these matters is an important starting point.

A history of who the main babysitters were and when and why they left is helpful. Not infrequently, children are more upset about the loss of a babysitter with whom they felt secure, valued, and loved than parents realize. It is also important to realize that babysitters and housekeepers often have a "favorite" among the children in the family. One needs to get the parent's sense of these relationships and alliances. Often there are cultural assumptions regarding male and female children, resulting in attitudes toward a child quite divergent from those of a parent. Or, simply for reasons specific to the caretaker's personality or the system of interacting that has developed, a housekeeper/babysitter may "favor" the family scapegoat and feel more negatively than most about the family "angel." Parents, when questioned, usually have some feeling about this. Since these attitudes are rarely expressed overtly, it is quite difficult for young children to articulate what they intuitively sense.

Frequently, because they depend on the caretaker, parents are loathe to recognize problematic interactions. Sometimes, the force of negative interactions only becomes apparent when the housekeeper is invited into the session. One babysitter, for instance, whom the parents felt "adored" their child, whom she had cared for since birth, responded extremely harshly to their little girl's tantrum in the therapist's office. This occurred in a session that included only the children and the housekeeper. When the younger, "adored" child (age 9) fell apart emotionally upon losing a game to her elder sister (age 11), the housekeeper reacted with a barrage of criticism about how this youngster always brags, provokes her older sister, cries at the slightest disappointment, and was never "embarrassed" or "ashamed." The housekeeper had the girls rigidly categorized as "sweet" and "selfish," and though she claimed to "adore" the "sweet" one, she also conveyed a good deal of exasperation and resignation in regard to the youngster's behavior.

Although children generally are more concerned about their parents' judgments of them than a sitter's, their identity and sense of self can be seriously affected, both positively and negatively, by the feedback they get from caretakers. Thus, we need to include information about these relationships in the complex equation of the system in which the child's troubles exist.

For example, one 9-year-old rarely let herself be hugged by her parents. Ever since she or they could remember this child seemed to be easily upset, angry, and irritable and seemed to her parents demanding, self-centered, callous, and unfeeling. When one parent was upset about a seriously ill relative, this little girl seemed completely unconcerned and bitterly resented obligatory visits to see her ill great-aunt. Nor did she have any sympathy for the parent's upset. Yet with the housekeeper this child seemed to melt. She showed warmth, love, and concern for this elderly caregiver and was regarded in turn by this grandmotherly babysitter as a "good child with a heart of gold."

Another child, age 10, the second oldest of four, was the sibling least demanding of attention. His younger sister had serious emotional problems and had been receiving therapy. The next youngest was an exceptionally cute 5-year-old who seemed instantly to charm anyone with whom she spoke. Although the 10-year-old had always seemed well adjusted, he began to exhibit difficulties (crying jags, stealing) shortly after a new baby boy was born. In a meeting alone with the parents, two additional pieces of information emerged which shed some light on why this birth might have disrupted his equilibrium so badly. It seems that a teacher who was very fond of him had been sick and out of school for 2 months. Most important, however, a housekeeper who had been living with the family for 5 years had been abruptly fired 6 months earlier. Because the parents had bad feelings and resentments toward the former babysitter, they did not arrange for the children to have continued contact with her in any way. Both parents agreed that the other children seemed unconcerned about the change in sitters, but this 10-year-old was quite upset. Apparently, she had related very well to this quiet youngster and he was clearly the child she liked the best.

USING QUESTIONS REGARDING TEMPERAMENT AS A SOURCE OF SYSTEMIC INFORMATION

It is now virtually common knowledge that babies differ in innate temperament. Although family therapists implicitly recognize the importance of different personality styles or temperaments in a family, they rarely (see Guerin & Gordon, 1986) address this factor explicitly.

A number of the dimensions of temperament described by Chess and Thomas (1986) provide a useful framework for inquiry about the children's dispositions. Discussion should include information about the child's current dispositional qualities as well as what and when changes occurred. Generally the easiest trait for parents to describe is the youngster's *activity level*. It is important to inquire as to whether the child can occupy himself peacefully for significant lengths of time or whether she seems to seek a good deal of activity. Some children get physically restless rather easily, and parents describe them as having what looks like a physical need to release energy. It is best to exclude television watching as an indication of a child's need to sit still; many very active children (and even hyperactive children) are calmed by the hypnotic effect of television. Activity level can be a sensitive sign of the child's psychic state. A noticeable change in activity level may be a sign of depression and parents should be asked to try to pinpoint when the change occurred.

Related to activity level is the child's attention span and ability to become engrossed in what he or she is doing (called *distractibility* by Chess and Thomas). Some children move rapidly from one activity to another. Others become so engrossed in what they are doing that they seem oblivious to what is going on around them. One must assess whether the child is simply absorbed or whether the child's absorption is a way of withdrawing from others. Of equal importance is information about the parents reaction to and way of dealing with the child's frenetic style. Some parents, for instance, try to settle children down with a video. Others get mad at the incessant "I'm bored," while still others try to amuse the child with an activity.

Inquiry about the child's *sleep patterns* also provides a wealth of information not only about the child's temperament but about some basic systemic interactions in the family. A noticeable change in sleep patterns is an important aspect of assessment. The situation of a 6-year-old child who has always joined his parents in bed at daybreak is very different from that of a child who only recently has felt a need to crawl into bed with his or her parents. Many parents do not mention until after a few sessions that their children join them in bed. Reticence about this behavior is probably due to a sense that this is psychologically "wrong" and will not be approved of by mental health professionals. American culture values independence and separateness and sleeping in bed with one's parents meets with cultural disapproval despite the fact that it is not uncommon in many other Western cultures. Of course, family structure and individual needs must in some sense be evaluated in comparison to the culture of which they are a part, and a child who relies on parents for self-comforting more than other children of his culture may have difficulty with what is expected of him or her outside the home.

One must not assume that parents who let (or even enjoy having) their children sleep with them for part of the night have marital difficulties and are triangulating in the child. Although this may, of course, be the case, many parents (as they reveal once they trust that the therapist will not be judgmental) simply feel that this kind of comforting is an appropriate aspect of parenting. Societal taboos about this pattern have created many "closet comforters," so to speak.

Although some very young children almost always sleep right through the night, most wake up several times nightly. The manner in which parents respond to a child's awakening has a great effect on the child's developing sleep patterns. Some children learn early to be self-comforting while others rely on parents to ease them into dozing off.

Inquiry about temperament should also include a discussion about the child's characteristic response to new events or people (called *approach–withdrawal* by Chess and Thomas). Some children seem to have been born fearless (Kagan, 1984). They experience little or no separation anxiety and approach new situations and people with enthusiasm. Others are cautious and somewhat slow to warm up to people. When inquiring about this aspect of the child's personality, it is extremely important to attend to how the parents feel about this trait. Cautiousness may elicit pride on the part of the parents in the child's good sense in sizing up situations before plunging in or disdain for the child's timidity. Conversely, a parent may endorse what others would consider inappropriately brazen behavior on the part of the child.

Generalizations about the fearlessness–timidity dimension can be misleading. Some children are absolutely comfortable in new situations as long as asserting their own opinion is not required. The parents of one very insecure 7-year-old were quite perplexed by how readily he volunteered to audition for a non speaking role in a television commercial being filmed at his school. Another child, age 5, who in many ways was outgoing and self-assured, withdrew from situations requiring him to perform at something he had not yet mastered. Articulating the nuances of approach and withdrawal help the parents have a more differentiated view of their children and counter the characterizations and pigeonholing of people to which it is all too easy to succumb. The importance of assessing a child's characteristic interpersonal stance is discussed further in Chapter 5.

Another of Chess and Thomas's temperament dimensions which seems particularly useful in learning about both the child and the system is *adaptability*. This is defined by Chess and Thomas as getting used to things "quickly" or as taking "a long time" to adapt. Another way to think of this dimension is to assess how readily a child is willing to participate and adjust to something that is not his preference. Teachers are referring to this temperament dimension when they describe children as "having trouble with transitions." Parents may describe a child as never wanting to leave the house and then hating to leave some place or activity once he has gotten there. A child may be described as a terrible dawdler who slows down the whole family whenever they are trying to go anywhere together. It is important to get a sense of whether the child is being "negativistic" or whether he becomes so intensely involved in an activity that it is hard to move on to something else. This is more readily determined by observing the child and family interacting than by parents' reports.

One 7-year-old girl had problems playing with other children. She would always resist their suggestions and wanted to play only the types of games she preferred. Another child of approximately the same age also had trouble playing with other children. In contrast to the first child, however, she had an extremely rich imaginative life, and after spending some time alone with her it became clear to the therapist that this child was *not* engaged in power struggles with peers but simply overwhelmed them with her almost manic enthusiasm and assignment of roles for fantasy play.

Some children (and adults) seem to be more sensitive than others to noise, visual stimuli, rough clothing, and so on. How the parents perceive and regard this characteristic (called *threshold level* by Chess and Thomas) is extremely important. Some parents regard such sensitivity negatively and see the child as overly complaining. Others try to accommodate to the child's needs.

Similarly, some children are highly expressive about what they feel while others have more modulated or low- key reactions to pleasing or disappointing events (called *intensity of reactions*). Inquire as to whether the child, when pleased, acts mildly enthusiastic or instead is the type that becomes ecstatic. When unhappy, does the child "fuss quietly or bellow with rage" (Chess & Thomas, 1986, p. 121). A highly expressive and emotional parent may feel disappointed in or even rejected by a reserved child's response to a surprise or treat. Conversely, less expressive parents may be alarmed by or critical of a child's "overdoing it." Of course, it is also often the case that an overly restrained, constricted parent gets a good deal of vicarious gratification out of the intensity with which his child reacts.

It is helpful to compare the child's temperament today with his or her temperament as an infant and toddler in order to determine whether the difficulties the child and the child–parent dyad are having are long-standing ones or whether they are a relatively new and uncharacteristic reaction to some current situation. Therapists sometimes assume that a difficult young child was a difficult baby, but this is often a mistaken assumption. Pinpointing when the child's temperament seemed to change gives us a clue to the systemic and psychodynamic factors that might be contributing to the child's current distress.

Inconsistencies in Manifestations of Temperament

Few of us behave "in character" all the time. Asking questions that help the parents think about ways the child's temperament is not uniformly consistent can be an important first step in changing rigid, locked-in definitions of family members. This is something that should be done with the children present as well as with the parents alone. The timid child may be more self-confident in some areas than the child who is regarded as outgoing and socially secure. Or, a child who is fearful when meeting new people may be quite willing to take risks with new activities, foods, and so on. Often these "uncharacteristic" behaviors have not, prior to therapy, been registered in a way that modifies generalizations about the child.

When talking about the temperament of the symptomatic child, parents often spontaneously compare that child to other members of the family. If comparisons do not happen spontaneously, it is helpful to direct the parents' attention to this question. In the privacy of sessions held without the children present, many parents are fairly overt about identifications and alliances between a parent and a particular child. Simply asking whether the child in question seems more like his mother or his father in "temperament" makes overt the systemic dynamics involving transference and distortions. A statement such as, "Johnny is a lot like his dad; he always prefers to lie around and do nothing rather than to be active," gives us a good sense of marital tensions and the systemic purposes the child's symptom may serve.

ATTENTION DEFICIT DISORDER, HYPERACTIVITY, AND LEARNING DISABILITIES

Parents with extremely active youngsters who have difficulty staying focused on activities often express worry that their child has an attention problem and is hyperactive. Care must be taken to give this concern serious attention. Yet, at the same time, we must be aware that it is all too easy to attribute difficulties to neurological impairment and thereby overlook the systemic, behavioral, and psychodynamic aspects of the problem. The younger the child, the more difficult it is to diagnose learning disabilities or neurologically based hyperactivity. It is beyond the scope of this book to address the assessment methods that can help differentiate true attention deficit disorder with or without hyperactivity from concentration problems and difficulty with impulse control which derive from psychological, rather than neurological, factors. Generally, before referring a child for an evaluation, I prefer to wait 6 weeks or so to see whether the child's behavior begins to change significantly as a result of family therapy.

It is important to keep in mind that many children have attentional difficulties without also being hyperactive. If a child persists in having difficulty concentrating and paying attention except in highly structured one-on-one situations, frequently asks to have instructions and statements repeated, or seldom engages in sustained activities I will refer the child for an evaluation. Similarly, when a child is always on the go, is extremely excitable, acts without thinking, has difficulty staying organized without a lot of attention, and continues to be this way despite changes in the family system and motivation on the child's part to do better, an evaluation for hyperactivity should be considered.

Therapists should also be alert to the role learning disabilities may be playing in the child's difficulties. Children who are having learning problems may act "silly" or uninterested in school as a defense against feelings of inadequacy. Highly aggressive children may be expressing the frustration that comes from struggling to master material that is harder for them than it is for their peers. Some children with learning disabilities are more concrete than other children and consequently do not process social cues as readily as their age-mates. A child's self-esteem can be profoundly affected not only by the academic difficulties he may be encountering but also by the problematic relationship with peers that can result from cognitive deficits.

BROADENING THE FOCUS

Thus far, this chapter has discussed ways to use meetings with parents to get a preliminary understanding of the child and the system. These meetings are also used to get to know each parent's family background and the concerns they have as individuals and as a couple. Each parent is asked to talk a bit about his parents, siblings, and grandparents. What is the nature of the current relationship with each spouse's family? How often does the family see them? Are they close? Is there friction between the spouses in regard to each other's family? Does the child about whom they are worried resemble or in any way act like someone in the extended family? How would each spouse compare family life in his current family with life in his childhood home? How did they each get along with siblings? With parents? What kind of student were they? It is particularly important to inquire about any serious emotional difficulties of family members. Schizophrenia, severe depression, or retardation in the family can cause parents to be hypervigilant or overreactive to a child's emotional difficulties.

It is also important to get to know some of the current concerns of each spouse. How satisfied are they each with their work? What are their interests? What is going well in each one's life? What upsets them? Is there anything about themselves that they wish were different? If they are in individual therapy or have been in the past, it is important to ask what made them go into therapy and what the status of these difficulties is at this point.

Not all this information is obtained in the first meeting or two. Each session with parents involves a mix of discussion of the current family situation and a deepening of our understanding of where the child's concerns and the parents' issues intersect. I have found that many parents who seek treatment out of concern about a troubled child are at first reluctant to talk about the quality of their marriage. After a session or two in which the focus has been on their concerns about their child, couples are generally more ready to talk about their relationship. It is at that point that I inquire about what goes well between them and what the areas of conflict and tension are. I ask for each person's views as to how the marriage has changed over the years? If the couple has ever been separated I ask for information about the conflicts that led to the separation and if and how they were resolved.

HELPING PARENTS LIKE THEIR CHILDREN

The initial meeting with the parents is not just for data gathering. From the beginning *therapeutic* processes are called into play as well. Family therapists are trained to notice positives and this orientation, right from the first meeting, can be a valuable asset in helping parents notice their children's strengths. In one instance, a parent reported that her son described "an evil feeling that takes over," which makes him act aggressively. The therapist responded by saying how remarkable it was for a child that age to be able to articulate his experience so clearly. In another, the therapist responded to a report of the child's remorsefulness after doing something wrong by noting that the child seemed to really *care* if the parents were upset with him and this is not always the case. In a similar vein, the therapist might say to the parents that their child must have a lot of personality or charm because, despite his aggressive acts toward other children, he seems to be extremely well liked.

Parents often tell funny anecdotes about something a child said or did. When the therapist laughs and genuinely seems tickled by the anecdote it helps the parents appreciate their child more. This thrust can be continued once the therapist has met the whole family and met with the troubled child alone. Warm grandparent-like expressions by the therapist of genuine pleasure in the things a child says and does in an individual session are a gift to the parents and a powerful therapeutic intervention. Of course, any feedback of this sort must be truthful. The more specific the compliment, the more believable it will be. Positive anecdotes about some of what transpired in the individual meeting provide the parents with an alternative and positive perspective to counter the negative self-images that are often being projected onto children. Just as an important ingredient of individual therapy with adults is the internalization of the experience of being liked and valued by the therapist, so too is the parents' self-valuation enhanced (and in turn the child's) by the recognition that the respected therapist, who knows many children, appreciates some of the qualities that makes their youngster special. Of course, it is important to remember that compliments and positive statements about a child will only be accepted if the parent feels that the therapist also perceives the child's problems and negative characteristics.

SUMMARY

Meeting alone with the parents for the first interview, and then from time to time throughout the work, has many benefits. Rather than furthering the scapegoating of the child as some fear, it enables the therapist to establish a working alliance with the parents and serves to minimize resistance. This chapter has provided some guidelines for the type of information one can obtain in meetings alone with the parents. The categories of inquiry presented should not be regarded as a hard and fast checklist. Nor should a therapist expect to obtain all this information in one meeting. The meeting with parents is *not* an intake interview. Thus, one should not delay meeting with the whole family or with the child alone until all this information is obtained.

It is important to have some sessions with parents alone throughout the whole course of the work. Soon after sessions that include the whole family I meet with the parents alone to give them feedback. The next chapter describes the types of information obtained from family meetings and how to share one's observations with the parents. Meeting alone with the parents enables us to inquire in depth about some of the interactions observed in the family sessions without being concerned that one child will feel singled out or overly scrutinized. Thus, for instance, when parents seem comfortable with a young child's inattentiveness in a session, or aggression, or physical clinginess, one can uses sessions alone with the parents to investigate the various parameters surrounding these behaviors? Does the child tune out at dinner? Is he attentive in one-on-one situations? Was the parents' tolerance for the child's way of acting in the session typical of how they react at home, or was it different? And so on.

Individual sessions are also used to give parents feedback about sessions alone with the child. Parents are eager for information about their children and in these sessions the therapist shares his hypotheses and provides some information about what the child has said and done that led to these formulations. Although the therapist does not share everything that goes on in individual sessions with the child's parents, there is no promise of confidentiality when working with young children as there is with work with adolescents or adults (see Chapter 4).

As the work proceeds, the focus of interviews with parents will expand to include collaborating on strategies and tasks that address the individual, systemic, and behavioral aspects of the problem. Parents will be given "homework" and specific interventions to try. Chapters 7 and 8 discuss interventions based on psychodynamic and behavioral understanding of the problem.

3

Getting the Most Out of Family Meetings

The bedrock of the integrative approach being described in this book is an understanding of the family's systemic dynamics and how they affect and interact with the child's difficulties. Attention to the relationship between systemic dynamics and individual perspectives (both behavioral and psychodynamic) pervades each and every chapter in this book. Thus, for instance, the use of maladaptive defense mechanisms in children (see Chapter 5) will be understood in terms of the way particular defenses are reinforced by family members and the way a child may be expressing issues that are conflictual for other family members as well. Even straightforward behavioral interventions (see Chapter 8) are utilized only in the context of attention to systemic factors.

In the previous chapter we looked at the way meeting with parents can be used both to learn more about the child and to develop some beginning formulations regarding the contribution of systemic dimensions to the child's difficulties. Questions, for example, comparing the temperament of the children in the family to that of each parent or inquiries regarding the relative degree of concern each parent has about a child's behavior furnish information for both individual and systemic hypotheses which are further explored in meetings with the whole family and the child alone. Thus, by the time we meet with the family as a whole we already have some ideas regarding possible systemic dynamics. We may already know, for instance, something about alliances, possible triangulations, and transmissions of three-generational patterns.

This chapter focuses on obtaining a more precise understanding of the family system through direct observation and interaction with the family as a whole. Its purpose is threefold. For experienced family therapists it is intended to give specific guidance on how to conduct family sessions with very young children. As discussed in Chapter 1, even seasoned family therapists often feel at a loss when it comes to meaningfully incorporating young children into ongoing family work. Although a good deal of this chapter is geared to the initial meetings with the family, it also includes material on the variety of ways family meetings can be used throughout the work.

For therapists who are approaching this integrative work from the orientation of individual child therapy, however, the aim of the chapter is somewhat different and perhaps more ambitious. It is intended to demonstrate how much information is gained not only when a child is known through individual sessions but when he is seen with his entire family. Many child therapists feel they are addressing the family component of the problem by meeting with the youngster's parents or perhaps even by having a joint session with the parents and the child who is their patient. Rarely, however, are siblings included. Yet one loses a good deal of information when one does not see how the family as a whole operates together. Individual child therapists who try this approach are likely to be quite surprised by what they see in these meetings. Thus, for example, a child whose fantasies involve extreme hostility to a sibling may in fact demonstrate more support and caring than was expected. Or, the "good kid" in the family may be more provocative than anybody has reported.

Finally, this chapter provides a brief overview of the types of questions a systemic assessment tries to answer. Although many readers will be familiar with systemic ways of thinking, it is hoped that they nonetheless find useful the particular organization of material suggested in this chapter.

The next section of this chapter reviews some of the ways therapist and families can interact in sessions so that a useful dialogue occurs.

THE FIRST MEETING WITH THE FAMILY

Many family therapists, from beginners to seasoned practitioners, gulp momentarily before going out into the waiting room to bring in a family with young children. Although they know it makes sense to meet with the whole family, it often seems so much more difficult than meeting with the parents or even the parents and only the symptomatic child. Experienced family therapists have told me in workshops that they feel uneasy about family sessions that include young children. Often they are concerned that they will not be able to engage the younger family members or that the younger family members will be disruptive and thus the session will not be productive. Young children often tell long, drawn-out stories that seem to have nothing to do with the matters at hand. Frequently they touch what they should not and open private drawers or closets. The most dreaded scenario, however, is that the therapist will, under the watchful and expectant gaze of the parents, fail miserably in her attempt to engage the children. Therapists are embarrassed when children refuse to say a word or, worse yet, act terribly bored and unhappy about being there. Parents hope that the therapist will help the child open up, and therapists, aware of this expectation, become anxious about proving themselves.

By explaining to the parents that the main purpose of the session is simply to give the therapist a chance to observe the family together and that it is not necessary for anything of much import to be revealed or talked about for the session to be extremely useful, both the therapist and the parents become more relaxed. Parents who worry about how the children will behave are reassured that just as much will be learned from sessions in which a child is uncooperative as from a session in which the child is communicative and well behaved. They are told that although the sessions are designed to be fun for young children, this cannot be guaranteed and that almost anything that happens will provide useful information. The therapist must keep in mind that sessions that go "badly" still provide invaluable information about parental reactivity, boundary setting, and power hierarchies.

INCLUDING SIBLINGS

Some parents feel quite concerned about involving the siblings of the child who is the identified patient. They feel worried that the child whom they regard as "uninvolved" in the problem will be angry at having to miss more desirable activities in order to come to therapy when it is not his problem. Parents are concerned too that the "nontroubled" child will be adversely affected by the exploration of problems. Frequently they state that there is already a good deal of resentment of the time and attention the identified patient gets at home because of his difficulties, and to require the other siblings to alter their plans to attend family meetings is to add insult to injury. As stated in Chapter 2, I do not assume that this is resistance on the parents' part but instead take the concerns at face value. Assurances are given that in our experience, family meetings generally ease tensions and resentments rather than increase them. Efforts are made whenever possible to accommodate the after-school schedules of all the children. Because the therapist has already formed a strong therapeutic alliance with the parents during sessions when they were seen alone, resistance is generally quite minimal after the therapist reassures the parents. Expressing the conviction that meeting with the whole family gives invaluable information about the child, without which the work cannot proceed, usually overcomes whatever reluctance the parents still feel.

THE TONE OF THE FIRST SESSION

A central premise of this book is that resistance is a response to anxiety and that anxiety interferes with the patient's really hearing what the therapist is saying. The more the therapist is able to put people at ease, the more they are able to hear and incorporate what she is saying (see P. Wachtel, 1993). Challenging, provoking, or intensifying conflict (Minuchin & Fishman, 1981) as a means of highlighting family dynamics is a method seldom used in this approach. It is particularly important in the first session to avoid, if possible, focusing directly on problematic interactions. One important goal of the initial meeting is to have the children experience the session as enjoyable.

Although parents have been reassured that crying, arguments, or other disruptive behavior is something they need not be concerned about, nonetheless, everyone feels better (including the therapist) if things do in fact go smoothly. The therapist can do a number of things that make a calm atmosphere more likely.

If a young child enters a room filled with tempting toys, she is unlikely to sit still long enough to engage in any family discussion or activity. Excited by the prospect of playing with a new toy, the young child, even if he can be disengaged from the toy, is eager to get back to playing with it. For this reason, it is wise to put toys out of sight or at least out of reach until the therapist is ready to have the children play while the adults speak. Similarly, markers, scissors, keys, and other small objects to which very young children would be attracted should temporarily be removed. Making the environment safe for small children as well as minimizing opportunities for distractibility helps adults and children relax.

Parents are often confused as to who is in charge. They may let their children do *anything* on the assumption that the therapist will take the lead in setting limits. Thus, it is important for the therapist to communicate to the parents early on that he is assuming that *they* will be in charge. This applies not only to setting limits but also to indicating to their children the degree of cooperativeness and participation expected. Thus, although the therapist takes the lead in trying to playfully engage young children and invites them to participate in family discussions or role plays, when a child is disengaged or disruptive the parents are asked to make their wish for the child's cooperativeness known to the youngster and to deal with his lack of participation in whatever way they think is best. In asking parents to take charge in this way, I not only learn a good deal about the system but divest myself of unrealistic expectations regarding my power to be a "magician" or "pied piper" who can work miracles with youngsters. Clear communication regarding who is in charge and what the parents expect, not surprisingly, generally leads to greater participation on the part of even very young children. Who takes charge and how the parents interact around the children provides invaluable information. Of course, one may find two parents who are at odds with one another regarding expectations. More details on what we can learn from these sessions are given later.

A good way to put everyone at ease is to start the first session by finding out what goes *well* at home. Although it is acknowledged that the family is here in order to help them get along better and because the parents have some concerns about the children, it is generally best to start by asking family members to talk about some of the things that go well in the family. Parents are willing to go along with this because, having had an opportunity to talk to the therapist alone in the first meeting, they know that the therapist is in fact quite aware that all is not rosy. Parents and children, even the youngest ones, are asked to tell about some of the things that happen at home that are fun. Young children, of course, will be very concrete. "I like it when Mommy buys me a toy," or "when we went to Disneyland." They may talk about when Daddy gives them a ride or Mommy brings cookies on the way home from work. This question could be followed up by more specific questions regarding some of the ways particular pairs in the family (e.g., two siblings or one parent and a child) enjoy one another and some of their memories about times that were especially enjoyable. These are questions that, when put in simplified language, even very young children can understand. Often there is a lot of laughter and excitement when reminiscing about good times. One problem that arises not infrequently, however, is that there may have been so much tension in a family that pulling for the positive simply does not work with all members of the family. Simply acknowledging that you understand there has been so much tension lately (or even for quite a while) that it is difficult to remember the good moments addresses the difficulty without immediately getting into the problem. One then shifts to family members who do have something positive to say.

Often I follow Chasin and White's (1989) suggestion and say, "I'd like to hear from each of you something good about yourself—something you're good at doing or something you are proud of" (p. 17). Asking other family members to add to what each person has described about himself generally gets lively conversation going and is informative regarding the capacity of family members to be supportive of one another. Parents are often surprised to see that siblings, competitive as they may be, frequently help each other out in saying good things about themselves. Of course, this question also highlights how people are regarded in the family and what is of particular importance to individual family members.

If there is so much anger and hurt in the family that talking about positives is simply impossible, the therapist must, of course, work immediately on what is going wrong. One or more family members (parent or child) may be scowling and simply unwilling to engage in any attempt to focus on positives about themselves or others. If this occurs, it is best to comment on the obvious unhappiness and invite that person to say something about what is bothering him. If that person refuses, other family members are asked for their input on what might be going on for the obviously angry or uncooperative family member.

ACTIVITIES FOR FAMILY SESSIONS

Skits, Plays, and Puppets

Role playing scenes from family life is an excellent way to obtain information while engaging children in active family play. Naming the youngest child "director," with the therapist or a family member as helper. is a playful way to engage children even as young as 2½ or 3. "Let's pretend" is an activity that even small children understand and enjoy. Shy children may prefer to use puppets or stuffed animals to represent family members rather than act out scenes using actual family members.

A variety of role plays are possible. The children can be asked, for instance, to put on a play showing what it is like when Mom come homes from work, when they all have dinner together, or it is time to go to bed. Of course, family difficulties will emerge, but it is important in the first session to pay relatively little attention to the *problems*, as many children, particularly those who are considered *the* "problem," will generally have a quite negative reaction to such discussions. Having fun as a family provides the foundation for further work and is in itself often a far too infrequent experience at home. An alternative to acting out scenes of family life is to have the family act out scenarios of how it would be if things in the family were different. Chasin and White (1989) give many interesting suggestions for getting even young children to focus on goals and to role play having their wishes come true.

Skits and puppet shows can be used in later sessions to enact some of the problems at home. At times these problem enactments occur in the first session, because it is what is really on the minds of the children, and it is what they spontaneously wish to demonstrate. Although, ideally, it might be best to save these negative enactments until future sessions, sometimes attempts to engage the family in positives, or even in neutral role plays, fall completely flat and the only meaningful thing to do is to immediately engage in a discussion of the family's difficulties.

Five-year-old Charles, for instance, having just had a tantrum on his way to my office, spontaneously started talking about how he "hated" his daddy. Rather than talking about what he felt or what happened he was asked to "show me" what had happened and used some big dolls to play out a scene that ended in his father spanking him. By asking Charles to have the doll talk and whine the way he had, and have the other doll talk, yell, and hit the way his daddy had, the child was able to convey a vivid sense of how he perceived the interaction.

Young children often choose the most current and immediate family situations to role play. One mother, for instance, was dismayed that her 5-year-old son portrayed her as lying on the couch when Daddy came home and portrayed Dad as waiting on her and the children. This was "accurate" only for the previous 2 weeks when the mother was recovering from some minor surgery. Accurate or not, these role plays vividly demonstrate what stands out for the child and even if the situation is an atypical one, a discussion of how this "skit" differs from most days is engaging and informative.

Board Games

I have found that parents and children alike are fascinated by opportunities to get to know each other's thoughts and feelings. As long as the discussion is structured so that expressing one's feelings is not in essence a disguised way to accuse one another, most children happily participate. There are many "psychological" or "therapeutic" board games that facilitate the nonaccusatory discussion of feelings and with some assistance even young children can participate in many of them. Families enjoy this activity so much that they often want to know where they can buy such games and occasionally have brought me some new ones to add to my collection. I am always on the lookout for games that will stimulate meaningful family discussions and consider these games absolutely essential office equipment. With some modification of the games children as young as 4 years old can play games such as the Talking, Feeling, and Doing Game; the Ungame (which has separate cards for child and adults); Family Happenings; My Two Homes; Scruples (separate cards for children and adults); Feeling Checkers; My Ups and Downs; and the Great Feelings Chase.[1] These games involve answering questions and doing things that range from silly (stand on one foot and count) to serious and psychologically revealing. (A boy was afraid to tell his father something—what was it and why? Or what is the worst thing a girl could say to her mother? Or what would you do if you saw your friend steal from a store?) No one has to answer any question, but those who do get chips or other rewards. With young children the cards are read and explained to them and only cards they are cognitively capable of understanding are used.

For most families, playing meaningful games such as these is a welcome relief from the problematic interactions that have brought them to therapy. The games are basically noncompetitive, although counting chips or points adds some incentive to participate. Young children can feel competent in these games because there is no right or wrong answer and the therapist (and it is hoped the parents) shows a lot of interest in the children's answers whatever they are. I have found it useful to announce that everyone must think seriously about their answer and that silly, quick answers will not result in points. Sometimes I have limited answers to things that have happened and feelings that relate to the family rather than to school, but this "rule" depends on the nature of the problem and the kind of answers the children are giving. The rule of thumb is that superficial, quick answers are not acceptable, but what this means will vary from situation to situation.

Drawing

Most young children love to draw. Zilbach (1986) has shown how children's drawings can be used as a way for them to communicate with parents in family sessions. Children are provided with appealing papers and washable markers and are asked to draw a variety of scenes such as (1) everyone in the family doing something, (2) something happy in the family, (3) the scariest thing they can imagine, (4) something sad, (5) how they feel when Mom and Dad fight, and so on. While they are drawing, the parents talk with the therapist about themselves—not the children. This arrangement gives the therapist a chance to observe something about how the family operates in a situation that in many ways parallels home life, where adults and children are engaged in separate activities. Do the children interrupt the parents a lot? Do they cooperate easily in sharing drawing supplies or do they argue? How does each parent react to interruptions? The therapist also gets a chance to see how each child deals with her instructions. Does the child comply with the request or does he draw something else entirely? Are the drawings revealing or guarded? The content of the drawings can be the starting point for a family discussion. For instance, one child drew everybody in the family doing something with the father off in a separate room asleep. This picture stimulated a discussion between the couple of how rarely they all do something together and how depleted the husband seemed by the time the weekend arrived. Samantha, age 10, drew her mother speaking on the telephone. Mother then talked about how angry she felt that her children never "let" her have a moment to herself once she came home. Issues of hierarchies and boundaries became the focus of the session.

A great deal of interesting material can also be obtained by using drawing as an activity for the whole family. A clipboard and paper are given to each person (young children seem to really enjoy clipboards) and each person is asked to draw something on a particular theme (e.g., the saddest thing that ever happened to you or the most frightening thing you can imagine). As many adults (and some children) are self-conscious about their inability to draw accurately, the instructions are that no one is to do a really good drawing because we want to spend only 5 to 10 minutes on each drawing, thus leaving time for the "guessing" part of the exercise. When the drawings are completed, each person shows his picture without explaining it. The other family members then guess what the picture represents. Each person's guess, of course, reflects his own concerns as well as an assessment of the concerns of another family member, and thus a great deal of projective material is revealed.

Family Discussions

Sometimes even young children are quite content to sit in a therapy room and just talk with their family. The experience of a focused family discussion with no interruptions or distractions can be very gratifying even to children as young as 4. Often, however, a situation arises where an older child is engaged by the opportunity to hear and talk with his parents and the younger child is restless or bored and wants to play. A good solution is to divide up the session between talking time and playing time. Knowing that an activity will follow shortly often enables the youngest family member to participate more patiently in family conversations. Giving the younger child some paper and markers, or even some quiet toys to play with "while he is listening," lets the child play and listen at the same time and avoids unproductive power struggles. Most children, given the opportunity to listen in on a family conversation without *having* to be fully part of it, will spontaneously join in and contribute to the conversation. When the child does *not* join in but instead does something to disrupt the flow of the discussion, the therapist is being given important information. Perhaps the child is feeling anxious about what is being discussed. Or perhaps she is feeling competitive with or jealous of the sibling who is the focus of attention. Or, conversely, the youngster may be helping out a family member who is on the hook by providing a distraction.

The content of what is discussed in family sessions varies greatly from case to case. In general, the aim of family meetings is to broaden the therapist's and the family's understanding of the context in which the child's difficulties exist. There are two separate but related aspects to understanding the child in context. First, understanding the context simply means sharpening our grasp of what takes place interpersonally within the immediate family as well as among family members, the extended family, and the larger community in which the family resides. Thus, for instance, if a child is having serious problems with impulse control and behaves in an overly aggressive manner, the therapist can use family sessions to explore questions such as the following: When do difficulties occur and, just as important, when do they *not* occur? How is the lack of impulse control handled at home, in school, by grandparents, etc.? How do the parents interact with the school around the problem? With other parents? With grandparents?

Much useful information can be obtained by asking questions that compare the reactions and feelings of each family member to those of the others (Penn, 1982). This technique often leads to a more precise and differentiated view of each individual in the family and the way each is perceived by the others. Questions of this sort can be used even with young children (Benson et al., 1991). The younger the child the more concrete the question should be. For instance, one might ask questions such as, "Who in the family was most afraid when Daddy got really mad last night?" "Does Mom worry about whether you will do well on a test more than Grandma does? Is it about the same? Or does Grandma worry more than Mom?" "Who is stricter about whining? Mom or Dad?" "Who in the family cries the most when watching a sad movie? Who cries the least?"

It can be helpful to have very young children "measure" the differences with some physical gesture. The child can be shown how to spread his hands wide apart to indicate a "lot" and to bring his hands close together for a "little." This gesture enables children as young as 3 or 4 to make comparisons. They can show that "Grandma worries . . . this much" (hands wide apart) whereas "Mom only worries this much" (hands closer together). By understanding the perception of *differences* of this sort, the therapist gets clues to who in the family may be reinforcing or encouraging behavior that is "officially" unacceptable.

The second meaning of understanding the child in context is to understand how the child's intrapsychic conflicts and unconscious concerns interact with the emotional issues and anxieties of other family members. Thus, for example, if a child reacted with rage to "slights" or, conversely, was stoically handling hurts, the therapist would raise as a topic of discussion in a family meeting how others in the family handle these concerns. The therapist might, for instance, ask the father how he acts when he feels injured and then ask other family members to comment on whether

Dad's self-assessment seems right to them. Inquiring into who in the family acts one way and who acts another makes the issue a family one and not just something only one child is dealing with. It also is extremely helpful to ask parents to relate these discussions to their family of origin. How for instance, did the mother's family deal with anger? How does Mom feel about it? What are the ways she wants her family to be different from her family of origin? In what ways similar?

OBSERVING SYSTEMIC INTERACTIONS

Much of what we learn about families from meeting with them comes from observing them interact. Although it is helpful to hear family members describe what goes on in the family, often the most valuable information comes from watching what might be thought of as almost "incidental" interactions. This section of the chapter is intended to help the reader organize the many observations that one inevitably makes.

The Family in the Waiting Room

When the therapist enters the waiting room and sees the entire family for the first time it is helpful to make a mental note of such things as the following: Are the children doing homework or are they playing? Have the parents brought any toys to amuse the very young children while they wait? Have they brought snacks for the children? How concerned are they about the eating habits of the child (e.g., do they care whether the children leave crumbs or wrappers)? Are any family members playing together or interacting while they are waiting? How do the adults interact with a shy child who will not say hello to the therapist? How do the parents interact with a child who refuses to come in? Or walks in still reading a book?

Careful observation of such events immediately gives us some useful information regarding the parents' expectations and the communication of these expectations to the children. A parent who comes armed with snacks and toys has very different expectations regarding children's capacity to delay gratification from the parent who has brought nothing and expects the young child to sit quietly until it is time to enter the office. This in turn is quite different from the parent who has brought nothing for the child to play with but interacts with the child while waiting, or the parent who never comes more than a few minutes early so that the children will not have to wait long.

When a child does not want to enter the office, some parents will firmly say, "You're going in and that's it," while others will explain, comfort, coax, or promise a treat afterwards.

Of course, it is important to notice the role each parent assumes. One may coax or comfort while the other is insistent and firm.

The parents' expectations regarding whether the child will behave "respectfully" to adults is often apparent at this point. Some parents make no mention of crumbs or candy wrappers or other debris that the children leave behind as they enter the waiting room. Others will communicate to the children that they are expected to clean up what they have left.

Similarly, some will demand that the child say hello appropriately while others seem accepting of behavior that others might consider rude — for example, not looking up when spoken to.

Upon First Entering the Office

It is not uncommon for one of the children to instantly claim the biggest and most comfortable chair. A squabble over who will sit in the "best" seat may occur. Although one might expect this squabbling between siblings, it occurs just as frequently between children and parents. I have seen many a little fellow push his Dad aside just as the parent is about to sit down. How this is handled is quite revealing. Some parents really do not seem to care and easily relinquish the good seat to the child. They tolerate this childish behavior with amused good humor. Others regard this as annoying behavior, and although they too may relinquish the seat, they experience themselves as engaged in a power struggle they are willing to lose. Still others insist that the child sit elsewhere. And not infrequently, the *other* parent intervenes, protecting the turf of the relinquishing parent.

It is important to observe not only how parents react to potential power struggles but also how the child responds to being told he may not have the seat. Does he easily accept parental authority or does he argue about it until the parent has no recourse but to threaten or physically remove the child? After such a confrontation, does the child recover quickly from this loss or does he stay in an irritable mood? Do either of the parents attempt to comfort him or calm him down after his defeat?

If the child is allowed to keep the "best" seat, it is important to observe the reactions of the other children. Do they seem resentful or tolerant? Are they indifferent to such competition or do they whine and complain about the unfairness of the situation? How does each parent handle the complaint of unfairness? Does he mediate (e.g., promise the other child a turn in the seat later) or does he say, "He's just a baby — let him have it"?

What the therapist observes in these initial interactions will be helpful as she gets to know the family and children better. For instance, the therapist may see that the father is overly reactive to challenges to his authority and easily engages in power struggles. The therapist may understand better an older child's resentment of a younger sibling if indulging the younger one is coupled with the expectation that the older child act maturely. The therapist may see that although the parents set limits, they inadvertently positively reinforce difficult behavior by comforting the child when he is upset. We must not generalize too quickly from such brief interactions, but these initial observations give us some hunches that may prove to be useful.

Physical Boundaries and Interactions

Young children are generally more physical with their parents than older children are. Most young children have a good deal of bodily contact with parents. The nature and quality of that contact, as well as the parents' reactions to it, are important to observe. Some young children will climb on their mother's or father's lap and snuggle in comfortably. Others, while cuddling, will poke, pinch, pull on, and kick the parent. Parents differ in their response to such behavior. Some parents seem to accept as "natural" what others generally regard as annoying or even painful physical intrusions. A little boy of 5, for instance, lay down on the couch with his feet on his father's lap and commenced to kick and pound his legs into his father's chest. The father mildly requested that the child stop doing this, but his tone indicated that he did not really regard the behavior as unacceptable. Similarly, a little girl of 6 climbed on her mother's lap and forcefully pinched her mother's cheeks and lips. The mother simply went on talking as if nothing even remotely annoying were happening. Only when the child kicked her shins did the mother begin to express some mild irritation with the little girl's behavior.[2]

Even physical expressions of affection can at times be intrusive. Fearful of hurting a child's feelings or believing it wrong to ever set limits on expressions of love and warmth, some parents ignore their own discomfort. It is important to assess, therefore, whether a parent *genuinely* feels comfortable with a child wrapped around his neck or cuddled in his lap or whether the parent is simply putting up with something he is not actually enjoying. In family sessions the therapist should try to assess whether there is congruence between the overt behavior and the feelings of both parents and children. Does the child's expression of affection seem genuine? For instance, if a youngster who cuddles a lot regularly hurts the parent in his embrace, one wonders whether the child is denying and simultaneously expressing some anger that he feels may be dangerous to express directly. One wonders too whether the parent who sets no physical boundaries actually feels comfortable with it or in fact harbors guilt over his wish that the child would go away. Is the parent being emotionally dishonest with the child and is the child picking up the parent's true feeling, which in turn leads the child to feel angry? These questions can be addressed in family sessions by asking the child to guess how a parent is feeling when embraced and asking the parent to comment on the child's perception. This kind of question must be asked with great tact and in a truly neutral tone if honest answers are to be given.

When a young child (less than age 6) has almost no physical contact with a parent in a session, it is in itself noteworthy. One wonders why the child keeps to himself so much. Some children as young as 4 or 5 will not allow parents to hug or kiss them. Sometimes this is an expression of anger. The child knows that this hurts the parents' feelings. She can deprive the parent of something most parents very much want. Some children keep a distance as a way of protecting themselves from physical intrusion. Many parents of young children will wipe the hair off the child's face, fix barrettes, wipe their mouths, and so on. For other children the lack of physical interaction with a parent unfortunately reflects a very early renunciation of dependency needs. It is as if the child were saying, "I don't care about being close to you."

Sexualized Behavior

On occasion a child may relate to a parent in physical ways that seem quite sexually charged. I have seen little boys kiss their mother's mouth and neck, caress her face, or stroke her breasts. Girls may wiggle around on their father's lap and whisper secrets in his ear. Some parents seem hardly to notice that this is happening, while others are uncomfortable but do not know what to do about it. It is important to observe too whether the "outsider" parent is distressed by this behavior or seems to accept it as natural. Some parents, "sophisticated" in psychoanalytic theory, assume that such oedipal behavior is natural and conclude erroneously (even by psychoanalytic standards) that the behavior should simply be accepted. Although, as Chapter 6 describes, an integrative approach does incorporate many psychodynamic formulations, we do not assume that *inevitably* there are oedipal issues in the family. Instead, observations of this sort are regarded as signals that alert us to the need to look more closely at what kinds of boundaries exist or do not exist at home. An increased awareness of just how frequently sexual abuse occurs in families leads us, of course, to look more closely at how the parents are relating to the children. No longer do we assume that sexualized behavior on the part of the child is always a manifestation of natural sexual drives that have not been appropriately checked and channeled. Instead, we must ask questions, both in sessions alone with the child and in sessions alone with the parents, that aim at giving us a clearer picture of what kinds of sexual boundaries are set at home. Does either parent feel uncomfortable about how the child looks at him (or the other parent) when he is getting dressed? Does either parent feel uncomfortable with the sleeping arrangements, bathing rituals, or degree of nudity in the family? By asking about differences in attitudes, we can obtain much information.

In cases where there is concern about overly eroticized behavior, I include in sessions alone with the child some opportunity to play with anatomically detailed dolls. In playing and talking with the child I incorporate questions about bathing, sleeping arrangements (particularly when one parent is away), and dressing. Of course, it is also important to observe the child's level of comfort or discomfort in answering these questions.[3] Although we must explore these concerns thoroughly, it is extremely important to keep in mind that we are not operating out of a presumption that sexualized behavior with a parent indicates abuse. We are simply exploring and gathering information: We are not conducting an investigation with which to indict the parents. Many families operate in ways that can be arousing to a child without in any way engaging in abuse. Sometimes, for example, a child may be allowed to behave in "sexual" ways with a parent because the parent is genuinely unaware of the sexuality inherent in the gesture. Thus, for example, Mrs. Jackson, a single parent who had raised her son Willie, age 7, from birth without a father, and who had not been involved with anyone romantically since his birth, genuinely did not experience the youngster's stroking of her breasts as sexual. Similarly, there are some families who, in their wish to make the child comfortable with nudity, walk around undressed and have no rules about privacy in the bathroom. Although many children are comfortable with an open attitude toward bodies, some children find such a milieu overstimulating. Generally, the rule of thumb I suggest to parents is that they stop walking around nude when they begin to feel uncomfortable about it. Usually the parents' discomfort reflects their sense that the child is looking at them and perhaps touching in a more eroticized way.

Clues to Coalitions, Alliances, and Roles

Careful observation of seating arrangements and patterns of movement in the session provide useful information about the role of family members and the structure of the family. Do the children sit next to their mother while their father sits apart? Do the parents sit apart from the children? How fluid are these arrangements? Does one parent seem more responsive to the children than the other does? Do the parents respond differently to different children? Does the parent who is the "outsider" seem happy to be left alone? Is he responsive when children initiate interactions?

It is particularly important to attend carefully to how the symptomatic child behaves toward each family member. Does the child behave in a rejecting way, saying, for instance, "No, I want Mommy to do it"? Does the child treat one parent as if she were not there?

If the child attempts to interact with a parent and is rebuffed, does the child become whiny? Aggressive? Withdrawn? Get engaged with a sibling? Play with toys? Become aggressive to a sibling? Become involved with some compulsive type of playing?

For example, the parents of a 7-year-old boy were considering residential treatment for their highly aggressive and difficult child. The mother, in an interview alone with the therapist, easily (and with no apparent guilt) stated that she believed this child was born difficult and that he had ruined their lives. She resented the fact that their cheerful, bright and "easy" 3-year-old daughter's life was being so disrupted by the disturbed older child, who from the time he was a toddler had, according to the mother, brought nothing but grief to this family. Although the father did not "denounce" the child as vehemently, he concurred wholeheartedly in his wife's assessment of the situation. In a family interview, the therapist was particularly interested in how these parents dealt with these feelings while the son was present and how the son in turn handled his feelings toward them.

What became clear in the family session was that the mother did seem to be totally disengaged from this child. The husband sat next to her in a way that essentially shielded her from the boy while the boy flung himself all over the father. The father showed much more affection for the boy than he indicated verbally and in fact they seemed to enjoy one another. Throughout the entire interview neither the boy nor the mother ever attempted to interact with one another in any way. The younger sibling mostly stayed apart playing with toys and only once in awhile interacted with the mother.

Reactivity and Standards of Behavior

Most young children are fidgety, fussy, inattentive, messy, and "impolite" by adult standards. Often they will not answer when spoken to. They may talk about something other than what they were asked. They may burp, pass gas, or get silly and "gross" with a sibling. Playful poking, pushing, shoving, and roughhousing between siblings often takes place even in a therapist's office. Sometimes this goes beyond playful horsing around. Siblings may get mad at one another and a shove easily becomes a smack. Families, and each parent within a family, differ tremendously in their tolerance for such behavior. What some parents find perfectly acceptable others react to negatively. Family interviews give important information about each parent's reactivity and tolerance level for these kinds of behaviors.

One mother, a single parent of an 8-year-old daughter, found it almost painful to be with her child. The child's "bad manners"—she would hold her cup of hot chocolate upside down hoping to get the last bit of chocolate, lick her fingers after eating ice cream, or sit with her feet up on the chair and fidget with her hair—simply drove this mother to distraction. In contrast, other parents hardly react at all to similar behavior. When a parent is very reactive to a child, it is important to watch carefully to determine whether the child is engaging in the annoying behavior in order to be provocative or whether the child is truly unaware of what he is doing. Equally important is how the child reacts to being told to stop. Does the child try to stop? Does he make a point of continuing to do it at least one or two more times? Does she seem annoyed or does the child try to stop without taking offense at the parent's reprimand?

Sometimes parents have extremely different expectations for children who may be only a year or two apart in age. Is the oldest child expected to control himself much more than his younger siblings are? Are the parents much more reactive to one child than they are to the others for reasons other than age?

It is important in observing family interactions to try not to let one's own preferences and style lead to a judgmental attitude. Our concern should be whether the parent's level of tolerance or reactivity is a problem for *this* family and *this* child. For example, the parents of two boys, ages 10 and 7, seemed quite relaxed about the wrestling and roughhousing these youngsters enjoyed with one another. It was clear that both parents took great pleasure in the boys' obvious closeness. They might mildly say, "Boys, now calm down," but basically they did not mind if the children fooled around a lot and did not seem to get nervous or tense about talking while this was taking place. Only when the fooling around resulted in one of the children getting hurt, and then enraged, did the parents get upset. They were concerned about the younger child's hot temper but had not thought to restrict the activities that resulted in so much excitement and reactivity.

VALUES AND ATTITUDES

Sessions that include the types of board games described earlier provide an opportunity to deepen the preliminary understanding of the parents' values that was obtained in the initial meeting. By listening carefully to each parent's answers as well as observing the attitude with which the game is played, the therapist begins to get a sense of what motivates and is important to each parent. For instance, responses to a question such as, "What is the most important thing a person can do in life?" run the gamut from an emphasis on achievement ("work hard at whatever you do so that you will be successful") to an emphasis on pleasure ("enjoy whatever you are doing") to an emphasis on morality ("look after those less fortunate than yourself").

Other questions in these board games give some indication of attitudes about aggression, hygiene, hostile feelings, and so on. "What do you think of a boy who sucks his thumb?" or "When was the last time you cried? What did you cry about?" are the types of questions designed to elicit attitudinal responses.

Perhaps more important than the explicit answers given is the atmosphere in which games are played. Some parents clearly enjoy competition and may playfully turn basically noncompetitive games into more exciting and challenging interactions. A child may be cheered on with statements such as, "Come on Doug, roll a good one, Nancy's catching up," or "Looks like Mom's the loser—Danny's winning!"

Competition between children or between children and a parent may be so strong that children call out an answer even when it is not their turn. Some children become quite frenzied when playing these games while others stay calm and unruffled. Some children voluntarily give extra help to the youngest family member or root for the player who is losing. Because these games are designed to be noncompetitive, the spirit in which they are played is a good index of the family's, as well as each individual's, general way of being in the world.

FOCUSING ON THE CHILDREN'S REACTIVITY, OPENNESS, AND METHODS OF COPING WITH STRESS

Although the purpose of the family meeting is to get a better sense of *family* interactions, the therapist also pays careful attention to the psychology of each child. For instance, as discussed earlier, we make note of how much the child seeks interaction with the parent or whether she keeps a distance. It is important to note how comfortable or uncomfortable each child appears to be with talking about emotionally sensitive material. Some children while going through the form of answering a question about feelings actually reveal very little. For example, there is a difference between a child who, when asked to state a wish, says, "I wish my mother was a teacher in my school," and one who says "I want all the money in the world." Although both children may be feeling a wish for more time with a parent, the first child is more comfortable expressing those feelings.

Most children are extremely uncomfortable hearing about problems in the family or about conflict between the parents. Some deal with this discomfort by trying to take control of the situation. They may tell long irrelevant stories without pausing to let anyone else say anything. These children cope with stress by diverting the family's attention. Others withdraw into a book or a game. Still others put a boundary between themselves and the parents by engaging (either playfully or aggressively) with a sibling. They can seem oblivious to the mood in the room or the tension expressed on a parent's face.

Conversely, some children seem extremely attentive to a parent's emotions. These children scrutinize faces for signs of what the parent might be feeling and anxiously ask such questions as, "What's the matter?" "Are you angry at Daddy?" or "Why are you looking at me that way?"

The therapist should also make note of how each child relates to her in terms of the desire for approval. Some children are obvious about wanting the therapist to think well of them. They spontaneously show something they are proud of and try to be engaging in a variety of ways. Others keep a great distance so that the therapist feels that they must be approached cautiously. If a therapist uses an affectionate term like "sweetie pie" some children warm up immediately while others look embarrassed or annoyed or may even say, "Don't call me that." Some children are very overt in rejecting any attempts at affection. They are not merely shy. Rather, they respond with hostility (scowling, insults, etc.) to friendly gestures.

Children display a range of reactions to the attention that a sibling may be receiving in the session. Some children seem comfortable and emotionally unthreatened by siblings. They do not seem to experience attention to a brother or sister as something that deprives *them* of attention. When a child does seem reactive to the attention a sibling is getting, her coping style should be carefully noted. Some children withdraw and start doing something of their own. Others become silly and annoying, thereby drawing attention to themselves. Others may interrupt, correct, or simply outtalk their brother or sister. Overt physical aggression may be displayed (pushing, pinching, etc.) or perhaps even excessive affection.

When working with young children it is important to be alert to when they seem fidgety, bored, or distracted. Is it defensive or is it simply a sign that the activity or discussion is not at a level appropriate for that particular youngster? Carefully noting the timing of the child's withdrawal gives clues to what may be making the child anxious or uncomfortable. Who was interacting with whom at the time? What topics were being discussed? What was the mood in the room?

Similarly, the therapist should make careful note of just when a child becomes disruptive. Often a youngster's disruptive behavior occurs when tensions between parents escalate. Some highly competitive children become disruptive when they find themselves losing even the noncompetitive board games described earlier. They may "accidentally" knock over the board or interrupt the game by doing something they are not supposed to do (e.g., peeking at cards, folding or crushing the box, leaving the room, or standing on furniture). They may bitterly complain about the rules or whine about the unfairness of someone else's success. Behavior such as this tells us a good deal about the child's lack of self-esteem and his need to prove his worth through winning.

It is useful to be alert as well to how the parents deal with this kind of reaction. Are they angry or comforting? Do they set limits? Do they remove the child and continue the game or do they let the youngster disrupt the family activity?

All these observations are useful in getting to know the child better as an individual. They provide the basis for formulating hypotheses about the child's conflicts, unconscious processes, and defenses which will be explored further in individual sessions with the youngster.

FEEDBACK MEETING WITH PARENTS

After an initial meeting with the whole family, parents are quite eager for some feedback. This meeting will be the first of many feedback sessions with the parents in which the therapist shares impressions and gives concrete suggestions. Throughout the work, but particularly in this first feedback meeting, it is important to include in one's comments statements that acknowledge the family's and the child's strengths. As discussed in Chapter 2, therapists do parents and children a great service if they can help parents see their children in a more positive light. When parents experience the therapist as having observed and appreciated aspects of their child that they may not have noticed or given much weight to, they often begin to have those feeling themselves. Both the parents' and the child's self-esteem is enhanced by the recognition of strengths and positive aspects of the child's personality. Helping families shift perspective through reframing and building on strengths is one of the hallmarks of family therapy, and never is this skill more important than when working with families with small children who are perceived very negatively by their parents.

It is important to preface positive feedback about the child with a statement that reassures the parents that you are well aware of the youngster's problems and how difficult he can be at times. The therapist's perception of strengths will not be accepted unless it is credible; by also indicating that the difficulties the parents worry about are very much understood, the therapist makes it possible for the parents to believe what she is saying. Even parents who do not see their children *particularly* negatively appreciate the underlining of strengths they may have taken for granted.

An example of what I am referring to might be the therapist's saying something about how involved the child became with new toys and how well he sustained interest and enthusiasm. Parents may be surprised by such a comment, assuming that all children play the same way. An elaboration that in fact some children lose interest very quickly, or need to continuously show the parent what they are doing, highlights that the quality of the youngster's engagement is in some way special, positive, and noteworthy. Similarly, the therapist might comment on how siblings play together and the ease with which they negotiate differences.

In general, the more specific the observation, the more impact it has. Repeating the answer a child gave in the Talking, Feeling, and Doing Game, for instance, and commenting on what made that answer interesting, has much more of an impact than a general statement about the child's giving interesting answers. Similarly, pointing out that the child had a thoughtful look before answering questions and gave serious thought to what he said may highlight behavior that the parents take for granted and do not notice as something to be valued.

Whenever possible, the therapist should try to convey respect, appreciation, and, if at all possible, affection for the child. In addition, the therapist must *learn* how to notice and spell out small positives. Although doing so may be consonant with a particular therapist's personality, it is nonetheless a skill that can be enhanced by training and practice (E. Wachtel, 1993).

Here are a few examples of the types of comments one gives in feedback sessions:

1. "Even though Cristie was shy and cautious, she clearly had a good deal of curiosity and wanted to communicate with the therapist. Her whispers to you seemed to be a way of communicating with me. She's shy but really *wants* to relate to others."
2. "It's clear Susie can be very provocative, but I'm struck by how interested she seemed when you were talking about your family?"
3. "Laura is really quite a tease. Sometimes it seems like she gets carried away by what started out as a joke. She's got a sparkle in her eye, and an adorable mischievous smile, which gets lost when she gets stuck in a power struggle."
4. "Danny is very direct. He lets you know exactly what he is feeling. He's really honest in his responses—nothing phony there."
5. "Johnny's quite a negotiator. I was impressed with how much he seemed to want to strike a deal."

6. "I was impressed by how patiently Ben waited while the instructions to the game were explained."
7. "It was impressive how Willie really likes a challenge. He wants to win a game fair and square and wouldn't accept the extra help you offered because then he wouldn't feel like he really had won."
8. "Evan's ability to describe what he is feeling is really impressive. His description of how he feels when his Dad is upset with him ('mad, and then sad') was amazingly clear."
9. "When you got annoyed with Sara, she was clearly bothered. She didn't just ignore you or have a 'who cares' attitude. Some children have gotten into such a negative stance with parents that they seem closed off to parental disapproval; that's not the case with her. She *cares* if you are angry at her."
10. "Tracy seemed extremely open and affectionate with her Dad."
11. "Johnny has a wonderfully expressive face. Every once in a while he showed his great smile."

Statements of this sort are followed by feedback regarding problematic interactions as well as suggestions regarding alternative ways of interacting with the children. Chapters 7 and 8 provide a full description of the types of interventions that might be proposed. For now, the focus is on initial interventions, which are the foundation for the collaborative planning and problem solving that characterize the bulk of the work. Positive feedback to parents generally (though not always[4]) helps strengthen the bond with the therapist, which in turn makes parents more receptive to suggestions.

After seeing for ourselves a sample of family interactions, we are in a position to explore further what we have observed. For instance, if we notice that the parents do not get firm with a 3-year-old youngster until they have reasoned with him for 5 minutes, we should describe and discuss this interaction. We may talk, for instance, about their feelings about being "authoritarian" or what they do at home when the youngster does not listen. Or, if we have observed that one child often interrupts when a sibling is speaking and seems to compete for attention, we should explore with the parents what happens at home in this regard and how they handle it. If the children have been huddled around Mom on the couch with Dad sitting apart, we should discuss this observation and find out from the parents whether this is typical and how they each feel about the role each parent has in the family.

The tone of these meetings is collaborative: Information is shared and together strategies are devised for tackling both individual and systemic difficulties. The initial interventions range from suggesting certain structural changes (i.e., that Dad be in charge of getting a child to school, or that Mom stops serving as the intermediary in family disputes) to working on the child's unconscious conflicts (see Chapter 7).

FAMILY MEETINGS AS PART OF THE ONGOING WORK

Thus far this chapter has focused on the initial meeting or two with a family in which the primary goal is to get to know the family in as relaxed an atmosphere as possible. Although later sessions with families continue in much the same spirit as earlier ones, there is a shift in emphasis to more direct work on resolving differences and planning new ways of interacting at home. The distinction between the early exploratory meetings and the later "working" sessions is not a hard and fast one, however. Throughout the whole course of treatment, meetings with the family are used not only to resolve problems but to expand our understanding of each person's needs and feelings.

Although each session with the whole family includes some follow-up on how any suggested interventions have worked, the therapist must make sure that the meetings do not turn into reports of failures and a litany of parental complaints and criticisms. Meeting with parents alone throughout the work generally enables them to use the family meetings productively because they have already had, and will continue to have, opportunities to discuss with the therapist "glitches" in strategies and interventions.

When meeting with the family as a whole, the therapist attempts to integrate into the family session the themes and concerns that have been illuminated in the meetings alone with the child and the meetings alone with one or both parents. For instance, one child told a story in which a baby elephant was afraid to grow up because the elephant family that had adopted her wanted a little elephant, not a big one. In a subsequent family meeting the therapist led the family into a general discussion of "growing up." Can one hold on to the old "baby" stuff? Could big girls use baby blankets or take their favorite stuffed bear to camp? Do the parents have any of *their* favorite items from childhood? Who (including adults) would like to be babied more? Who would like more independence?

With young children the sessions are very concrete and often involve actively demonstrating something rather than just talking about it. A young child might be asked to *show* how Daddy takes care of Mommy or how Daddy might like to be treated like a little boy. With somewhat older children, a more verbal mode may be employed. Thus, when it became clear that 9-year-old Tommy's overly aggressive behavior was based on feelings of extreme vulnerability, the topic of fearfulness and sensitivity to being hurt was raised with the whole family. How did the parents respond to slights or overt acts of hostility? What had they been like as children? Who in the family lets things roll off his back and who feels wounded easily? How do the parents feel when they know that one of their children has been slighted or emotionally wounded? How emotionally tough are the parents? What kinds of hurts have they experienced? Do they hold grudges? Do they show their hurt or anger or do they cover it up?

Although the first one or two family meetings should include all family members, subsequent meetings do not necessarily include all family members each time. Sometimes it is important for particular pairs or groups in the family to have an opportunity to discuss their relationship only with one another. Consistent with the integrative orientation of the approach described here, the therapist looks for ways to widen the discussion so that it includes not just systemic dimensions but also topics that are psychodynamically relevant. For instance, a father was frequently infuriated with his 6-year-old son, who was quite oppositional. Although the session started by focusing on the way the two interacted, the therapist broadened the discussion so that it included conversation that touched on the disturbing feelings of vulnerability, which seemed, from the information obtained in sessions alone with him the child (see Chapter 4), to lay beneath his refusal to go along with what was asked of him. The father was encouraged to talk about what it was like for this child when he and the child's mother separated. He was asked too to talk about the times in his own life that were most emotionally painful. How did he deal with the pain? Did people know he was upset or did he hide it? How does he deal with hurt now? Does he try to be very independent? Does he allow himself to be close and then feel rejected?

A discussion of this nature moves away from directly dealing with the symptomatic behavior and instead attempts to address the psychodynamic issues that lay beneath them. Chapter 7 describes many other ways to utilize psychodynamic formulations in family systems work.

Family sessions may also include a discussion of each parent's family history in relation to the particular issues relevant to the child and the family. For instance, one might ask what the attitude was in the father's family toward showing fear. How much was adventure valued? Closeness valued? Independence?

Generally, more detailed discussions of family history are reserved for sessions alone with the parents. This is the case both because parents are often guarded about revealing the extent of hostile feelings in front of their children and because doing detailed genograms is time-consuming and involves more "talk" than young children can generally sit still for.

In sessions alone with the parents, the therapist is able to explore more fully the extent to which parents may be acting out with their children unconscious agendas from their own history. Having met with the child, the parents, and the whole family at least once, the therapist has some idea about what issues need to be explored with the parents through discussion of their family history. In one case, by speaking with the father in some detail about his own childhood, it became clear (see the case of Mickey described in Chapter 9) that the child's extreme aggressiveness was covertly encouraged by his father, who had felt tremendously victimized by four older brothers. In another instance, it became clear that the mother's submissiveness to her tyrannical 6-year-old daughter was an acting out of the feelings of victimization she had had at the hands of her truly tyrannical mother.

Chapter 7 on utilizing psychodynamic understandings describes in detail some additional ways that family sessions can be used to address intrapsychic issues and defense mechanisms. The therapist may, for instance, work with parents in advance so that they can use a particular session to tell stories or reveal aspects of themselves that address unconscious concerns and defense mechanisms. Or, a session may be used for "Positive Reminiscing," which can reassure the youngster that his baby self is still known, or "Negative Reminiscing," the purpose of which is to interfere with maladaptive repression.

USING FAMILY SESSIONS FOR PROBLEM SOLVING

Throughout the work, family sessions are used to help the family plan new ways of doing things that will address the needs of all family members. Even children as young as 3½ or 4 can be engaged in finding concrete solutions to family problems. Four-year-olds are often delighted to be asked for their ideas on how things could go better at home. The problem, of course, must be stated very concretely. The therapist might say, for instance, that it seems that everybody gets pretty angry at one another around dinner time and that sometimes leads to tantrums, hitting, and punishments. What ideas do people have for how that time could be more fun? What could Mommy do to make things better? What could Daddy do? And what can the *child* do to make things more enjoyable at that time?

Children, of course, sometimes propose solutions that the parent does not want to agree to, although interestingly, this occurs much less frequently than one might imagine. When the child suggests something unacceptable to the parents, the therapist helps them to come up with some compromise or some alternative with which all parties are satisfied. Each person's suggestions are regarded as the beginning of negotiations and family brainstorming. When children are enlisted in problem solving of this sort, they feel proud of their ability to come up with some good ideas. This in turn makes them much more invested in actually following through on agreements.

The process also provides a model for problem solving which the child and the whole family can use in other difficult situations that may arise. The therapist encourages each family member to offer some suggestions regarding what he as well as others in the family could do to make things better. Once a plan is agreed on it is restated by the the therapist to make sure that everyone understands and is in agreement with the proposal. The family is also encouraged to anticipate and plan for difficulties they might encounter in actually putting the plan into effect. Consequences for not following what has been agreed on should be clearly spelled out. Sometimes rehearsing through role playing is helpful. Six-year-old Dawn and her mother role played how Dawn would greet Mom when she arrived to pick her up at the after-school center and how Mom would act in return.

Children often come up with creative solutions to problems and take great pride when they actually work. Nine-year-old Alex wanted everyone to tell a joke at dinner, and although that was not always possible, it highlighted the need everyone felt for a more lighthearted atmosphere. Eight-year-old Sally "solved" the problem of how upset her father felt by her refusal to eat what he had cooked for dinner by agreeing to plan menus with him and promising to try one new thing a week. And 5-year-old John thought a note (with a picture on it, as he could not read) in his lunch box telling him if it were a candy day or a fruit day would help him stop nagging his mother for candy on the way home from school.

As simple and concrete as these suggestions are, they really do help alter repetitive problematic patterns of interaction and increase children's feelings of control and conviction of the efficacy of talking out difficulties. The "solution" works not only because the child is asked to be an active participant in problem solving, but also because many of the issues surrounding the problem have been addressed. Thus, in the case of Tricia, she was willing to give up control battles over food in part because she no longer had to fight her *mother's* battles and in part because she was getting the *emotional* nurturance she craved. Contracting must always be thought of as just one aspect of the work and will not be effective if the related systemic and psychodynamic issues are not also attended to.

WORKING ON BOUNDARIES AND ALLIANCES

An important part of the ongoing work with families is to help them make some structural changes in the way the family operates (i.e., boundaries, alliances, communication patterns, and hierarchies) so that the needs of both parents and children are better met. Suggestions with regard to structural changes are based not merely on an understanding of the role of the symptom in the system but also on the behavioral and psychodynamic analyses that are part of a multifaceted approach. For instance, if a child's anxiety about doing school work "perfectly" is in part a reflection of a parent's anxiety around this issue, the therapist might suggest that the other parent be in charge of the homework and that the "anxious" parent engage, instead, in activities with the child in which both can have fun without trying to do it well. Or, if a child is enraged at his toddler sibling of whom he is expected to be tolerant, the parents might be asked to find ways to establish some boundaries between the children so that the older child has some private time with the parent. Or if a youngster's caution and anxiety relate to the expectation that he is mature enough to look after a younger sibling, sessions may focus on how to "deparentify" the child.

Not infrequently, parents inadvertently interfere with the development of a child's problem-solving skills because the parents are overinvolved or overprotective. In cases of that sort, sessions might be used to discuss what each child could begin to do autonomously and the ways the children might tempt parents to become reinvolved. How should parents handle the obsessive worry of a child? Could the parent leave it up to the child to do his own homework? What would make that possible? What kind of reassurances would the parent need? What if the child requests help?

If a child's power struggles with a parent stem from a need to separate from what the child is experiencing as an overly close relationship, more productive ways of becoming more separate are planned in family sessions. In some instances, for example, the parents have stopped relating to one another as romantic partners and are looking to their children for the support and nurturance they are not getting from one another. Family sessions might discuss how the parents can reestablish a grown-up, private relationship instead of relating entirely in their role as parents. How would the children react to not being included in some outings? Do the children respond positively or negatively and how should their reaction be handled?

When a child's difficulties with impulse control stem in part from a lack of clear limits, family sessions can be used as an occasion for clarifying rules and determining who will enforce them and how. Usually it is best to meet with the parents privately first so that different expectations can be clarified and negotiated. If agreement still cannot be reached, the family session could be used to discuss how these different rules could be incorporated into the family.

When a child's need for greater independence is an issue, family sessions might be used to set up different obligations and privileges for each child depending on his age and capabilities. Differentiating more between children based on their ages is often quite effective in helping with sibling tensions.

Sometimes, however, parents need to alter expectations of *younger* children so that they are more in line with what is expected of the older ones. Older children resent what they experience as too much license for the younger one to do what he pleases simply because he is young and thus regarded as less capable of understanding rules and being disciplined. Although young children notoriously overestimate the "culpability" of their toddler-age sibling, parents may in fact be underestimating the extent to which a toddler can learn to respect an older sibling's boundaries. Family sessions can be used to discuss what it is fair to hold each child responsible for. Once parents are open to discussing these issues, older children often become a lot more reasonable in regard to what should be expected of their younger siblings.

ESTABLISHING RULES FOR COMMUNICATION WHEN PARENTS ARE DIVORCED

When parents are divorced or separated, each family is generally seen separately. Often, parents need to accept that they simply cannot control the operation of the ex-partner's household and that children will need to adjust to each parent's way of doing things. If, however, widely divergent expectations and rules are having a negative effect on a child, the therapist needs to make it clear to each parent that efforts must be made to establish somewhat greater consistency. It is beyond the scope of this book to discuss exactly how to get warring parents to declare a truce, but often it is helpful to confront them with detailed evidence of the negative impact their adversarial relationship is having on their children (Isaacs, Montalvo, & Abelsohn, 1986).

Family sessions with each family should include a discussion of expectations regarding the child's communication with the other parent. Frequently children are confused and conflicted about what is permissible to talk about when they are with their other parent and stepfamily. I have worked with children who in order to protect a parent, or to protect themselves from hearing disturbing negative statements, do not talk at all about any aspects of their life with the other parent. When in one home, it is as if the pets, stepsiblings, and family friends in the other home simply do not exist. Such strong prohibitions against open communication lead to anger and a sense of isolation. Explicit discussion of this is-

sue in family sessions is a relief to children and they welcome the chance
to tell their parents how they feel about the hostility that is expressed
(often subtly rather than explicitly) toward the other parent. Explicitly
spelling out what the parent feels he can emotionally handle is helpful
in freeing up excessively inhibited children. Other common issues that
need to be resolved with both the child and each family and between the
divorced parents themselves if at all possible are (1) frequency of telephone calls to the other parent's home when the child is away from that
parent, (2) handling child's complaints about the other parent or stepparent, (3) the reluctance or refusal of a child to visit with the noncustodial
parent, and (4) the child's feelings when both parents attend an event.
A discussion of these issues, as well as other concerns children have about
divorce and separation, can be facilitated by playing board games with
their parents (My Two Homes or Family Happenings) that ask questions
about situations that arise for children who are dealing with divorce, separation, and blended families.

OVERALL DYNAMICS OF THE FAMILY SYSTEM

It will be obvious to the reader that in any particular case different aspects
of the family system are of central importance or relevance. If one can
step back from the specifics of any given case and consider the broader
set of concepts and considerations that bear on the difficulties children
and families encounter, it is helpful to reflect on the entire set of considerations that the therapist should have in mind when meeting with
the family. In the final section of this chapter I present a brief overview
of what I regard as the key foci that the therapist needs to bring to bear
in examining the systemic dimensions of a child's difficulties.

The reader should keep in mind that in the work being described
in this volume, the distinction between evaluation and intervention is a
somewhat artificial one. Although the first few sessions are generally spent
just getting to know how the family operates, assessment of family dynamics does not proceed in a linear fashion. The methods used to ascertain and appraise family dynamics are in themselves often therapeutic.
Moreover, assessment of evolving family dynamics continues throughout the whole course of treatment. In fact, many of the assessment issues
about to be described cannot be addressed until some interventions have
been attempted.

Perhaps the most important consideration when thinking about the
child's problems systemically is to determine how the family interacts
around the child's symptoms. The therapist must try to ascertain not only
what other family members gain from the child's symptom, or what the

child might be expressing that other family members cannot express for themselves (see Chapter 1), but also what specific behavior on the part of the parents implicitly encourages or accepts the child's symptoms. Similarly, the therapist must always be alert to how the family's attempted solutions to their problems might inadvertently be making them worse.

In assessing the role of family dynamics we try too to determine what events may have shifted some stable pattern in the family or what might be going on developmentally in the lives of the children that is affecting family interactions. Understanding the effect of developmental or other changes on the family system involves having a well-articulated sense of the predominant transactional pattern of the family (see Minuchin, 1974). We notice, for instance, whether there are strong alliances between particular dyads in the family and whether the ways of relating are flexible or rigid. If, for instance, a mother and child are extremely close and the father is treated like something of an outsider, can the system readily shift if the father expresses dissatisfaction with this arrangement or the child begins to feel a need for more contact with her father? Perhaps the most important boundary issue in working with families with young children is whether the parents have a relationship separate and apart from their role as parents. Often, one or both parents are feeling a good deal of frustration and deprivation because they are overwhelmed by the demands of parenting. When both parents juggle careers and family life they frequently feel that there is little or no time for themselves or for the relationship. Detailed inquiry into schedules and exactly how nonwork time is allocated is helpful in understanding what sorts of changes in the structure of the family might alleviate some of the tensions being expressed through the child's symptoms.

Understanding how the psychodynamic issues of the child relate to those of other family members is another important aspect of a systemic assessment. From information obtained in family meetings, meetings alone with the child, and meetings alone with the parents we learn what feelings are easily expressed in the family and what feelings are expressed with difficulty or not at all. Transference distortions, in which the child is being responded to with feelings from some other relationship, are of particular importance. So too is information from parents about unacceptable aspects of themselves which are possibly being denied and then projected onto the child.

A systemic assessment also involves making some determination regarding what methods of intervention are likely to be most effective with any particular family. Some families come to therapy looking for behavioral suggestions while others are much more interested in exploration and insight. We must ask ourselves, therefore, whether this is a family that is likely to respond well to tasks, or explicit suggestions.

Whenever possible, it is best to begin in a manner that will most readily be accepted by the parents and that fits with their unarticulated expectations about the way therapy will work.

Last, and perhaps most important of all, we need to be able to articulate the strengths of each family member and notice and underline each person's motivation and ability to change his part in problematic interactions.

4

Knowing the Child in Depth:
A Clinical Guide
to Effective Individual Sessions

S ix-year-old Anna sat on the couch with her head buried in her mother's shoulder. As she vigorously sucked her thumb she would surreptitiously raise her averted eyes to glance at me and a slight smile began to emerge as I waved and made funny faces. As I talked with Anna's mother, the shy little girl and I continued our nonverbal flirtation. But with each question or comment directed to her she burrowed into her mother's armpit. Mrs. McDonald implored Anna to talk, but the pixie-faced youngster remained steadfast in her preference for thumb sucking.

Seven-year-old Andrew was quite happy to leave Mom in the waiting room. He strutted solemnly but confidently into my office, pulled up a chair, stood on it, and reached for Chutes and Ladders. My statement that he could not play that game just yet but that there were some other fun things I thought we could do together was met with a terse, "I don't want to do anything else." Andrew sat silently as I described some of the things we could do. "I want to play Chutes and Ladders, I want to play Chutes and Ladders, I want to play Chutes and Ladders," he repeated over and over again.

Another child, John, age 9, started talking to me before he even entered the room. Without a moment's pause he offered a nonstop stream of commentary on Ninja Turtles and the pros and cons of various Nintendo games. Attempts to slow him down or to engage in conversation served only to trigger monologues on new topics.

It is the feeling of helplessness that scenarios such as these evoke that is probably the source of many therapists' feeling that it is not useful, necessary, or even possible to meet individually with troubled youngsters. This chapter aims at giving family therapists the tools they need to foray into the largely uncharted territory of including individual sessions with children as part and parcel of family therapy. Like "choose-your-own-ending books," there is no *one* correct answer for what to do next in such scenarios. But it is hoped that this chapter will provide the reader with ideas on how to engage little children and use the time with them productively.

THE PURPOSE OF MEETING ALONE WITH THE CHILD

Children are more difficult to get to know than adults are. When seen only in family sessions, it is easy for the therapist to overlook their idiosyncratic characteristics and perceive them in simplified, noncomplex, categorical terms (parentified child, acting-out child, good child, baby of the family). Unlike adults, who even in family sessions are very much known to us as individuals, children often remain essentially unknown because they do not easily talk about themselves and their feelings. One reason, then, for individual sessions with each child in the family is simply to get to know them in something approaching the depth to which we get to know the adults.

When I first began to meet with children alone I limited my role almost exclusively to getting to know better their concerns and unconscious conflicts. My purpose was simply to understand the child more deeply so that I could better incorporate an understanding of child's concerns as an individual into the work with the whole family. I used the sessions to try to answer such questions as the following: What is the child worrying about? What are his fears? Are there unconscious conflicts that might be contributing to a child's difficulties? What is his coping style? Does he withdraw from difficult tasks, or is he able to persist even when frustrated? Is the child emotionally open, or is he cut off and detached? Does the child seek a lot of approval? Is the child cooperative, or does he create a tug-of-war? What are his social skills?

Over the years I have found that such a narrow definition of purpose was unnecessary. In addition to better understanding children's concerns and needs, the time alone with them could be used to directly help them change their part in troublesome systemic interactions by playfully coaching them on ways to be more effective in getting what they want from parents. It could also be used to do some direct work on social skills, impulse control, or anxiety reduction.

Individual sessions with children should be held only after rapport with the parents has been established. It is crucial to convey to parents that their concerns have been heard and that individual meetings with the child will enable the therapist to further explore the issues they have raised.

When I began to experiment with direct therapeutic interventions in individual sessions, rather than limiting my role to enhancing my understanding, I was concerned that working directly with the child might undermine my relationship with the parents. This concern has proven to be unwarranted. By carefully maintaining a strong bond with the adults, I ensure that the child's pleasure in our meetings is not threatening to them.

Although direct therapeutic interventions with the child are sometimes incorporated into the first one or two individual meetings, these sessions are generally used primarily for the purpose of establishing rapport with the youngster and getting to know him better. For the sake of clarity, this chapter focuses primarily on the methods used with children in the first one or two meetings. Chapters 7 and 8 provide guidelines and suggestions for how meetings with children can be used to directly work on their difficulties.

SOME GUIDELINES FOR INDIVIDUAL MEETINGS WITH CHILDREN: DIFFERENTIATING THESE MEETINGS FROM PSYCHODYNAMIC PLAY THERAPY

Seeing children alone enables the therapist to include an understanding of the child's psychodynamic conflicts in the family work; however, it is important that therapists be clear, in their own mind and with parents, that they are *not*, by seeing the child alone, embarking on "child therapy." A brief detour at this juncture to review some of the differences between psychodynamic child therapy and the integrative child–family approach being described in this volume may help prevent therapists who try this approach from inadvertently slipping into traditional roles, which are not appropriate to this way of working.

The Relationship with the Therapist

In individual psychodynamic child therapy, the relationship between child and therapist is regarded as the vehicle through which change takes place. The therapist becomes a "developmental facilitator" with whom developmental tasks are completed (Chethik, 1989). Many child therapists feel that by responding to the child in more caring ways, the therapist demonstrates new ways of relating and alters the child's unconscious expectations regarding interactions with adults. Anna Freud (1964) described the analyst as becoming a new love object for the child and substituting herself for the parents as the child's ego ideal: "They obtain from the analyst what they have up till now expected in vain from the original love objects" (p. 41).

In contrast, the therapist in the approach described here studiously avoids substituting for a parent in any way. Although an affectionate and warm relationship with the child is essential, the focus at all times is on improving the relationship between parent and child, not on giving the child a corrective emotional experience with the therapist. A central assumption of working with young children in the context of family therapy is that a relationship with a therapist can never have the impact on a child of the actual interactions with family members. The aim is to help the child have a corrective emotional experience *within the family,* and individual sessions with the child are directed in a variety of ways toward that end.

Needy children who bond quickly to a therapist can evoke strong nurturant feelings in therapists. The therapist must carefully avoid becoming the "good parent." Instead, the warm relationship with the child should be used to influence the youngster's behavior in ways that will change his interactions with his family as well as with other significant people in his life. It is an underlying assumption of this book that new experiences provide a much more powerful and comprehensive corrective experience than the brief time spent alone with a therapist.

Interpretations and Transference

An important aspect of the work of psychodynamic child therapy is the uncovering of unconscious or traumatic material so the child can discard unhealthy defenses (Winnicott, 1971) and accept forbidden impulses. The child's unconscious wishes and conflicts become known not only through his play but through the transference relationship that develops in the unstructured, accepting atmosphere of long-term therapy. It is believed that a nondirective approach fosters the development of transference which is the basis for insight and interpretation. A fundamental assumption of traditional psychodynamic therapy with children is that the child, in the transference, repeats and eventually corrects his difficulties in relationships by acting them out with the therapist. The child may repeat with the therapist aspects of specific past relationships, may transfer onto the therapist global assumptions expressed with many people (Chethik, 1989, calls this character transference), may displace onto the therapist feelings about current people and relationships, or may attribute to the therapist feelings that the child has been unable to accept in herself.

The child therapist, in time, begins to interpret to the child the meaning of her behavior. According to Holder and Holder (1978), "The therapeutic work proper, which gradually leads to fundamental intrapsychic changes, only begins with the verbalization and interpretation of the unconscious mental processes that find surface expression in the child's play. For example, Chethik (1989), describing the therapy of a 6-year-old child with elective mutism, says that "he began to point out to Amy that she was showing him that she felt sometimes that her mouth was like a cutting or biting thing" (p. 116) and wondered aloud whether the child got mixed up that when she would talk it would be like biting or hurting someone.

Psychodynamic child therapists generally assume that a good deal of time and frequent contact with the therapist are necessary to unearth the child's unconscious fantasies. Once they are understood, much time is spent letting the child "work through" in play his concerns. In the child-in-family model described here, the therapist *also* tries to understand the psychodynamic dimension of the child's difficulties. This is done, however, through occasional meetings with the child in which the therapist directs the activities of the session in a way that maximizes the likelihood that unconscious concerns will be revealed. The directiveness of the sessions, combined with the fact that the meetings are only occasional and interspersed with family meetings, minimizes (although by no means eliminates) the intensity of transference reactions. In the approach being described in this volume, it is *not* assumed that it takes a long time to understand what is bothering the youngster. Nor is it necessary for the child to reveal every nuance of his unconscious fantasies. Usable psychodynamic formulations, though perhaps not of the same depth as those obtained in psychoanalytic treatment, may be gained in just a few meetings.

As in individual therapy, helping the child become less afraid and thus defended against unconscious material is also a goal of the family–individual orientation. This goal is achieved, however, primarily through the work with parents and family and not through the relationship with the therapist.Unlike psychoanalytically oriented individual child therapy, interpreting unconscious motivation and concerns to the child directly is almost never a part of the work. Instead, the therapist provides insight *to the parents* regarding the meaning of the child's behavior and helps them use this insight to interact with the child in therapeutic ways.

The question of how important insight is if therapeutic change is to last is one that is still being debated. It can be argued that without insight the child does not have the tools to handle other problems that might arise. On the other hand, most children, never having been in therapy, proceed fairly smoothly through the developmental tasks of childhood with no specific attention to insight into what may be unconsciously motivating them. The therapeutic approach being presented here aims to help youngsters and their families get back on track. New experiences presumably will alter feelings without it being necessary for the child to confront and articulate directly heretofore unconscious concerns and feelings. The approach described here is based on a view of psychodynamic conflict (cyclical psychodynamics) (see P. Wachtel, 1987, 1993) that does not regard unconscious anxieties and wishes as existing in a world apart, impervious to influence, but instead sees both sides of the conflict as kept alive, if unconscious, by the individual's way of being in the world and the responses this invokes in others.

Susan Harter, who has done extensive research on the cognitive developmental aspect of children's ability to understand emotions (1983b, 1986), describes the difficulty children have in accepting the coexistence of contradictory affects (e.g., happy and sad):

> Children first deny that such feelings can co-occur, then acknowledge that they can occur *sequentially,* and eventually appreciate the fact that they can simultaneously co-occur. It is suggested that the most difficult conceptual task is to realize that one can have two opposing feelings, e.g., love an anger, toward the *person* at the same time. (1983b, p. 52)

Even apart from the question of what kind of insight is actually possible for young children, knowing when and how to make interpretations is something that is difficult to do without a great deal of one-to-one experience with young children. Children can become quite frightened by interpretations, that interfere with what might be rather fragile defense mechanisms. Brody (1964) points out that those who work with latency-age children know "how irritable a child may become if we merely remark upon the presence of a barely conscious conflict. . . . The technical problem is delicate, since children tend to regard all signs of internal conflict with distaste" (p. 391).

There is much good work that can be done in individual sessions with a child without risk to the delicate balance the child may have achieved. There may be occasions, however, when it is difficult to get the child to try out new behavior without some limited addressing of unconscious motivation that might be getting in the way.

The Role of Play

The purpose of play in psychodynamically oriented child therapy is twofold. Through play the child both expresses her concerns and works them through. A significant (though not sufficient) component of psychoanalytically oriented child therapy is the use of play as a way for the child to abreact troubling experiences (Sarnoff, 1987).

Generally, psychoanalytic treatment of children involves letting the child play in an undirected fashion. The therapist carefully avoids influencing the child's play so as not to interfere with the validity of the projections. Gradually the child's working through of the fantasy begins to change. Though this may provide some relief in itself, many analysts feel that without interpretations the improvement in the child obtained simply by play is not likely to last.

In the child-in-family work being described here, the child's play is viewed not as a way for the youngster to abreact troubling emotions but rather as a way to get to know what is bothering the youngster. In contrast to child therapy, the play is often directed. The therapist actively explores certain themes by steering the play toward concerns he wishes to investigate. Thus, the therapist might say, "Let's pretend this guy here is a bully and these are little boys who are afraid of him." By directing the play toward specific concerns, the therapist is often able to get material that would otherwise take a great deal of time to emerge (Winnicott, 1971).

Chasin and White (1989) in contrasting "play" in family therapy from "play" in child therapy encourage therapists to use play that is more factual than imaginative. Whereas imaginative techniques focus on fantasies about animals, monsters, and other invented characters, factual play "documents the actions and feelings of real people as they are now or could realistically be in the future" (p. 9). In their work with families with young children, the child plays out family scenes (enactments) or uses hand puppets to communicate "emotionally engaging information in an intelligible way" (p. 9) that requires little interpretation.

In the individual–systemic approach being described in this book, both types of play are important. When sessions include the whole family, factual enactments of the type described by Chasin and White are extremely useful. Even the youngest of children are engaged by such play, and the enactments often highlight problematic systemic interactions. When children are seen alone, however, it is important to allow the play to go beyond directly factual material. Factual, role-playing types of play generally reveal very little about the child that differs from what has been said or enacted in family sessions.

A WORD ABOUT CONFIDENTIALITY

In my experience, young children *expect* therapists to talk with their parents. Unless the therapist alters this expectation by promising confidentiality, which I do not, children are generally not bothered by my sharing some of the content of the session with parents. Often, in fact, they want to run out to the waiting room to show a picture or to tell Mommy or

Daddy about what we are doing. Or they might tell me to "tell my Mommy about the story I made up." Sometimes in a meeting with a child I might suggest that we ask a parent to join us in an activity or a discussion. On occasion, in a playfully conspiratorial spirit, I might say, regarding a particular strategy I am suggesting to a child, "Let's keep this our secret and see if Mommy and Daddy notice what is different about how you are doing things." This type of intervention is described further in Chapters 7 and 8.

Occasionally a child asks me not to tell a parent what he has said. This request, in itself, may reveal a great deal about what is going on with the child and family. Perhaps the child is angry at his parents and expresses this anger in withholding, or passive–aggressive behavior. Or perhaps the child feels intruded upon and is attempting to set some boundaries. Or the child may be afraid that her parents will be angry if they know that she has revealed some family secret or may feel guilty for some thought or action that was confessed in a meeting with the therapist.

The child's wish for confidentiality must be handled with great tact. Generally I respond to the child's concern with reassurance and support but make no promises I cannot in good conscience keep. By talking to me about the topic, the child is clearly indicating a wish for help in dealing with that issue. Rarely has a child rejected my offer to help him talk with his parents about something. Assurances that I will not repeat his exact words but nonetheless must let his parents know about his worries usually give the child enough of a feeling of control that a possible power struggle between us is averted. I also let children decide whether they prefer to be present when I discuss their concerns or whether they prefer for me to first speak with their parents alone. This too gives the child some sense of control and safety.

Negotiations such as these, however, are infrequent occurrences, because most children do not come into a meeting with me with the expectation that I will be their confidante. Parents need some guidance on what to tell their children about the meeting with the whole family and subsequent individual meetings with the children. The simplest and most understandable explanation for family therapy is that the therapist is a person who helps families get along better, feel happier, and have more fun together. The child who is the identified patient should also be told that the parents are concerned about some difficulties he is having and that by meeting as a family they will be able to work together to find some ways to help both him and the family as a whole. After meeting the children in a family session, the therapist should tell them that he will be meeting with each of them alone just to have a chance to get to know them better. Further sessions with a child who needs additional help are explained as an opportunity to have the therapist help them with some difficulties.

Within the approach described here, neither the parents nor the therapist should say to a young child, "You may have some things you'd like to talk about in private." A statement such as this may set up an expectation of a secret alliance which can be threatening to both parent and child. Further, it may inadvertently reinforce the child's feeling that what he is feeling is a guilty secret that he rightly should not reveal publicly. It is important to treat the individual meeting as matter-of-factly as possible and to convey to family and child alike that these meetings simply give an additional perspective to the family work. Parents often expect the therapist to get the child to "open up." In order to avoid pressure on the child and the therapist as well as the disappointment and possible disillusionment of the parents, it is helpful to explain that there is much to be learned about the child just by interacting with her and that young children seldom open up in direct, conversational ways. Rather, they reveal in their stories and play activities some of their concerns, many of which they would not be able to articulate consciously.

When giving parents feedback on the session, the therapist must caution them not to discuss with the child too directly what has been said. They are asked to be discreet in what they relate to the youngster. The reason for this is to avoid making the child self-conscious about everything she relates to the therapist. Although the child does not expect confidentiality and knows that I will be talking to his parents about him, it is nonetheless important that he not feel that everything he says to me is reported verbatim to his parents and will result in a direct discussion with them about the topic.

Parents often want immediately to talk to a child about the youngster's concerns. Such a discussion can be counterproductive, however; if the child feels that he will have to elaborate on, discuss, or defend everything he has said to the therapist he will understandably be more cautious about what he talks about. If, for instance, concerned parents were to go back to the child with, "I hear you think we love your brother more than we love you," the child might feel embarrassed and overwhelmed. The parents' wish to quickly *do something* about the child's upset is of course understandable, and the therapist works with them to address this issue without raising it with the child as something he reportedly said in the individual meeting.

THE FIRST MEETING

Separating from Parents

The child and I are not strangers when we meet for the first time alone. Already, we have had some fun together. In a prior family meeting, the child, with my help, has orchestrated some playful family enactments. Almost always we have shared some laughter in that first family meeting. Some children have already let me tease and perhaps even hug them. Always, I try to say something in the family meeting that aims at making the youngster feel proud. Generally the session has been fun and the child has a positive association to me. Often the child has already given me a drawing or showed me a cherished toy.

If a young child seems anxious about coming into my office alone with me, I start the session by having the child and a parent come in together. Most children, even those as young as 2½ or 3, eventually are eager to have the parent wait in the waiting room. While the parent is in the office, the child may be asked to talk with us or, if that seems too difficult, he will be given some paper and drawing materials to occupy himself while I am talking to the adult. The child is told that soon we will ask Mommy or Daddy to wait outside while he does some fun things with me. This approach has the benefit not only of alleviating anxiety, because the child feels more secure in the presence of a parent, but of heightening the child's wish to spend time alone with me since play is delayed until the parent leaves. There is, in effect, a paradoxical benefit to requiring the child to wait for the therapist's full attention. It is generally best, therefore, not to engage in an activity with the child while the parent is still present, as this will eliminate an incentive for having the parent leave.

There are some young children who simply are too anxious to separate from their parent on a first visit. Reassuring parents in advance that it is not *crucial* that the child spend time alone with me helps both parent and child relax about the meeting. Parents should be told that the session will provide useful information even if the child frets, fusses, and is generally uncooperative. It is important for the therapist not to set herself up for failure by giving the parents the impression that she will probably be able to win the child's confidence.

Some parents unconsciously identify with and encourage the child's ability to resist and defeat the "experts." Resistance of this sort is minimized by not rising to the "challenge." The therapist's attitude when parents express concern about the individual meeting should be something like, "It can be very useful; should we give it a try?" If the parents give their assent, it is helpful to ask their advice on what they think might make it possible for the child to be comfortable with an individual meeting. Engaging the parents in a collaborative effort in this way minimizes any resistance the parent might feel.

Creating a Playful Atmosphere

Even the most confident of children may feel somewhat apprehensive in those first few moments alone with the therapist. T-shirts, lunch boxes, baseball caps, and backpacks often serve as entrees into some casual and friendly conversation with the youngster. One need not be an expert on pop culture to engage a little fellow in a discussion of some bizarre-looking figure printed on his shirt. "Who's that guy?" gives the child an opportunity to talk about something he probably knows much more about than the therapist does, and this temporary shift, in which the youngster is in a sense the authority, can do much to put him at ease. Or, with very young children, some concrete questions about the lunch box such as, "Is it new? What kind did you have last year?" or "What did you eat for lunch today?" help them relax, in that answering my questions seems fairly easy.

Occasionally, of course, one encounters children who are so timid that although their parents wait outside they nonetheless do everything possible to avoid contact with the therapist. These children keep their head down, avoid eye contact, and remain silent when spoken to even about neutral subjects such as those just cited. Faces frozen with fear, these youngsters seem to be feeling almost tortured with anxiety. "Hello there, little boy. Won't you play with me?" said in a squeaky "rabbit" voice by the big stuffed rabbit that is an essential piece of equipment in my office, often elicits a smile straining to emerge and a tentative peek. "You look like a very nice little boy," says my stuffed friend. "Please, please, please, won't you play with me?" Children of all ages almost always respond to such obvious ploys.

A cozy, friendly, furry friend is an invaluable assistant in making these meetings seem like fun. Giving the youngster another stuffed animal to hold, and talking, for example, to "little bear" instead of to the child directly may break the ice. It is good to sit down on the floor with all little children, but especially with those who seem very frightened. The less formal the situation seems and the more the adult is down at his level, both figuratively and literally, the more relaxed the child will feel.

If the child continues to seem very frightened and frozen, the therapist should consider asking the parent to join the session. Deciding whether or not to do this involves assessing whether the child is showing some signs, albeit slight ones, of adjusting to the situation, such as exploring accessible toys or holding the animals proffered. If the youngster really seems only to be suffering and enduring the time, the parent should by all means be brought in. Though information has not been obtained in the way the therapist had hoped, experiencing the child's anxiety directly and noticing the interactions that take place when he is reunited with the parent provides important information for future interventions.

TALKING: FROM FACTS TO FEELINGS

Although I might try to engage the very fearful child by immediately taking out some toys and inviting the child to join me in playing, generally,

I prefer to start the meeting by talking to the youngster a bit. I tell the child what I already know about him from the family meeting (e.g., that he is in second grade, is good at drawing, and likes to cook with his Mom) and follow up on some of what I know by asking very neutral and concrete questions. The younger the child, the more concrete my questions will be. With a 5-year-old, for instance, I might say, "So, I know you are in kindergarten and that you go to school on the bus. So, tell me about some of things you do in the morning before you go to school." With young children it is helpful to include some "doing" in the "talking together" part of the meeting. I might, for instance, take out my "friend," the big stuffed rabbit, and say, "Let's make believe this rabbit is you, and let's place the rabbit on the couch and pretend he is you asleep in your bed. Could you show me how Mommy or Daddy wakes you up? You be the grownup and the rabbit will be you. What happens next?"

Once I have engaged the child in relatively nonthreatening conversation, I try to directly discuss the difficulties I know she has been having in order to get a sense of how willing she is to acknowledge the difficulties. I try to couch the problem in a way that does not make the child feel blamed. For instance, I might say to a 4-year-old, "Mommy tells me that she is unhappy about how she yells at you a lot and that the two of you get mad at each other almost every morning." Abstract questions like, "What do you feel about that?" generally lead to dead-end answers. Instead, I might say, "Did you and Mommy have a fight this morning? Do you remember what she got mad about? Let's act out what happened this morning?"

Or, if a youngster is not concentrating in school, I might say something like, "Your Dad says that you seem to be having trouble paying attention and learning things in school. Do you know what he means?" I might go through the child's school day step by step and ask him to rate when it is easiest to concentrate and when it is most difficult.

Or, if the main concern is that the child has extremely aggressive outbursts I might tell her that I understand she can get really really mad sometimes and that she gets into some trouble with her parents and teachers when she has what they call a "temper fit." Could she tell me about what got her mad the last time she had a fit and what Mommy or Daddy did when she got upset?

Often, it is from very concrete descriptions of events that we learn most about the child's feelings and experience of the world. Even the most verbal of children, however, frequently have a difficult time narrating events in a coherent chronological fashion. Young children do not have the cognitive capacity to organize numerous and complex facts into a temporally correct sequence. Thus, stories told by children are often very confusing. Exactly what happened and when are jumbled together into an incoherent tale that can leave even the most attentive of adults bewildered. Furthermore, like adults, children often do not *know* what exactly happened that led to an upsetting interaction.

If, for instance, you ask a youngster about a recent tantrum, he might simply say, "I was mad, I didn't want to leave the park." Tantrums, however, usually are the culmination of numerous small preceding frustrations and disturbances which are often unconscious or too subtle for the child to articulate. Helping the child give a step-by-step narrative of the course of a disturbing event is one of the best ways for therapists to get some clues as to the child's deeper feelings. In order to get a moderately accurate description of an event, the therapist must be active in helping the child tell her story.

Generally I try to hear the parent's version of an event first so that I have some guidelines for my discussion with the child and do not have to guess what she may be omitting. For example, the mother of 7-year-old Norene reported that the child had been very whiny and complaining when playing ball with three other children and the other children's father. According to the mother, after half an hour of the child's complaining about injuries and unfairness to her in the game, the mother said angrily, "If it's not fun we'll have to leave." Shortly thereafter, when it was in fact time to leave anyway, the child had a tantrum that was quite extreme. The conflict escalated with both mother and child losing control until the mother slapped Norene and dragged her, kicking and screaming, all the way home.

In a session alone with Norene, I explained that I wanted her to tell me very very slowly what happened so I could really understand what made her so upset. As children are wont to do, she summed it up simply. "I had a tantrum because I didn't want to leave," she said, "Mommy got very mad, I cried a lot but the next day I stopped crying and we didn't fight any more." Questions about what she had been doing in the playground elicited a confused story about how she kept getting hurt while she was playing ball with her friend, the friend's father, and each child's younger sibling. It is important to be persistent in the pursuit of clarity while at the same time being careful not to make the child feel badgered or inadequate in his ability to communicate. To help Norene, and to make the whole interaction a little more enjoyable, I asked her to act out for me parts of the narrative. Together we blew up a balloon that would serve as our make-believe ball and put some large dolls on the couch to serve as representatives of Norene's mother and other women who were sitting on the park bench. With these props Norene was able to act out the sequence of events that had occurred. She demonstrated how she had gotten hurt and role-played, by talking to the doll, just what she had said to her mother and the tone of voice in which it had been said. By acting out responses to my inquiries (e.g., What did Mommy say to you? What happened next?), it emerged that Norene felt she was getting hurt a lot in the game and believed that the other children's father (it is important to note that Norene's parents were divorced) was not being fair in how often he threw the ball to her. Finally, I asked the youngster to role play what she wished Mommy would have done when Norene complained to her about getting hurt. From this role playing it became apparent that the child felt unable to change the game to something she would have enjoyed more and wished her mother would have said to the other children's father, "This game seems too rough. How about if you play something else with them?" Her repeated complaints to her mother about being injured were her attempts to get her mother to help her cope with what she was experiencing as a difficult situation.

On a psychodynamic level, the detailed narrative from Norene's perspective of the events that preceded the tantrum made it clear that her upset was not so much about leaving the park but was, rather, a manifestation of feelings of deprivation and of not being sufficiently protected. These feelings had to do with the relatively little time Norene spent with her father as well as the fact that Norene's interactions with her mother were not gratifying. She did not know how to express her needs in a way her mother could respond to, nor did her mother know how to decipher the real meaning of Norene's whining.

Using Drawings to Help the Child Present a Coherent Narrative

When a child is having a difficult time narrating a complicated series of events in a manner that is clear to the therapist, it can be helpful to ask the youngster to help draw or sketch what happened in the sequence in which events occurred. Concretizing the child's words with a rough sketch can help the child express with clarity the time sequences he is describing. For instance, when 8-year-old Doug tried to explain the sequence of events that occurred the night he returned home from a 1-month stay at sleep away camp and stole $50 from his mother's purse, he became quite frustrated with my failure to understand exactly what transpired. The specifics of the events of that evening were important because they could provide clues to the feelings that led to the "theft." Only by my translating his words into some quick diagrammatic drawings was I able to piece together a complex series of events in which Doug and his brother were picked up at the bus stop by his father and stepmother, visited briefly with his paternal grandparent, was dropped off for dinner at his mother and stepfather's house and picked up by his stepmother after dinner for the start of a 2-week holiday with their father. Simple drawings of the camp bus, each house, his siblings, and the car trips between each visit greatly clarified the events that preceded Doug's taking his mother's money. As Doug described the events, it became clear that it was hard for him to once again leave his mother after having been away for a month and that this feeling was exacerbated by the fact that dinner with her felt very brief and was interrupted by the presence of a 6-month-old half brother.

WHEN THE CHILD SEEMS SERIOUSLY DEPRESSED OR IS BEHAVING BIZARRELY

If a child is exhibiting signs of depression or is behaving in a manner that seems paranoid or bizarre, it is important to talk to the child in a way that elicits information about these concerns. Though we want to build on strengths and as much as possible avoid "pathologizing" a child, nonetheless, we must not shy away from inquiries that might reveal serious disturbance. Family therapists need not become experts on child clinical assessment and psychopharmacology. It is our obligation, however, to make an informed decision as to whether a psychiatric/psychopharmacological evaluation is appropriate.

Depression

The younger the child, the less likely he is to directly express the feelings of sadness, hopelessness, and low self-esteem that characterize depression in adults. Instead, the child's dysphoric mood may manifest itself in a diminished wish to socialize, a change in attitude toward school, extreme fluctuations in mood, deterioration in school performance, sleep disturbance, loss of usual energy, somatic complaints, weight loss, self-deprecatory ideation or an increase in aggressive behavior. (Rehm, Gordon-Leventon, & Ivens, 1987; Rutter, Tuma, & Lann, 1988.) Even very young children *can* talk about their dysphoric feelings if they are given a method to concretely describe how they are feeling. A simple and often informative method of helping children discuss their feelings is to ask them to place their feelings on some gauge embedded in a physical metaphor such as a speedometer. Clasping my hands together in front of me, I tell the child that this is like the "speedometer" of a car. "When I put my hands all the way over to this side, it is the most unhappy anybody can get, and when my hands are all the way over to the other side, it is the happiest feeling a person can have; show me how I should put my hands so that they will show how you feel most of the time. Show me how I should put my hands when you are feeling very sad and when you are feeling very happy." The child might also be asked to indicate on the gauge how happy or sad she has been feeling in specific circumstances (e.g., in school, when she is home alone with Mommy, and at the playground).

Some children readily reveal what they are thinking when they are extremely upset. It is not uncommon to hear children say things such as, "I'm stupid," or "I hate my body," or "I wish I were dead." When a child makes statements such as these, or when a youngster places himself at the extreme end of the continuum on the "emotional speedometer," therapists should take such statements seriously. Many therapists feel uncomfortable asking a child about suicidal thoughts for fear that such questions will seem strange, or that it will give the child dangerous ideas. Clearly great tact and care should be used when embarking on such an investigation, but therapists must force themselves not to shy away from this responsibility. It is important to inquire whether the child is ever so unhappy that he sometimes feels like hurting himself. Affirmative answers should be followed with questions regarding how he has imagined hurting himself and when such feelings have occurred.

When there is concern about a child's being depressed, it is important to find out from teachers and parents whether the child's mood changes in reaction to particular circumstances and environments. A child who seems consistently flat and constricted is very different from a child who, though unhappy at home, is lively and enthusiastic at school. Some children complain to parents about hating school, yet the teacher may report that the child is a lively and engaged participant most of the day. Conversely, some children who seem to teachers to be quiet and constricted are outgoing and rambunctious at home. When a child's negative mood seems consistent across situations, it is of greater concern. We look, therefore, at how readily the child's mood changes if circumstances change. One also needs to get a sense of whether the child's mood has changed recently or whether the predominant affect reflects a long-standing characterological adaptation.

Thought Disorder versus Normal "Lying"

Young children often talk about fantasy and reality in one breath. Adults, not accustomed to this blending of fact and fiction, can easily become confused and concerned about the sanity of the youngster who is relating an improbable story. Primary and secondary process thinking are not as clearly separated in children as they are in adults. Many children make such extravagant claims about their abilities and prowess that one wonders whether they are capable of distinguishing their wishes from what is really the case. "I played at Jimmy's yesterday and we buried six dogs." "Six dogs?" "Yes, they were poisoned by the stuff that was sprayed to get rid of the gypsy moths and we buried them?" "Who buried them?" "Me and my friend." "What did the dogs look like?" "They were big and black." "Did any grownup know about it?" "No, we found them in a secret spot where nobody knew they lived."

A dialogue such as this can be alarming and bewildering to adults. Though many children mix fantasy with reality, most by the age of 3 or 4 have some, though by no means complete, ability to differentiate between actual and invented events and by age 6 or 7, children should clearly be able to distinguish between fantasy and reality (Simmons, 1987).

In talking with a child it is important to assess whether the youngster can distinguish between reality and fantasy. Directly inquiring about the child's understanding of what he is saying can tell the therapist whether the youngster is able to differentiate between primary and secondary process thinking. If the child telling the "dog" story described above was 4 years old, he should be able to acknowledge that some parts of the story *really* happened and some were "just fun to think about." Goodman and Sours (1967) point out that some very peculiar and fantastic verbalizations a child might make are more comprehensible once questions such as, "Where did you hear that?" or "Who said that?" (p. 63) are asked. Often, children who have been insistent that the story they are relating *really* happened will shift away from their adamance when a comment is made that perhaps their story is similar to something they heard or read. Young children may feel that something they read or heard *really* happened and the therapist's highlighting the distinction between "stories" and actual events enables them to reflect on their narrative without questioning their integrity.

Sometimes the question arises as to whether the child is confusing fantasy and reality or is "making something up" or lying. Anna Freud distinguishes between a variety of types of lying in which young children engage. Some lying (which she calls "innocent") occurs when children have not yet made the full transition from primary to secondary process and thus cannot clearly distinguish between inner and outer reality. "Fantasy" lying, on the other hand, may occur in children who can make these distinctions but who are coping with intolerable realities by means of regression to infantile forms of wishful thinking. The child, for instance, who feels abandoned by a parent who does not maintain contact with him may engage in a compensatory fantasy that the parent is someplace where there are no telephones; if asked, however, he can clearly distinguish between fantasy and truth. Finally, some lying (which Anna Freud, 1965, calls "delinquent" lying) is motivated by the desire to gain material advantage, fear of authority, escape from criticism or punishment, or wishes for aggrandizement. Although young children engaged in delinquent lying of this sort may temporarily convince themselves that their fibs are true, there is no loss of reality testing and unless they are afraid of the consequences of confessing, inquiry usually makes clear that there is no thought disorder.

Parents or teachers may report behavior that could be a sign of schizophrenia, delusional (paranoid) disorder, or autism. If, for instance, a child is described as extremely socially isolated, "almost in a trance" and "muttering to himself," the therapist should ask the child what she is thinking about at those times. Most children will simply say, "I don't know," or will give some specific and concrete answer. If a child looks distressed or distracted when asked these questions, or when asked questions about wishing to hurting himself when he is upset, further inquiry regarding delusions or hallucinations is called for. Did he ever hear a voice telling him to do something? Was the voice his own voice which came from inside him, or was it a voice from outside? What did the voice say? What did he say to the voice? Was it hard sometimes not to listen to the voice?

Similarly, if a child's fear is so extreme that preoccupation with it interferes with normal functioning, one should inquire into the child's thoughts regarding the possibility of harm. Does the fear have a delusional quality? Does the child believe that someone is trying to hurt him?

Though we can try to ascertain the young child's level of reality testing, the younger the child the harder it is to come to firm conclusions. What we would regard as signs of a thought disorder in an adult are far less significant in young children, whose sense of what is possible and not possible in the world is still in the process of developing. The younger the child, the stronger the belief, for instance, that in some unknown way the physical universe will punish you for wrongdoing (Piaget, 1932b). It should also be noted that in young children even very bizarre behavior such as twirling and talking to oneself may be a coping mechanism which does not signify psychosis. Notwithstanding an overall reluctance to "diagnose" children, there are some circumstances under which a referral for psychiatric or psychological evaluation seems warranted. When signs of a possible thought disorder are detected, or the child seems potentially suicidal or severely depressed, a psychiatric consultation should be arranged. When and whether medication is called for are complex questions, but at a minimum, parents should discuss this option with a psychiatrist and/or psychopharmacologist.

It is important at this juncture to note that *generally* diagnostic classifications play little role in the child-in-family approach being described here. Rather than classify and categorize the type of disturbance the child is manifesting, the child's specific vulnerabilities, deficits, and anxieties are worked with in the context of the family. There is a good deal of overlap in diagnostic categories and the fine distinctions necessary for accurate *Diagnostic and Statistical Manual* (3rd ed., rev., DSM-III-R; American Psychiatric Association, 1987) classifications do not seem relevant to effective therapeutic intervention of the sort being described in this volume. Instead, interventions are tailor-made to match the individual issues of the child and the systemic dimensions of his family life. Categorizing the child, for instance, in terms of such classifications as "borderline," "schizoid," or "narcissistic" may even be harmful in that it may limit the therapist's quest for creative interventions and solutions to disturbed behavior. Many children who say and do bizarre things respond extremely rapidly to family interventions and soon look "normal."

PLAYING, TELLING STORIES, AND DRAWING

Almost all young children are eager to engage in some activity and have a relatively low tolerance for sitting still and talking. Children will become fidgety, look bored, or ask outright, "When can we play?" Though such reactions are completely natural and expectable, therapists should nonetheless make note of just *when* the child changes the topic. It is important to consider, for example, whether the child is avoiding some uncomfortable topic which is beginning to emerge. One of the goals of a session alone with the child is to get a better idea of the defense mechanisms this particular child uses. Chapter 5 reviews some of the typical ways children avoid awareness of troubling feelings. A child who suddenly becomes distracted or inattentive, or talks about something totally unrelated to what has just been said, is quite different from one who says directly, "Can we play a game soon?"

The primary reason for "play" (I include in this term telling stories and drawing as forms of play) in the context of this approach is to elicit projective material from which one obtains a deeper understanding of both conscious and unconscious concerns. Games that are not primarily geared toward the stimulation of meaningful discussion, such as Checkers or Chutes and Ladders, are not used unless a child is so anxious that it is only possible to engage him around this type of neutral material. Games of this sort are best kept out of sight until they are needed: Once a child fixes on these simple and familiar games, getting her to shift gear to more meaningful play may be difficult.

Initially, when selecting play activities for young children, the rule of thumb is that one wants to get projective material as quickly as possible while relating to the child in a way that he experiences as a game. Thus, as described earlier, it is best to be "directive" in the play, not only in limiting the child's choices to meaningful games but also in participating in the games in such a way that one's "hunches" about what might be going on for the child are explored. It is helpful to have a variety of special games and materials (to be described later), although even with simple materials one can turn an easy activity into an interaction that reveals a good deal about the child and his concerns.

Though most children definitely prefer to play than to talk, there are some children who by age 8 or 9 or even younger are quite articulate about their feelings and seem not only willing but eager to talk about themselves in a conversational manner. Although eventually one wants to use projective material to get at feelings that may as yet be unconscious, it is important to follow the child's lead in regard to the pacing of this shift. For instance, one 7-year-old girl with whom I was meeting for the first time seemed to prefer to talk rather than to play. With the most minimal encouragement she talked about memories of the time when "Daddy still lived with Mommy" and what she missed about their being together (crawling into bed with them). She eagerly recounted the events of the day 2 years ago when her parents announced to her the decision to separate and described how she felt at that time. When children talk with such ease about feelings, one wonders whether they have simply learned to verbalize but are emotionally detached from what is being said. It was clear from later meetings with each parent that this child had not in fact ever spoken of these matters to either of them and that she was grateful to have an opportunity to speak about these memories.

"FEELING" BOARD GAMES

Most children love structured games. In the context of a game, children will do a lot of things they would not otherwise do. "Freeze," "Take two giant steps forward," "Go back three spaces," "Spin," "Give one chip to the player on your left," and "Answer the following question," are commands easily complied with once a child has agreed to submit himself to the rules of a game. It is as if games induce a somewhat altered state of consciousness in those who choose to play. Both adults and children surrender their normal inhibitions and objections to the rules of the game. When playing games, one steps outside one's usual self. Perhaps there is something comforting about the clarity and objectivity of "the rules of the game." Even children who generally have a great deal of difficulty around compliance will often willingly follow the simple commands of board games.

The pleasure children take in playing board games can be put to excellent use in enabling them to describe feelings and events of importance to them. A child asked by a card in a game to tell about the scariest thing that ever happened to him is much more likely to answer such a question than if asked outside that context. Even rather guarded youngsters will reveal a great deal about themselves if it is ostensibly for the purpose of accumulating points or chips. It is not that children are easily fooled. As with "animal" stories that really pertain to the child, the youngster is generally quite aware of what the adult is up to. The magic of the game or story allows the child to indulge the adult. Children willingly but not naively play along with the adult.

There are a variety of games that are designed to elicit self-revelations. The Talking, Feeling, and Doing Game (created by Richard Gardner) is an easy game that children seem to enjoy a great deal. As the child goes around the board, she picks cards from the three categories of talking, feeling, and doing. The cards vary greatly in how provocative they are and a child is allowed to pass if she does not want to answer a particular question (but then does not get a chip for answering). There are no right and wrong answers. Points or chips are accumulated simply for expressing one's thoughts or feelings.

Whenever I play this and other similar games with children, I tell them that they only get a point if they think seriously about a question and give the best answer they can. Without this instruction, many children would give glib, meaningless answers in their eagerness to quickly win through the accumulation of chips. When it is the therapist's turn to answer board game questions, she must carefully choose answers that may stimulate greater self-revelations on the part of the child. For example, if a child is struggling with denied anger at a parent, the therapist might answer the board game question "What's the worst day you can remember?" by talking about something the therapist's parents did that made her very angry. Or, if a child may be feeling stupid or inadequate, the therapist's answer to a question such as, "Tell about the scariest thing that ever happened to you," might describe an event in which the therapist felt scared that he would not pass a test or remember a speech that he was supposed to deliver. If the child then chimes in with some similar feeling or incident, the therapist may give the youngster an extra chip for volunteering information even when it was not his turn.

The Ungame is a commercially available game which, like the Talking, Feeling, and Doing Game, poses stimulating questions to children as well as to adults. This game is totally noncompetitive. Many children and adults are made uncomfortable by the fact that one just goes around in circles. There is no clear end point toward which all players move. In order to use this game (which has the benefit of specialized cards for different age groups including adults), I have had to devise ways to make it mildly competitive and more goal oriented.

Another board game that is very similar to the Talking, Feeling, and Doing Game is the Family Awareness Game. Although this game is designed to be played by families, it can easily be adapted to play between the therapist and youngster. An advantage of this game is that the cards are coded so that the therapist can preselect cards relevant to the particular circumstances of the child (alcoholism in the family, abuse, remarriage, stepsiblings, etc.).

Feeling Checkers is a game in which, in order to take an opponent's piece when jumping him, the player must first talk about the feeling named on the underside of the checker. I have found it best to make this rule a bit more concrete and demanding so that glib responses are not offered. The child is asked to talk about a time in the last week or so that he felt that feeling at home or in school. If, for instance, the checker selected said "Sad," the child could only claim that checker if he told about something that happened in the last week that left him feeling sad. It would not be enough for the child to say, "I'm sad when Mommy won't buy me a toy." Instead, the child should be encouraged to tell about a time when that happened.

Card games like My Ups and Downs, in which a child must talk about the feeling illustrated on the card before using it, is another variation on the theme of talking about a particular feeling.

A simple wooden cube with names of feelings etched on each side (Feelings Cube, Project Charlie, Edina, Minnesota) can be rolled back and forth between the child and the therapist. Each player gets a point for talking about a recent event that relates to the feeling named on the side of the cube facing him. As always, the therapist tailors her response in such a way that it fits with the child's concerns. Children may be given extra points for talking about feelings that they have not themselves rolled.

Learning about the Child by How He Plays the Games

Careful observation of the child during the course of playing these games provides the therapist with much useful information. Some children seem anxious about their ability to answer questions correctly. Because the questions in these games have no right or wrong answer, the persistence of this kind of anxiety after "successfully" answering some questions is an indication that the child feels quite insecure about her abilities. Paradoxically, sometimes a child's *overenthusiasm* for these games may be a sign of low self-esteem and insecurity; some children seem almost too thrilled at their success and indicate by their self-laudatory statements ("I'm good at this, I've got 12 chips!") that the feeling of competence they are having is somewhat of a novel experience.

Despite the instruction that they must really think about their answers, some children talk a lot but say little that is self-revealing. When a child seems reluctant to be open, it is best to give chips for whatever *has* been volunteered and to switch to a game that is less demanding of self-revelation until trust develops.

Waiting for the game to be set up and explained can be a taxing task for some children. These children seem so impatient and frantic that they create a feeling of tension in those who interact with them. They grab at the playing pieces, spin, roll, and say, "I know . . . I know . . . let's play," leaving the therapist with hardly enough time to catch his breath. One needs to determine whether this is a true impulse control problem or whether it is simply a manifestation of anxiety, over-enthusiasm, or an intense wish to compete. By warmly but firmly asking the youngster to wait, one gets a sense of how much self-control the child possesses and how willingly he responds to limit setting.

Competition is so important to some youngsters that they will turn these essentially noncompetitive games into fierce contests. Counting their chips, they may gloat about how much they are winning. A throw of the die that leads to a loss of chips is very upsetting to some children and may result in a desperate attempt to "win" by cheating. Intensely competitive play in low-key games such as these is an indication of an ego sorely in need of bolstering.

Sometimes one sees the reverse of the excessively competitive child — one who worries about the player who is losing. These children actively hope that the other player will have some good luck. They seem to feel guilty about winning and change even mildly competitive games into ones in which there is no winner and no loser.

However the child reacts — whether with enthusiasm, caution, competitiveness, or generosity — one learns a good deal about both his interpersonal style and his level of security and self-esteem.

TELLING STORIES

Through stories children reveal their concerns, defense mechanisms, and coping styles. Stories can be told as direct narratives or they may be part and parcel of some fantasy play using plastic figures, dolls, stuffed animals, or puppets. Though most children enjoy creating stories, there are a variety of techniques one can use to make the process of story telling seem more like a "game" (Gardner, 1971). There are also methods of providing "provocative" stimuli for stories that minimize the possibility of guarded and facile narratives.

Squiggles and Embedded Pictures

I have found it useful in working with very young children to use a variant of Winnicott's Squiggle game. In this game, the therapist or child draws a squiggly line and the other uses the line as the starting point for a picture. The instructions are simple: "I shut my eyes and go like this on the paper and you turn it into something, and then it is your turn and you do the same thing and I turn it into something" (Winnicott, 1971, p. 12). This technique was used by Winnicott in brief consultations (which he distinguishes from psychoanalysis) with parents and young children. Through the child's simple drawings the child communicates his concerns and Winnicott replies with responsive drawings as well as direct interpretations to the youngster. His interpretations to the child are based on a theory of emotional development rooted in an object relations approach and are by no means obvious or self-evident from the drawings themselves. In addition to Winnicott's direct interpretations to the children, he uses the drawings as a means of communicating the child's concerns to the parents.

I have found that children as young as 4 or 5 years of age can "make something" out of the simple squiggly line I draw. The drawings I do in return are intended to address specific themes and issues that I think may be of concern to this particular youngster. Often this leads to pictures that are more self-revelatory than the initial ones produced by the child. When an informative picture is drawn, I do not interpret the meaning of the drawing to the child but instead ask the youngster to make up a story using what he has drawn. Often with very young children they need help in getting started and I have found Gardner's (1971) method of prompting the child with neutral connective material quite effective.

A variant of the Squiggle game, which older children enjoy, involves making an elaborate squiggly design that covers the page. The task then is to make a picture out of a shape inadvertently created and embedded in the scribbled patterns. As with the simple squiggles, the child and the therapist create stories, often collaboratively, about the discovered pictures and through these stories gain an increased understanding of the child's experience. Tailoring one's discovered picture and story to the child's psychodynamic issues is a fast and effective way to stimulate informative projective material. One might, for instance, find an angry face of a monster in the child's squiggle and might make up a story about a monster who acted like a monster but really felt very frightened. Often, children respond with some story of their own or a real-life event which in essence is their free association to the dynamics described in the therapist's story.

Observing how the child approaches this game may be as informative as the actual material elicited. Some children are extremely tentative or constricted in their responses. They see only the most obvious things in the squiggle and may find the same figure in each drawing. Some children will not risk creating an original story. They parallel or imitate the therapist's story almost exactly. For instance, if the therapist tells a story about a whale that was lost, the child might tell almost the exact story about a fish. Inhibited children such as these need the active participation of the therapist in creating stories. Starting the child off with a few neutral sentences which she is then encouraged to complete (e.g., "Once upon a time there was a . . . ? who lived . . . ? and who felt . . . ?") and encouraging more by saying, "What happened next?" often lead to richer stories.

If the child with this kind of assistance cannot really tell a story, the therapist has learned something important which needs further clarification. The therapist might consider whether the child is frightened and defensive or perhaps has an inadequately developed capacity for an active fantasy life. Children who behave impulsively and aggressively often seem to have a less than average capacity to sustain fantasies (Sarnoff, 1976).

Divorce Story Cards

Divorce Story Cards (Shapiro & Thiobdeau, 1987) are designed to be used like Thematic Apperception Cards. They are black and white drawings of provocative situations which can be interpreted in a variety of ways. These cards serve as a useful stimulus for children regardless of whether or not there has been separation and divorce or even marital conflict. The scenes depicted are quite varied; they include scenes that almost all children can relate to, such as pictures of children and parents in playgrounds, children interacting with teachers, daydreaming youngsters, and so on. To make the story telling seem more of a game, I present children with a few of these 9″ × 12″ cards as if they were a giant hand of cards and ask them to close their eyes and pick one. I preselect the cards that seem most relevant to this particular child.

I then ask the child if she can make up a really good story about the picture on the card. The child is encouraged to make up a story that has a beginning, a middle, and an end, and I ask the child questions that gently push him for more depth. If a child is hesitant to tell a story based on the card, I will start the child off or may even tell a complete story myself in order to make the child more comfortable with the task.

The Divorce Story Cards are useful too in stimulating discussion of important events and occurrences in the child's life. Very often, young children will spontaneously discuss an incident in their own life which is similar to what is depicted on the card. They may even discuss the picture as if it were literally a picture of them and their family. One 4½-year-old, for instance, said, "That's me with the bow, that's Mommy, and that's my Daddy leaving the house. Mommy cries when they fight and Daddy leaves."

Sometimes a child ignores the main event in a card and focuses only on the background. This may be a sign that what is stirred up by the picture is too troubling and that the child is defending against acknowledging the feelings evoked. At times, the child may in fact be drawn to the background scene because it is particularly meaningful to her. One little girl, for instance, ignored the foreground figures of an angry-looking mother pushing a child on a swing and instead only talked about the happy looking threesome in the background as "my mother when she was a little girl, with her mother, pushing my mother's little sister who is a very happy baby."

Bag of Toys

Another playful way to encourage children to invent stories is to let them pick a small toy from a grab bag and use the object picked as a stimulus for their narrative (see Gardner, 1971). The bag should be filled with small objects, animals, and people. If the child picks an elephant, for instance, he must try to include the elephant in a story. A variation on this game which many children enjoy a great deal is to have them pick two or more items which they must then try to weave together into a narrative. The silliness of this task lets many children relax and leads to looser and more fantastical stories than they might otherwise create. Miniature egg beaters, mice, hats, guns, motorcycles, food, stairs, drums, and so on are combined to make fanciful stories which nonetheless express something about the child's concerns and unconscious wishes and anxieties. The therapist can join with the child in the game, picking an object and adding it to the story in a manner that may stimulate the child to address her concerns in the next portion of the story. For instance, even an egg beater can be used to introduce a variety of feelings: rejection (e.g., "it was discarded and uncared for"), anger ("the egg beater is used as a weapon"), or a need for independence ("the egg beater wished it could do all its work on its own; it didn't want anyone to hold it or turn its handle").

Spontaneous Stories

Many children spontaneously start to speak about some favorite fantasy superhero. Unless one happens to be familiar with the common stories and mythologies of current superheros it is difficult to distinguish the child's projections from stories he has encountered in books and media. One must not assume, therefore, that because the child is "free associating" the content of what is being said necessarily reveals unconscious concerns. Monologues are a common way for children to defend, ward off, and effectively block communication. When a therapist feels "trapped" or impatient with what seems like nonstop chattering, the feeling may reflect some sense that the story is being used defensively. One should listen, however, for a moment or two before concluding that the child's retelling of some story is not pertinent to the uncovering of unconscious conflict. Buried in the confusing and seemingly disconnected gush of words, the therapist may find themes that seem related to the issues and concerns with which the child is struggling. Although using the child's spontaneous stories is not the *optimal* way to get projective material, the therapist can add elements to the child's script which, in effect, serve as invitations for projections. The therapist does this by introducing events that then, like the drawings in the Divorce Story Cards, serve as stimuli from which associations arise. One might, for instance, playfully introduce a monster who is so scary that even the child's superhero "wants his big brother to protect him." It is important to note how the child reacts to the therapist's change of script. Some children enter into a dialogue with the therapist in which they each participate in elaborating the fantasy. Other children continue their monologue nonstop without any indication that they have even heard the therapist's comment.

THE CHILD'S REACTIONS TO HIS STORY

Observing how the child feels about the stories he has produced and whether the child wants to share the story with the parents is in itself very informative and deepens one's understanding of the youngster. We may in fact learn as much about the child from how the child acts in relation to this activity as we do from an analysis of the themes and conflicts embedded in the stories themselves. For instance, some children really become engaged by story telling. They seem to put their whole self into it and exhibit true pleasure in their creation. These children may want to take the squiggle drawings home or may ask me to write their story down for them so they can take it when they leave. Some children want to make their stories into a book with illustrations that they will draw. Children like this are demonstrating, at least in this realm, a high level of self-esteem and enthusiasm. This is an especially positive sign if the child is having a very difficult time in school or is in great conflict with his parents. The capacity to engage and enjoy one's creative productions is a good measure of the resiliency of the child. Furthermore, the child's wish to show the drawing or story to a parent is a sign that despite the problems in the relationship, the youngster is still engaged with the parents and wants their recognition and approval. In contrasts some children will show the story to a parent only reluctantly.

There are children who cooperate in story telling without really engaging in the process. Some children are obviously insecure about their ability to perform well and experience the request as a task. Such children are very cautious in their responses and the stories they tell tend to be repetitive and imitative of the therapist's.

Other children, unsmiling and tense, produce only the most superficial of stories. There may be a flatness to both the story and the manner in which it is told. Generally the meaning of this sort of constrictedness is best determined in the context of other information we have about the youngster. Lack of affect may reflect, for instance, angry withdrawal, depression, or severe doubts about ones ability to produce something worthwhile.

A WORD ABOUT TELLING STORIES

Thus far story telling has been discussed as a means of helping children reveal unconscious concerns. The stories told are not neutral in that they may be stimulated by provocative stimuli such as the Divorce Story Cards or the therapist's comments. Yet the specific and highly individualistic ways children respond to emotionally loaded stimuli reflect their particular anxieties and intrapsychic as well as interpersonal concerns. Story telling as it has just been described above is primarily a diagnostic rather than therapeutic activity. The goal is to get the child to *tell* stories rather than telling stories *to* him. It is important to remember, however, that telling stories *to* children is also an important part of the work being described in this volume. Chapter 7 discusses the use of Eriksonian storytelling methods (see Mills & Crowley, 1986) in individual sessions with a child as a means of bypassing the child's defenses. Chapter 7 also describes a method of having parents tell stories to children that embody the child's concerns and normalize feelings about which the child feels shame.

DRAMATIC PLAY WITH PUPPETS, DOLLS, AND TOY FIGURES

It is helpful to have a variety of materials in the office which the child and therapist can use to act out scenarios. Scenes can be acted out with miniature plastic figures and props (such as the type found in Playmobil sets), with cardboard cutouts and backgrounds, with family hand puppets (anatomically explicit or not), dolls, or even stuffed animals.

The materials used should not include superheros or other popular figures about which the child already has numerous preformed fantasies and stories. Materials that lend themselves to more factual realistic play rather than "fantastic" stories give more immediate and comprehensible information about the child's concerns. Monsters, witches, genies, and robots should not be included in the available props. Of course, a child may imbue even "realistic" figures with supernatural powers. When this is done, however, the story is likely to have more psychological significance than if a magical figure is used simply because it is there.

Some stimuli have such strong associations that the child's response will in effect be predetermined and have little personal or idiosyncratic meaning. For instance, almost all children faced with guns or tanks invent aggressive play. Objects with a strong valence toward aggression should be eliminated from the toy box. If a child wants to express aggression he can easily invent weaponry from neutral materials. Aggression expressed this way is far more meaningful than the automatic anger and hostility that children describe when the materials seem to call out for that theme.

In suggesting materials for play scenarios, therapists should keep in mind that the more defended the child, the more threatened she may be by very realistic play. When children seem guarded and frightened, it is best to suggest material that allows a safe distance from reality. Stories that involve stuffed animals or somewhat unrealistic puppets allow the child more psychological distance from the fantasy play than do dolls or realistic figures.

As with all the forms of play thus described, here too much useful information is obtained by actively participating with the child in the creation of a fantasy. The therapist can start the child off by suggesting a pertinent situation. "How about if we pretend these are boys and girls in the playground at school." If the child assents, he is asked what role he would like me to take. The child often replaces the suggested scenario with one more to his liking. I will interject into the youngster's script some characters and issues that I think might evoke self-revelatory statements or actions. For instance, with one little boy who felt so inadequate at school that he hid rather than do challenging work, I played the role of several puppet children taunting a little boy for not being able to swim. In response to the taunting, this timid little boy had his plastic character punch the taunters.

Young children rarely develop a sustained and elaborated script in dramatic play. Rather, they jump from one bit of action to the next and frequently do not articulate what is happening unless pressed to do so. Often when I ask a child what I should say or do as a "character" in the drama, the child insists that *I* make something up. Though they obviously know that it is me talking, youngsters are nevertheless enthralled by dolls and animals which "talk." Once I get a drama started, they are almost inevitably drawn into it and start directing my actions. When creating a scenario, it is important to incorporate, yet sufficiently disguise, the child's concerns. Plays that are too close to the child's real situation will not be perceived as fun and will increase the child's resistance.

It is important to make note of the manner in which the child plays with these materials. Some children become intensely involved in the drama they are creating. They talk aloud and seem completely absorbed by the fantasy play. How involved the child is in his own fantasy life does not directly relate to how ready he is to interact with me around what he is doing. There are children who, though intensely involved in their play, give a running report of the action they are creating and invite my participation. For others, I do not exist while they are in their world of fantasy.

Some children seem to have a more limited ability than others their age to engage in fantasy play. They act out very simple occurrences rather than stories of any sort. They may, for instance, simply push a doll on a swing rather than make up a story about what is happening. When given puppets or dolls without props or background scenery, some youngsters are inventive while others seem bored or look to me to make something interesting happen.

USING CLAY

Clay is an extremely good medium for helping constricted, guarded children produce fantasy material. The child is given a lump of soft, moist potter's clay, a board on which to work, and an assortment of "tools" such as a garlic press (for making hair and worms), a rubber mallet (for smashing enemies), various shapes for making designs, a knife, a corkscrew, a rolling pin, or anything else that might intrigue a frightened and defended youngster (Oaklander, 1988). Although very soft plasticene can also be used, I have found that working with soft ceramic clay (and perhaps a bit of water) has a dramatically relaxing effect on children.[1] Even children who are initially uncomfortable with the sticky, messy feeling of clay generally feel comfortable when they realize that the amount of water they add affects how messy it will be and that when it dries, it flakes right off their hands. I usually give children a short while just to play with the clay and see what emerges. I then might ask the youngster to describe what he has made, or, if the child is hard to engage, I make a game of trying to guess what he has sculpted. With some children I might then suggest that we make up a story using the object they have created and volunteer to help them make some of the characters that they need for the story.

In addition to using clay to construct (quite literally) a story, it can also be used to inquire directly into some of the things that may be bothering a child. For instance, one could invite the youngster to make something scary out of the clay, or to make somebody he is mad at, or to make a scene of people in his family. Clay can also be used to enable children to express unconscious or unexpressed aggressive feelings. This is discussed in Chapter 7.

DRAWING

Most children love to draw. Much information can be gained simply by asking a child to draw pictures on specific themes. Suggestions for what a child could draw can range from the very specific to the very abstract. For instance, the therapist could ask a child to draw everyone in his family doing some activities, or he could give a more vague direction, such as, "Draw a picture of your anger." Generally, younger children are more engaged by concrete suggestions. I might ask a child to draw something that made him angry; something he remembers doing when he was little; a time that he felt shy, embarrassed, or scared; or the worst thing that ever happened in his life or the best thing that ever happened.

When the child has completed the drawing, I usually just ask him to tell me about his picture. When children are anxious and reluctant to talk, I make a game out of trying to guess what the picture is about, and this usually results in the child's explaining and correcting my erroneous guesses. One can also use the drawing as a stimulus for obtaining even more projective material. After the child has drawn a picture of his family, for instance, he could be asked to make one statement about each person in the picture or to say something to each person in the picture or have the person in the picture say something to him (Oaklander, 1988).

Oaklander (1988) has numerous suggestions for combining guided fantasy and drawing (e.g., draw an inside place, a place you dream about) and for utilizing Gestalt methods to get the child to express feelings or various aspects of himself by talking about the various parts of the drawing (e.g., "What is this circle thinking? What will happen to it? Have the . . . in the picture talk to the . . . in the picture.").

UNDERSTANDING THE CHILD'S PROJECTIVE MATERIAL: SOME GENERAL CONSIDERATIONS

Our understanding of children's fantasy material is not divorced from what we know about events in their lives and the family situation of which they are a part.[2] Generally, a young child who has had some difficult or traumatic events with which to cope, is likely to enact them in one form or another in play scenarios (Simmons, 1987) Irwin (1983) has described well the complexity inherent in children's projective scenarios:

> When a child spontaneously enacts a story in a therapeutic setting, she or he is simultaneously playwright, actor, director and critic. Projecting something from his or her inner world into the play sphere, the child sets the scene, becomes the various characters in the story, and through action, speech, gesture, and pantomime, acts it out. . . . The drama reflects an admixture of things experienced and imagined, an amalgam of past and present, impulse and defense, will and counterwill. (p. 149)

In understanding the meaning of the stories and fantasies the child creates, one must keep in mind, however, that the material will incorporate the psychosocial conflicts that are characteristic of particular stages of development as well as the child's unique and idiosyncratic psychodynamic conflicts. Therapists utilizing projective material must look for both the real-life situations that are reflected in the youngster's stories and the child's idiosyncratic way of processing and coping with these situations. For example, 10-year-old Samantha did a drawing of a very dressed-up rock star who had come to the Grammy awards expecting to win. The singer was extremely disappointed when her rival won instead and vowed that she would get the best songwriters in New York to make sure that she would win the following year. In this simple story we see something about Samantha's extreme wish for approval and her fluctuating sense of self-worth. On the one hand, the singer is so certain of how good she is that she comes dressed to receive the prize. But, by telling a story in which the protagonist is humiliated by her overconfidence, Samantha reflects her uncertainty about her own self-worth. This conflict makes sense when one realizes that Samantha's mother (who not incidentally, in terms of understanding this story, was well-known in the arts) regarded her daughter as a precious gem to be admired, stroked, and protected almost continuously, while, in contrast, Samantha's father, recently remarried, felt that when the youngster made her biyearly visit (he lived across the country) she should fit into the household routines and not expect so much attention. It is important to note that the story not only tells us something about the child's confusion regarding self-worth but also reveals her coping style. The singer in the story actively keeps trying to be the best rather than, for instance, congratulating herself on what she has achieved, retreating from the business, or blaming unfair judges,

In another instance, Marla, age 6, paired the family puppets up so that the Mommy and Daddy would be together and hugging and the boy and girl would also be hugging. "They love each other," she said. Knowing that this child's home life was filled with violent strife made it clear that the play scenario was clearly representing the child's strong wish for harmony.

Johnny, age 10, did a drawing in which a bully was pushing someone off the World Trade Center viewing deck. As the boy fell he realized that the only person there to catch him was a teacher who hated him. The boy died. "It happened because the teachers weren't paying attention," Johnny said. This story seemed to relate to a change in living arrangements at home; Johnny's older half brother, whom, according to the parents, Johnny "adored" and "looked up to," had come to live with the family. Though Johnny expressed no objections to sharing his room and parents with this older half sibling, the story he invented provided a clue for further exploration of the supposedly problem-free relationship of the two brothers. It seems that Johnny's parents had not noticed that the older boy, angry at feeling abandoned by his mother, had been taking out his feelings on his trusting younger sibling. This case is described in detail in Chapter 9.

The content of a story can be deciphered more easily when we have the child's associations. The therapist might ask a child, for example, "Who, of all the people (or things) in the story, would you *most* like to be, and, who wouldn't you want to be?". Gardner (1971) asks the child the lesson or moral of the story or whether the story reminds him of anything he has seen or heard before. One can also ask the child how different characters in the story feel about events that take place.

Though we can learn a great deal about a child by examining the content of his fantasy life, care must be taken to see this fantasy material as just that, fantasy. The therapist must be careful not to overgeneralize from the fantasy material in a way that pathologizes the youngster. One must keep in mind that we are "pulling" for unconscious material. It is all too easy to forget that what we are seeing is the child's fantasy life and *not* how he thinks and acts when he is utilizing his normal defense mechanisms and relating in the real world.

In utilizing projective material to evaluate degree of disturbance, certain formal characteristics of the child's fantasies may be more significant than the content per se. Formal characteristics of the story (e.g., whether it is original or stereotyped, whether it is disorganized or finished, static or fluid) give clues about the child's internal state and degree of organization. One looks for how the child copes with emerging impulses, feelings, and fantasies. Some children become distracted and never finish a disturbing story or the story may become disjointed, illogical, and fragmented. Other children become quite agitated by their fantasies and seem to have difficulty separating themselves from the pretend story. Still others are very tight, constricted, or bored.

Simmons (1987), in describing the use of projective material in psychiatric evaluations of children, states:

> Qualitatively, fantasies that deal with real life problems indicate a reasonably healthy use of fantasy as a coping device in both healthy and moderately neurotic children. Such phenomena are seen in children who use doll play to act out, perhaps ventilate their experiences. On the other hand, fantasies replete with sadism, sexually symbolic behavior and megalomanic world destruction with little or no relevance to the child's reality situation, are seen in borderline psychotic and severely neurotic children. (p. 83)

Simmons (1987) describes how in early latency (ages 6–8) children commonly produce fantasy material that contains amorphous, scary figures such as monsters or ghosts. As they mature (ages 8–11) the frightening characters in their stories become more humanlike (i.e., witches, robbers, and bad guys) and less amorphous. As a child's symbolization capacity increases, he enjoys elaborating on details.

When an older, latency-age child produces fantasies that have a great deal of noise and fighting and very little detail and when he uses symbols such as fire, shadows, and floods which are "affect-porous" (Sarnoff, 1987) he may be having some serious difficulty with aggressive impulses and persecutory fantasies.

Even when a child's fantasies fall outside expectable parameters, the import of this must be weighed against everything else known about the child. As is discussed in the next chapter, even serious-seeming symptoms in a child are not necessarily a sign of severe disturbance (A. Freud, 1965).

DEALING WITH THE CHILD'S HOSTILITY

Some children, despite valiant attempts to alleviate their anxiety by being friendly, affectionate, and supportive, treat the therapist not merely with indifference but with hostility. A youngster may attempt to demonstrate his hostility by being physically destructive or aggressive; he may throw things on the floor, purposely knock into things, or even attempt to act out physically against the therapist. With a solemn look and strong words I make it clear to the child that although he is welcome to tell me what he is feeling, behavior of this sort is not permissible in my office. I empathize with his feeling that he is unhappy being here and wonder aloud if he would tell me why he is feeling mad. If at this point the child does not desist, I invite the parent into the room and conduct the rest of the session with the parent present. It is important to ask the parent to take charge of limit setting. Many children calm down when a parent is with them. The aggressive acting out may indicate extreme feelings of vulnerability which are alleviated when the parent joins the meeting. If a child continues to be agitated and aggressive even when a parent is present, it does not make sense to attempt to see him alone at this point in the work. Rather, the first priority is to work with the whole family, both on the control of aggression, and on the sources of frustration which have resulted in the child feeling so angry.

When a child is expressing anger through silence, curt answers, or rudeness, it is often helpful to take a one-down position in which you let the child know that you have no power to *make* the child talk, play, or have fun. Acknowledging one's own limitations may enable the child to give up a power struggle.

On numerous occasions, dramatic shifts in the child's manner of treating me took place simply by giving the child feedback regarding how *I* was feeling. I might say to a youngster that I feel bad that he won't play with me and is acting as if he is angry at me or doesn't like me. Or, if the child is being very provocative, I might let him know that I am feeling annoyed and not having fun being with him. Children are often quite startled by the candor of my reaction; it is as if it had not occurred to them that I had feelings or that my feelings about them were dependent on how they treated me.

The aim of this chapter has been to provide some guidelines for making the best use of individual sessions with children. Through games, activities, and story telling that invite the child to be self-revealing, the therapist has obtained a good deal of information about the intrapsychic and interpersonal life of the child. In the next chapter, we will use this material (as well as what we have learned about the child in family sessions and from the parents' and teacher's reports) to evaluate the youngster's coping style and defense mechanisms in the context of the family system in which he lives.

5

Anxiety, Adaptational Styles, and Defense Mechanisms

Having met with the parents, family, and child, the therapist has obtained a wealth of information about the individual child which needs to be synthesized and understood in ways that can be integrated into systemic work. Although being open to reports from parents about what they regard as disturbed behavior, as discussed in Chapter 2, and obtaining projective material in individual meetings with the child provide invaluable data which supplement systemic perspectives, therapists must be careful that information of this sort does not lead them to see the child as being more troubled or having more deficits than he in fact has. This chapter will help the therapist organize and evaluate the information that has been obtained so that the child is neither pathologized nor too readily pronounced "fine." To this end, we look at the range of possible adaptational styles and defense mechanisms children typically utilize and discuss how to determine whether a particular youngster's choices are maladaptive.

A basic premise of this book is that a detailed understanding of the child as an individual does *not* necessitate *individual* interventions; rather, a well-articulated description of the child's difficulties is an essential component of helping the *family* help the youngster. Thus, last, and perhaps most important for eventually formulating interventions, is a discussion of the relationship between the child's coping and defense mechanisms and the family system. Later chapters discuss the way systemic interactions relate to the *content* of the child's concerns, but for now the focus is on understanding how the family operates to contribute to useful or maladaptive modes of dealing with intrapsychic and interpersonal stress.

We also take a look at the problem of underdeveloped defense mechanisms and the way family interactions contribute to or, conversely, correct this problem.

Children, perhaps more than adults, need ways to deal with both internal and external sources of anxiety. Their world is full of new and often stressful situations over which they have little or no control. Even children growing up in the most secure and stable family (something of a rarity in our modern world) must cope with a great deal that is frightening and distressing. First, they must learn to conform to expectations and gradually to control urges and impulses that are not acceptable to others. As they mature they are expected to give up childish behavior and increasingly master challenging tasks. Furthermore, children must cope with one another. Young children can be alarmingly hard on their peers. Adults are often horrified by the cruel things children say and do to children they dislike and even to those who but yesterday were dear friends. And, of course, children have little or no say over such crucial aspects of their life as the teacher or babysitter who will be with them all day, or whether their parents separate, or whether a parent on whom they depend is depressed, or whether they will have to move or share their parents with a sibling. Furthermore, young and childlike dependence is not unusual for this age group.

Even when a child's difficulties are not uncommon for children of her age, one must be careful not to dismiss or minimize their importance. How the child and the family deal with various emotional stresses, even those that are in some sense "normal" ones, is at least as important as the anxiety itself. Thus, family therapists must learn to assess not only the relative severity of the child's problems but also the effects on family, peers, and teachers of the child's adaptational style and defense mechanisms.

ADAPTATIONAL STYLES

A child's temperament (see Chapter 2), as well as his characteristic ways of dealing with new and possibly difficult situations, has a great interpersonal impact and may have extremely significant positive and negative consequences for the formation of relationships. Having met with the child alone as well as with the family, the therapist is now able to formulate some clear and specific notions regarding the child's manner of relating to the world.

Approach–Avoidance

Meeting with the therapist is, in itself, a new situation with which the child has to cope. The first thing to notice is whether the child avoids the unfamiliar or approaches it, if even in a counterphobic manner. Some children cope with their uncertainty by working hard to engage and charm the therapist. These youngsters approach the unknown head on. An extreme example of this was Bennie, a recently adopted 4-year-old who had been given up by his mother at age 18 months and had been in two foster homes before finally being adopted. This little boy had learned early in life to be unusually friendly and engaging. Within minutes of meeting me he successfully captured my attention and won my affection by asking questions, standing close to my chair, and initiating physical contact by gently leaning against me while showing me a toy he had brought with him. Bennie had the knack of turning strangers into nurturant old friends.

Others are much more cautious, and even while being compliant try to avoid or block out the anxiety-producing therapist by ignoring her presence. Averting his eyes, the avoidant child tries his best not to make eye contact. These children may quickly engage in an activity with an intensity that excludes the therapist. Seven-year-old Mickey, for instance, complied with the therapist's request to draw his family but drew his picture with a yellow marker on yellow paper and offered only one-word responses to the therapist's queries.

Some children cope by retreating into fantasy. Using dolls, animals, or fantasy figures, these children amuse themselves in fantasy play and make no attempt to share their mumbled scenarios with the therapist.

The approach–avoidance dimension can also be assessed in terms of the physical distance the child puts between himself and the therapist. Some children take the most distant seat possible and move away if the therapist, joining them in play on the floor, gets too close. Other children seem excessively in need of physical contact. Hannah, for instance, when sitting next to the therapist on the couch, moved so close that the therapist felt physically crowded and uncomfortable. Behavior that is cute in a 5-year-old can be very off-putting when displayed by an older child of 8 or 9. A child who feels clingy and overly familiar at the first meeting is not only expressing dependency needs but also demonstrating a coping mechanism that has significant interpersonal ramifications.

Some young children stoically walk into an unfamiliar situation, while others are more apt to express their concerns and ask for help in coping. Very young children typically turn to a parent for reassurance. They may want the parent to stay for awhile, may request that the door be left open, or may start the interview by whispering comments to the parent, who is then expected to say aloud what the child wants to communicate. When a young child marches in without a glance backward at a parent, one wonders whether the youngster has learned to cope by denying fear and renouncing dependency. It is a good prognostic indicator when a child who at home is having a difficult time with a parent, nonetheless feels comfortable asking for some assistance in this new situation. It is important to note carefully how able the child is to acknowledge anxiety and how comfortably he asks parents or other adults for help in mastering a new situation.

Praise and reassurance that they are doing well may be actively (or even compulsively) sought by some children. For instance, Ethan, age 9, after each nearly identical drawing of a shark, would expectantly ask, "Isn't that good?" Some children, on the other hand, seem uncomfortable with praise. Jeremy, age 5, would frown and squint when something nice was said about him. Renouncing any need for approval is unfortunately a not uncommon way that some young children have of coping with concern about expectations and judgments.

Similarly, some youngsters at an early age are indignant about being called by "pet" names, or by being referred to as a "little" boy or girl. Rachel, for instance, at age 5 would assert, "I'm not a little girl! I'm my Mommy's *first* baby!" Of course, sometimes the rejection of affectionate, adult-to-child gestures is merely a matter of a child's adoption of a coy or "macho" style and does not reflect a true discomfort with dependency. The child's verbalizations are evaluated in the context of her overall manner of relating to parents as well as to strangers. A child may not be receptive to friendly overtures on the part of the therapist yet may be perfectly comfortable with dependency on a parent.

There are some youngsters who "approach" by being avoidant or hard to get. Coy smiles, furtive glances, whispered communications to the therapist through a parent all say "come and get me!". These little ones want to be pursued and won over. Although they may at first appear to be shy and withdrawn, they let the therapist know that they in fact are eager to be engaged. They cope by acting in a way that in effect elicits reassurance and active involvement on the part of the therapist.

Compliance–Opposition

This dimension, perhaps more than any of the other ways of relating that the child has developed, has enormous interpersonal consequences. An avoidant, reticent child evokes very different feelings in adults than does the child who approaches new situations by being oppositional. There is a big difference between retreating into an intense private activity, which though it excludes the therapist does not *feel* hostile, and *stubbornly* refusing to participate, which generates anger in others. Occasionally it may be difficult to distinguish between the two, but generally the child's facial expressions, gestures, and body language enable the therapist to determine whether the child is simply withdrawing or attempting to cope with (and protest) what he regards as demands. Some children withdraw or become oppositional only while a parent is in the room and soon after the departure of the parent actively interacts with the therapist.

Equally noteworthy is the child who seems to be overly compliant and cooperative. These children cope with the anxiety of this new situation by trying very hard to please. They may be hesitant to assert their own desires and when asked to choose an activity leave the decision entirely in the hands of the therapist. Such a child may even wait for the therapist to tell him when he has done enough on a drawing or story rather than concluding it when he himself is satisfied.

In assessing the child's adaptational style, the therapist must keep in mind that the coping mechanisms a youngster uses often differ with the particular nature of the situation in which he finds himself. A child who is hesitant to relate to the therapist may not be avoidant at all when confronted with a new game or puzzle that taps his cognitive abilities. Often children cope differently with intellectual challenges than with interpersonal ones. When a child's adaptational style at school is an issue, it is helpful to give the youngster a task that simulates academic challenges. A young child could be asked to write his name in script or to demonstrate certain mathematical skills. The therapist can use books with puzzles and word games for older children. By giving the child activities similar to the intellectual tasks faced in the classroom situation, the therapist has an opportunity to observe how she copes with the stress of a demanding learning situation. Some children demonstrate a tremendous capacity to concentrate and persist until they succeed. At the other end of the continuum are those who will not even try something they perceive as difficult. Most children, of course, are in the middle range. One should observe with these children *how* they cope with the pressure of a new learning situation. Does the child plunge right in without listening carefully to the therapist's instructions? Does the child ask for help, and how does he respond to assistance when offered? How much effort will the child make before giving up? *How* does the child give up? Does he just become interested in something else or is he more actively rejecting of the task, perhaps saying something like "this is stupid!". Does the child change the task so that he shows what he *does* know? A detailed understanding of the child's style is helpful in formulating behavioral interventions to help the child develop coping strategies for cognitive challenges.

DEFENSE MECHANISMS

After meeting with a child alone once or twice, the therapist should have a fairly good idea not only of the child's intrapsychic conflicts but of the mechanisms he uses to ward off the anxiety that results from these unconscious forces. In planning systemic as well as individual interventions, it is important to have a clear idea not only of *what* the child fears but of *how* he defends against those concerns.

Younger children generally utilize more primitive defense mechanism than do older ones. The younger the child, the easier it is for frightening feelings to intrude on his consciousness. Anna Freud (1946) points out that small children ward off their unconscious wishes not because they conflict with their conscience (superego, in psychoanalytic terminology) but because the expression of certain feelings is prohibited by parents and society. With increasing age, the child experiences unconscious impulses, wishes, and feelings as a threat to her maturing self and her ability to cope with the demands of reality. Thus, for instance, a child who cannot adequately defend against regressive urges may find it extremely taxing to muster the maturity necessary to function in an age-appropriate way at home or at camp. Furthermore, certain feelings are best kept unconscious because they conflict too much with opposing wishes. Children, like adults, seek some sort of harmony between conflicting and opposite tendencies. Awareness of wishes for dependency, for instance, may conflict with strong urges for autonomy, and thus the strength of one of these affects needs to be minimized and perhaps even excluded from consciousness (cf. Horney, 1945).

Latency-age children[1] tend to be more well defended than younger children, and if they are not, the lack of defenses against impulses and fears is a problem that needs to be addressed. Sarnoff (1987) has called the particular cluster of ego mechanisms characteristic of latency-age children the "structure of latency." When these defense mechanism (described shortly) are not sufficiently developed, there is a breaking through of impulses which interferes with the state of emotional equilibrium necessary for the child to behave well, stay calm, and be receptive to what he is being taught.

The defense mechanisms most typical of very young children (but used by older children and adults as well) are denial, reaction formation, avoidance of stimuli that would stir unwanted feelings, and projection. By noticing just when these defense mechanisms are used in a session, the therapist can learn a good deal about what may be bothering the youngster. The frequency and strength of the defense mechanisms a child uses are an indication of just how alarmed the child is by unwanted feelings.

Reaction formation, in which impulses are changed into their opposite, is often seen in family sessions when a young child has an infant sibling. Poking, followed by a good deal of kissing, is not uncommon. It is important to assess whether the child (and the family) is able to accept negative feelings toward the newcomer when *explicitly* asked about those feelings. Four-year-old Connor, when asked to say some of the good things about having baby Nelle in the family, responded easily. But when asked to say some of the things that he did npt like he remained silent and started instead to try to make the baby laugh by making funny faces. Although reaction formation is a normal and useful defense mechanisms for young children, if it is too rigidly employed, the child does not learn that his negative feelings do not make him a monster.

The use of reaction formation in less common situations should be noted. Six-year-old Kristen, for instance, often was "too busy" to talk with her mother when she called home from the office. One must be careful, however, not to confuse a wish for mastery with a reaction formation against dependency needs. Kara, at age 6½, rejected being read to and vehemently insisted that she preferred reading to herself. Although this behavior *could* be regarded as a reaction formation against regressive wishes and jealousy of her 3-year-old brother who loved nothing more than cuddling up to a good long story, other aspects of Kara's behavior made it clear that reaction formation was not at work here. Her rejection of being read to reflected her pleasure in the newly acquired skill of reading; she had little trouble expressing jealousy and regressive wishes in other ways.

Reaction formation is of course used by older children and adults as well. What is an obvious defense in young children may have become incorporated into the character of the older child and may represent an ego ideal rather than a defensive operation.

Denial involves the distortion of the perception of reality in order to protect against uncomfortable feelings. One of the most primitive of the defense mechanisms, it is typically used by young children whose ability to distinguish between fact and fantasy is not yet consolidated, although it can be used by older children as well. Once a child knows clearly the difference between reality and make believe, denial does not work quite as well. Simple, straightforward denial is at work when, for instance, a child, shown a picture of a woman with a very angry expression on her face describes it as a woman yawning.

Children under the age of 6 or 7 may tell rather elaborate "fibs" for the purpose of denying some reality that is evoking disturbing feelings. Suzanne, who had little contact with her father, replied to a question about him with an elaborate description of the wonderful places he was taking her on her vacation. A private chat with Suzanne's mother revealed that in fact no vacation plans whatsoever had been made.

The fact that a young child uses denial is so expectable that it is not in itself of concern. It is helpful, however, to notice under what circumstances the child feels the need to use this defense. When an older child

(7 and older) uses denial to a substantial degree, the use of the mechanism itself is of more concern. Older children should have ways to cope with disturbing feelings other than the extreme and outright distortion of reality characteristic of denial.

When unpleasant affects arise, young children often use *avoidance* as a defense mechanism. The child diverts the conversation or game away from a troublesome topic. Rachel, age 5, no longer wanted to play the Feeling Cube game when her sister, age 3, in response to what made her "angry," talked about Rachel's pinching and hair pulling. Somewhat similarly, 9-year-old Steve got interested in the pictures on my wall when asked to include his father in the picture of everyone in the family doing something. As with denial, the use of this mechanism with young children is quite normal. Again, the important thing is to note carefully when this phenomenon occurs, as one can assume that the diversion created reflects anxiety stirred at that time. When avoidance is the predominant defense of an older child, it is maladaptive and not appropriate to the child's age.

Repression is a mechanism in which the individual has no conscious awareness of a disturbing internal state. Unlike denial, in which the child feels something and then distorts in order to make the feeling go away, repression is a mechanism in which the disturbing feeling is put completely out of awareness. Denial and avoidance are often used as adjuncts in the service of bolstering repression. For instance, Jenny, age 10, was excessively sweet and oversensitive. She was easily frightened by stern teachers and was very disturbed by raucous boys in her class. This child had no memory of any interactions between her parents who had divorced when she was 4. When shown the Divorce Story Cards, Jenny used denial and distorted a scene so that instead of fighting, a couple was putting on a play. Each of Jenny's parents in separate meetings revealed that prior to separating they had had some violent fights which were serious enough that on one occasion a neighbor called the police. Although no one had ever been physically harmed, there were dents in the wall from their fights and furniture and dishes had been broken. In order to maintain the repression of these events, Jenny avoided all potentially aggressive situations. Chapter 9 includes a full case study of the treatment of this child and her family and describes the use of Negative Reminiscing to help the child work through previously repressed material.

Perhaps one of the most important defense mechanisms for therapists to keep in mind when talking with young children is *projection.* By changing the source of the unwanted impulse or feeling to something that is occurring *outside* oneself rather than owning it as one's own, the individual preserves psychic equilibrium but often at a considerable cost. Understanding the mechanism of projection enables us to make sense out of the child's stories and fantasy play. Imaginary friends and animated animals frequently express the child's projected feelings.

Although fears and phobias in children may be based on some actual frightening experiences from which the youngster has overgeneralized, they are often based on the projection of the child's own unwelcome impulses. Four-year-old Jennifer spoke of being afraid that someone "will steal me and throw me in the garbage." This fear could readily be understood as a projection of the child's own wish to similarly dispose of her 1-year-old sister. Many of the typical fears of childhood such as fears of monsters or of being bitten by animals can be understood as the projection outward of the harm and destruction the child's own wishes could cause.

Displacement, though often used in conjunction with projection, is a somewhat different phenomenon. When using displacement, the child feels and acknowledges a negative feeling but substitutes someone more acceptable for the source of the feeling. A common form of displacement seen in children is their antiauthoritarian reaction to teachers or schools. Some children who do not complain about parents express exaggerated and inappropriate anger toward teachers, caretakers, or other adults. Of course, one must be very careful not to dismiss fears or negative feelings as groundless. We have come to understand that child abuse can occur in situations assumed to be safe, and a child's fear of, or dislike for, an adult should *always* be taken seriously. When, however, we have investigated the reality components of a situation and are assured that the "offending" adult is in fact benign, we can then consider whether the child's difficulties with an adult may be a signal that there are problems with a parent that are being displaced.

The therapist should keep in mind that it is not only negative affects that can be displaced. Some children experience a teacher, babysitter, or therapist as the "good parent," whom they try to please and with whom they express their wishes for comforting and nurturance. Of course, before we call this displacement, we must be sure that the child's perception of the parent as one who is critical and demanding, in contrast to the supportive "other," is not in fact accurate. Katie, who was 8½ years old, for instance, insisted on being very babyish with her rather stern, but loving babysitter. When her mother wanted to cuddle or read to her, however, Katie would want only to show how mature she was and how well she could read by herself. Katie correctly perceived that her mother had an extreme need to foster competence and high achievement in her daughter. Wanting to be what her mother valued, she displaced her wish to be babied by her mother onto the housekeeper. She had split her needs for nurturance and for competence between the two women. Actually, however, although Katie's mother did strongly value competence, she was also comfortable with, and even desirous of "cozy" times with her little girl. Katie, however, could not tolerate having "baby" needs with her mother. Perhaps they felt too threatening to Katie's growing sense of maturity and self-reliance. Katie did not keep from awareness her regressive urges (as in projection or repression) but rather displaced them as something she felt only with the sitter.

Isolation, intellectualization, and rationalization are methods many children use to cope with disturbing events. A child who is using isolation, intellectualization, and rationalization talks about events in a way that is devoid of appropriate affect. Nine-year-old Ethan, for instance, talked calmly and dispassionately about being disliked by the children in his class. He repeated verbatim some of the comments children had made about him regarding nose picking and "weird" behavior. At no time did he show signs of being disturbed by these occurrences, and it was only when his mother was given a report of this by another parent that the seriousness of the situation in school was understood. Never a tear was shed by Ethan when talking about how the children would not touch things he had handled. Ethan used intellectualization to reinforce the isolation of affects and truly believed that he "understood" that the children were "immature" and jealous of how well he did in school. He also strongly believed that he *preferred* playing by himself.

Obsessional defenses are perhaps the most commonly used mechanisms employed by latency-age children. Often these defenses serve the purpose of binding aggressive and sexual impulses so that the child does not act them out inappropriately. Latency-age children spend a good deal of time and effort in such activities as collecting cards, stamps, or coins; playing board games with complex rules; or following the blueprints for model planes or complex Lego structures. This defense mechanism, though frequently used to bind aggression (Sarnoff, 1987), is also used to help the child isolate affect. As in the case of Ethan, a child who intensely focuses on some "obsessional" activity has a greater ability to not feel hurt, rejection, or other forms of psychic pain.

Undoing and compulsive behavior is closely related to obsessional defenses. Here, a child needs to perform some particular act in order to avoid a feeling of anxiety. Young children have many rituals to help them cope with difficult feelings. Children become very set in their ways and often insist on predictable routines. Rituals that involve doing and undoing have more dynamic significance. When a child erases and redraws a picture over and over again she is both avoiding and communicating something about a troubling feeling that arises from the drawing. Five-year-old Rachel, for example, when asked to draw a picture of her whole family doing something, kept redoing her mother. Over and over again she crossed out what she had drawn and added something in its place.

She would alternate between putting her mother in the kitchen and having her leave for work, until the distress of having to choose led to a tantrum. When a child draws only one thing over and over again even when asked to do something else, he is engaged in compulsive behavior that binds the feeling and may also simultaneously express it. When Ethan, described earlier, first met with me alone, he was negative and oppositional. Nonetheless he agreed to cooperate by drawing some pictures. He literally drew dozens of separate pictures, each one a variation on an open-mouthed shark.

Identification with the aggressor is a defense mechanism often seen in children. The child incorporates an expected rebuke, projects the offending action onto someone else, and in turn rebukes that person. Youngsters often imitate people who have been aggressive or critical toward them. They transform themselves from the person threatened into the person who makes the threat. According to Anna Freud (1946), the child using this defense internalizes the criticism of the adult, but instead of it being transformed into self-criticism, it is dissociated and turned back on the outside world. Eight-year-old Lynda, for instance, criticized her friend Sarah for bragging about abilities she did not in fact have. In reality it was Lynda who did just that, and who had been chastised by her parents for "lying" and pretending competencies that she had not yet acquired. Instead of being self-critical, Lynda had dissociated the "reprehensible" part of her self and projected it onto her friend whom she then criticized.

An understanding of the impact on the child's functioning of the types of defenses she uses enables us to determine, with the parents, what should be encouraged and what discouraged. When a decision is made to intervene in any way with the youngster's coping style or defense mechanisms, it is essential that the feelings, impulses, and needs that made the defense necessary are simultaneously addressed. For example, if a child's use of reaction formation against aggression is to be addressed, it is important that the circumstances that led to the child's strong aggressive feelings be dealt with simultaneously. Or, if a child's macho behavior is actively discouraged, we must be sure that the environment is accepting of increased dependency needs and more attuned to rewarding more appropriate attempts at mastery and competence. Children's defenses may be overutilized because of family situations that overstimulate them in one form or another and thus require the child to ward off impulses that circumstances have allowed to get too strong. For example, a daredevil, counterphobic youngster may be living in a situation that evokes more than the average level of fear.

The registering of new experiences can be interfered with by defenses that are no longer necessary. In order for a child to experience a change in the way people in the family are acting, it is sometimes necessary to actively work with the child and the family to help the child "see" the changes that are occurring. Chapter 8 discusses behavioral methods that reduce the use of defenses that are no longer adaptive.

The remainder of this chapter focuses on the ways that defense mechanism are both a product of and affect systemic interactions.

WHEN DEFENSES AND COPING STRATEGIES ARE MALADAPTIVE

The determination that a child's coping and defense mechanisms are maladaptive is based on an assessment of the extent to which the methods the child uses to cope with anxiety interfere with the development of age-appropriate skills, satisfying personal relationships, curiosity, and the capacity for pleasure. If, for instance, a child who initially copes with an intellectual challenge by withdrawal can readily be induced to try, we need not be nearly as concerned as we are about a child who continues to use avoidance even when he gets encouragement, reassurance, or assistance. Similarly, oppositionalism can seriously interfere with exposure to and mastery of new experiences. The frustration of dealing with a child whose first response is negative can lead to a "why bother" attitude on the part of adults and the child is, consequently, offered fewer options for new experiences.

Often, defense mechanisms that do not create problems when used in the family may have serious negative consequences when used with peers. For instance, 9-year-old Cathryn made great use of reaction formation to control angry feelings. She took pride in being mature and responsible and was lauded by her parents for how much they could rely on her. They often talked about how kind and protective she was toward her younger sisters and how she always inquired about the well-being of an elderly great-aunt. Both her parents were quite volatile and had come to rely on Cathryn as a parentified child who could calm the others down. They were delighted with their youngster and were puzzled and troubled that she seemed to be so socially isolated. Further investigation revealed that Cathryn had a lot of trouble with the "cattiness" and "meanness" of children her own age. Because her defenses did not permit her to be aware of angry feelings, she did not fight back and was, according to the teacher, perceived by her classmates as a "goody-two-shoes" to whom they could not relate. Thus, although Cathryn's "good nature" was highly valued in the family, it interfered with the development of friendships and the assertiveness necessary to get along with others.

Almost any defense mechanism used to excess can have a negative impact on relationships and interfere with cognitive and social development. Tommy, age 7, channeled his feelings of anxiety into compulsive, perfectionistic behavior. He was extremely orderly and both play and work had to be done just right. This led to several difficulties. First, it was hard for him to play with other children because he had very rigid ideas of how games should be played; his assigning of roles and scripts and his putting toys in order as they were being played with did not endear him to his playmates. His compulsiveness crossed over the line of personal preference to being domineering. In school, Tommy's compulsiveness made it difficult for him to complete projects in the time allotted. His need to do his work meticulously led to struggles and frustrations when the teacher asked him to finish up. When prevented from completing a task in the way he wanted, he would burst into angry tears.

When negative feelings are not "owned" but instead dealt with primarily by projecting them onto others, the child may develop a "chip on his shoulder" and a paranoid stance that, of course, greatly interferes with the ability to form trusting relationships. Children such as this can easily fly into a rage at perceived assaults. Sometimes children like this are the object of a good deal of teasing in that their peers enjoy being able to make them have a "fit." At other times they are simply ignored and isolated from their peer group.

A related issue to what has just been described is whether or not the defenses used seem to be fragile and impulses and feelings break through inappropriately. When defense mechanism are fragile, the child will suddenly, and without provocation, fall apart. He may sob for no apparent reason or may erupt in anger. Four-year-old Sara, for example (who is described in detail in Chapter 9), was attempting to repress memories of her father who had suddenly terminated contact with her. As part of the effort to repress the memory of her father and the painful feelings of abandonment, she repeatedly insisted that she had another name and was many years older than her actual age. These defense mechanisms were fragile and the child began to have violent outbursts in which she would destroy the work of her classmates and fall to the floor with uncontrollable crying.

If a child's defensive and coping style is maladaptive, the therapist should enlist the parents in the task of helping the child establish new modes of behavior. Redirecting a child's defense and coping mechanisms is no easy task. Before embarking on such a course the therapist must thoroughly discuss with the parents just how the particular defense and coping mechanisms the child is using are interfering with her development. Defenses that are acceptable at home may be having a negative effect on the child's functioning in the world at large and it is the therapist's job to clearly explain the link between the defenses and the problems of concern to the parents.

UNDERSTANDING THE BEHAVIORAL AND SYSTEMIC REINFORCEMENTS FOR MALADAPTIVE DEFENSE AND COPING MECHANISMS

Having determined that a defense is maladaptive, the therapist and parents must analyze together how the child's defenses are being reinforced by the family or other significant adults. Often the child's maladaptive defensive posture is being encouraged in ways that are quite inadvertent and completely at odds with what the parents actually intend.

For example, 6-year-old Arthur was an extremely frightened and avoidant youngster. He would withdraw from any situation that presented even the mildest of challenges. In school he refused to participate in group activities and games. Only with a good deal of support and individual attention could his teachers get him to focus on the rudimentary age-appropriate academic material he was intellectually capable of mastering. Not infrequently, even with a teacher's undivided attention, Arthur would withdraw from a challenging task by tuning out or simply getting up and wandering off. At home, similar behavior occurred. Teachers and parents alike found, however, that with a good deal of support, reassurance, and coaxing, Arthur could be induced to try a new activity, and sometimes he would even stick with it and get pleasure from the feeling of competence that ensued. The occasional success parents and teachers had with coaxing reinforced this style of dealing with Arthur's avoidant behavior. Unfortunately, however, the pleasure in mastery that these experiences gave Arthur was not strong enough to overcome his tendency to avoid. The implicit theory behind the coaxing was that eventually Arthur would learn from experience that in fact he could overcome anxiety and master new challenges. Though certainly a valid approach for many youngsters, Arthur's tendency to avoid was so massive that encouragement and support simply were not working fast enough. Although he was of above-average intelligence, his school was concerned that he could not be worked with in a normal classroom setting. A detailed behavioral analysis of the transactions occurring between Arthur and his teachers and parents revealed that in fact coaxing was serving as a positive reinforcement for avoidance. Instead of minimizing the child's tendency to avoid, the adults in Arthur's life were actually positively rewarding, with a lot of individual attention and support, the very behavior that was so problematic. Furthermore, Arthur seemed to be learning that he could *only* do new things with a great deal of support and guidance and had not learned any ways to deal with his anxiety by himself. A systemic analysis of the situation revealed that Arthur's mother interpreted his avoidance as a "strong will" and took a good deal of pride in the fact that "no one could put anything over on Arthur; he *knows* when you are trying to get him to do something."

Reaction formation is a defense that often receives a good deal of positive reinforcement. It is hard for most adults to experience a child as being "too good." What parent does not bask in the feeling of well-being when an older child just seems to adore a new sibling? When children dissociate themselves from their wilder or more rebellious classmates, it is a rare parent who feels any need to intervene. When reaction formation has become excessive and maladaptive the therapist usually needs to explain in great detail why it is problematic if he is to enlist parents' cooperation in tasks that help a child feel more comfortable with aggressive and "dark side" feelings.

Sometimes, however, a reaction formation is so excessive that it does become extremely annoying to parents. When Sara, age 4 (described earlier), repeatedly said "I love you" to her mother, the mother became so irritated that her reassurances, tinged with anger, no longer worked. The interventions employed in addressing the excessive use of reaction formation by this child are discussed in detail in the full case study of Sara in Chapter 9.

Frequently, young children are quite obsessive. Obsessive and compulsive activities, while serving the purpose of warding off unwanted impulses and feelings, also play a big role in making the child's world more predictable. There is great comfort to be had in *knowing* and being able to anticipate what will be happening next. Many young children want an exact timetable of when and what will be occurring. They may insist on knowing *to the minute* when a parent will be leaving and returning. Or, perhaps they insist that there be no variation whatsoever in the route driven to school or develop long and detailed rituals not only for bedtime but for numerous aspects of daily life. Although in some circumstances such behaviors may be adaptive, they may readily become problematic and interfere with normal functioning.

Five-year-old Rachel, for instance, would have severe tantrums when family routines were in the least bit altered. If her mother walked on a different path to the playground the child created such a commotion that Rachel's mother felt she had no alternative but to retrace her steps and walk the way the child wanted. In the morning, this little girl needed a great deal of time to get ready. On her insistence, *everything* in her room had to be left in an exact place and there were set and detailed routines for eating breakfast and getting dressed. On evenings when Rachel's parents left her with a babysitter, she would howl with upset unless given exact information as to what restaurant her parents would be at, when they would arrive, when they would leave, where they were going afterwards, and what time *exactly* they would return.

The parents were at a loss regarding what to do. In order to keep Rachel calm, they provided as much information as they possibly could.

But their doing so kept the child from learning that she in fact would be safe even if she did not have exact and detailed information. By accommodating to the child's obsessiveness, her parents inadvertently reinforced her belief that this kind of information would in fact protect her from harm.

Perhaps the most common way parents contribute to the formation of maladaptive defense mechanisms is in their encouragement of repression of painful memories. The wish on the part of many parents to spare their youngsters undue emotional pain often leads them to studiously avoid the mention of highly disturbing experiences. By so doing, parents not only give the message that some things should not be talked about, but actually may help the child "forget." As discussed earlier, total repression of negative memories often becomes maladaptive in that the youngster has to cut off many perceptions and feelings in order not to be reminded of the excised emotion.

Not talking about painful experiences is particularly common in situations in which one parent, after a divorce or separation, has failed to maintain contact with a child. The remaining parent may shield the child simply by avoiding mention of the missed telephone calls and visits. Another common situation in which repression is frequently encouraged is when parents have been engaged in intense emotional and/or physical battles. Once the couple has patched things up, or perhaps separated, they act as if the frightening episodes never occurred. Mention of these events by the child may be met with what is intended as a reassuring minimization of what the child experienced. When specific painful situations are being avoided, the parents can be coached on ways to open up communication about disturbing events. When a child has repressed the memory of troubling experiences, sessions may be used for some "Negative Reminiscing" (see Chapter 7).

Repression of particular disturbing emotions and experiences is also encouraged when parents themselves find an experience or feeling difficult to handle. One family, for instance, did not tell me of the father's having been the victim of a brutal and violent crime which the children witnessed (at ages 3 and 5) until their now 10-year-old son's overreaction to slights and perceived assaults had escalated to the level of paranoia. They explained that the episode (an armed robbery in their home in which the father was tied up and threatened), having taken place 7 years earlier, was largely out of their minds, and that they saw no point in dwelling on an experience in which they all had felt terrorized. Although the parents could now readily understand the contribution of this experience to the child's difficulties, they were so disturbed themselves by the memories of the event that they first needed some help in working through their own feelings.

INSUFFICIENTLY DEVELOPED DEFENSE MECHANISMS

Unlike many of the children discussed above, whose defenses have become overly rigid and generalized, many young children need help in *developing* rather than *relaxing* defense and coping mechanisms. These youngsters do not yet know how to modulate intense feelings. For instance, a child of 5 who feels terribly anxious when separating from his mother can be thought of as having insufficient defenses against the intensity of his dependency needs. Nor has he developed ways to calm his anxiety. Some young children may feel intensely, and express too readily, sexualized feelings toward a parent (e.g., Sam, age 6, would passionately kiss his mother on the mouth and stroke her breasts). Or, the angry and even sadistic urges that many youngster's feel may be given too ready expression, especially in regard to a younger sibling. Children whose jealousy toward their younger sibling is so extreme that the feeling dominates their thoughts and disrupts their functioning (whether or not they actually act out their hostility is not always the criterion to use) have not yet developed the defense mechanisms necessary to cope adaptively with what they are experiencing as a highly stressful situation.

Of course, in all cases of inadequate defense mechanisms, it is a crucial part of the therapy to address and remedy the situations that led the child to have such intense feelings. Chapter 6 discusses both the intrapsychic and interpersonal aspects of overly intense impulses and feelings.

A common reason for referring a child and family to therapy is that a youngster is too impulsive in school situations. These children "act out" what they feel rather than control themselves in ways that are considered age appropriate. When angry, they may react with such extreme aggression that other children are endangered. Frustration, even with themselves, may lead to tantrums, destructiveness, and a temporary loss of the child's ego capacities (e.g., reality testing, delay, anticipation, or memory of future gratifications). For instance, a child who, when frustrated with his inability to add one more block to his tower without its tumbling, destroys what he has already pridefully built, has had a temporary lapse of ego strength.

Of course, it is important to keep in mind that the sufficiency of a child's defense and coping strategies must be judged according to the youngster's age. Generally, by the time a child enters latency, defense mechanisms have sufficiently developed so that the child more often than not is in a state of equilibrium (Sarnoff, 1987). The use of repression, obsessive compulsive activities, doing and undoing, reaction formation, and sublimation of impulses into fantasy, when not used to excess as described earlier, results in a degree of calm and emotional comfort which permits the child to concentrate and learn. When, however, learning disabilities make the mastery of academic material quite difficult, a latency-age child's defenses might be fragile and maladaptive. It is not uncommon for regressive dependency wishes to resurface when a child is feeling inadequate in the academic arena. To help these children, we must understand the deep blow to their self-esteem that many learning disabled children feel as a result of the difficulty with the learning and mastery that are the main tasks of that age.

We evaluate the sufficiency of a child's defense mechanisms not only by the reports of parents and teachers but also by what we observe of the child's behavior in both individual and family sessions. Some children become very upset if they are losing a game and may even knock the board over so others cannot play. Or a child may become very distressed by a discussion of certain issues and simply fall apart in the session.

How well a child can play is an indication of the adequacy of his defense mechanisms. When a child's defenses are not sufficiently developed, anxiety may be breaking through to such an extent that the youngster does not have the patience and calm to learn a new game or even to concentrate on self-directed play. Some children play with something for just a couple of minutes and then get up to see what else they can do. Even when the therapist makes active attempts to engage them directly in an activity, their concentration span may be quite limited. The child may be easily distractible and move from one toy to another in rapid succession. Conversely, some children seem to be listless and bored. They may be mildly engaged for just a short while and then seem to lose interest.

In sessions alone with a child, we get a chance to see how frustrated she gets when a task is difficult and whether she has developed mechanisms both to reassure herself and to persist in trying something new and difficult. Always, of course, we must evaluate the child's level of attention and restlessness in relation to what one generally expects from children of that age. Parents' complaints that a child cannot or will not play on her own may be based on expectations that are not age appropriate. In the therapy office, a 4-year-old's capacity, for instance, to play the Squiggle game described in the previous chapter and then to create either alone or collaboratively "stories" about the squiggle, will be completely different than the 7-year-old's ability and willingness to be engaged in such an activity. For therapists who have not yet accumulated sufficient experience with young children to judge with confidence whether the child's attention span is within the expectable range, it is helpful to talk with the youngster's teacher to get a sense of how the child compares to his age group on that dimension.

The nature of a child's stories and fantasy play is also revealing with regard to the adequacy of his defense mechanisms and ego structures. Children who have difficulty controlling themselves often use puppets or dolls in a global, unarticulated way rather than creating a "story" in which the action makes sense. When playing, children carry on *monologues intérieurs* (Piaget, 1962a), through which they act out and express at a symbolic level what they cannot act out in reality. An insufficient capacity to engage in symbolic play through which feelings are worked through is associated with greater acting out of impulses (Chethik, 1989; Irwin, 1983; Sarnoff, 1987; Singer, 1975; Willock, 1983). As Irwin (1983) said: "To the observing adult, pretend play seems effortless, artless. And to most children, it is. But there are some youngsters, many of whom come for treatment who cannot play so easily. Their play doesn't 'hang together'; it may seem a disconnected, fragmented puzzle" (p. 153). When a child's capacity to fantasize and use symbolization is not sufficiently developed for his age he is unable to use play to redirect impulses and to master difficult situations.

UNDERSTANDING THE BEHAVIORAL AND SYSTEMIC COMPONENTS OF INSUFFICIENTLY DEVELOPED DEFENSE AND COPING MECHANISMS

Just as we looked at family interactions for clues to behavioral and systemic contributions to the development of maladaptive defenses, so too it is important to understand what interactions may have contributed to the insufficient development of necessary coping and defense structures.

Overstimulation

First, it is important to notice whether there may be things going on in the child's environment that are overstimulating him so that his defenses are simply not adequate to handle the level of arousal to which he is being exposed. For instance, Sam, age 6, could not stop kissing and touching his mother. In school he would try to pull down girls' panties and would, in play, climb on top of other children (boys and girls) in a sexually suggestive way. Although some sexual curiosity is common at age 6, Sam had become preoccupied with sex to the exclusion of other sorts of play and activities.

After discussion with Sam's parents, it became clear that this child just could not handle the level of sexual openness that was acceptable to the parents. It seemed that when Sam's stepbrother, age 15, came for weekend visits, he often brought a girlfriend of the same age, and the parents were comfortable with allowing the teenagers to sleep in the same bed and spend days watching television curled in each others arms. Sam often hung around with this older sibling and his girlfriend and was stimulated by the adolescent passion he sensed but had probably not (as far as the parents knew) directly witnessed.

Similarly, when a child seems filled with rage we must not only help the child get control of his anger but also understand what might be *provoking* anger so intense that she has not developed expectable levels of self control. We must evaluate the level of aggression the child has witnessed as well as, of course, what he himself has been subjected to. Are there violent arguments at home? Has the child been the victim of physical or verbal abuse? Is there excessive control and discipline leading to constant battles or internalized hostility.

Although a youngsters' anger may be the result of high levels of parental hostility, it is also important to look closely at sibling relationships. Younger children can feel helpless and overwhelmed by anger from the teasing, bullying, or physical assaults they may be subject to at the hands of an older child in the family. The child's parents may be unaware that what to them is a normal degree of fighting between siblings is experienced by the younger child as absolutely infuriating and that his defenses are inadequate to the task of controlling the degree of anger that is evoked.

Being Overly Supportive

Another way that parents may be inadvertently contributing to a child's lack of development of coping and defense mechanisms is by being too comforting and supportive. Some parents are so responsive to a child's anxiety that they quickly do whatever it takes to make the child feel better. These parents often identify with the child's feeling of distress and have difficulty tolerating the temporary upset children have to go through as part of the process of developing coping mechanisms. A great many parents of children 5 or 6 years old, for example, have gotten into a pattern with their child in which they have responded to the child's crying when put to bed by attempting to calm him with their presence. After a time, they come to feel that staying in his room until he falls asleep is a necessity. When this happens, the child will develop few or no self-comforting devices on which to rely.

Although such a pattern may have significant systemic meanings and repercussions, it can also result from the parents' overidentification with the child around feelings of abandonment and isolation. It is interesting to note and to point out to parents that a child's ability to be self-comforting and to cope with anxiety on his own may be well developed in some areas while in other areas the youngster seems to have inadequately developed coping strategies. This generally occurs because, in particular situations, for one reason or another, parents have been more insistent on the child's overcoming anxieties without much parental assistance.

There are many other ways that parents who are too empathic and helpful may fail to encourage the development of mastery over emotions. Often, for instance, parents sit with children while they are doing homework assignments. Many children just cannot settle down to their work unless a parent sits with them. Although working at the kitchen table certainly evokes warm images of hearth and home, children, if not encouraged to work on their own may not develop the internal capacity to stay calm and focused. Simple changes in structure (see Chapter 7) can make a big difference in enabling children to gradually cope with anxiety and calm themselves down so that they can stay focused when stressed.

Failure to encourage self-control and mastery over emotions is not necessarily related to the degree to which the parents themselves possess these qualities. Frequently parents who have considerable ability to be self-comforting and to channel intense feelings of frustration and anxiety in productive directions do not think (or do not know how) to educate their children in what they take for granted. Feeling at a loss to know how to handle the child's anxiety, parents may choose to directly reassure their youngster rather than help her develop the coping skills necessary for self-modulation. For instance, when 8-year-old Elliot, the son of two highly successful and self-controlled individuals, had full-blown tantrums (complete with crying, kicking, and breaking things) when he was losing at a board game, both his parents would offer comfort and reassurance that he would have many other opportunities to win. They felt so badly about his distress that all they could think to do was to be supportive. Although of course one must understand why this youngster cared so much about winning, it is essential to focus on helping the parents teach the youngster the mechanisms of coping and control that they themselves possess.

Giving Mixed Messages about Impulse Control

Perhaps the most common contribution of the family to the difficulties some children have with impulse control is the mixed feelings one or both parents may have about asserting their wishes over those of the child. One source of this ambivalence is the erroneous assumption some parents make that controlling a child involves "breaking his will." Others simultaneously feel angry, worried, and *pleased with* the child's expression of aggression. As discussed in Chapter 1, they may vicariously identify with the child and take pleasure in the youngster's being able to express emotions that they themselves cannot express.

When one or both parents have mixed feelings about how much control they want or expect the child to have, it is important both to discuss their concerns and to look at just how this ambivalence is actually communicated to the child. For example, Mickey, age 7, had a violent temper. He had come close to causing serious injury to playmates both at home and at school. Mickey's father, Roger, the youngest of four boys, had learned at an early age to hold his own against the aggression of his brothers. He described himself as someone who never let people get away with hurting him; he would get back at people even if it took years. Mickey's mother, on the other hand, was a very controlled person who, when angry, dissolved in tears. For a variety of reasons including the fact that Mickey had been born with a mild congenital difficulty, both parents saw this youngster very much as the "underdog" in comparison to his older, more robust brother. Understanding how they might have been subtly supporting Mickey's ferocity when angry needed to be translated into concrete terms which they could then alter. For instance, it was important for them to notice how they laughed with affection and wonder when they told the story in front of both boys of how one time, Mickey, wielding a bat, had terrorized a whole gang of older kids. The interventions used in this case are discussed in detail in the case study of Mickey in Chapter 9.

Reinforcing Upset and Negative Perceptions

Many parents are committed to relating to their children differently from how their parents related to them, and thus they try extra hard to be attentive to their children's feeling and to encourage their youngsters to express every feeling. Although, in general, encouraging children to speak about what is on their mind is a sound and positive policy, it can on occasion become excessive and may ironically lead to increased levels of distress. For instance, Mrs. Hughes, a single parent, wanted very much to be close to her 8-year-old daughter, Janine. When the youngster complained about a fight with a friend or said she did not like her teacher, Mrs. Hughes would stop what she was doing to listen and encourage the child to say more about what she was feeling. Mrs. Hughes, who was herself depressed, was in effect reinforcing dysphoric feelings in her young daughter. The child was learning that every negative experience was to be taken seriously; conversely, she was not developing an attitude that sometimes it is best to shrug off a feeling or to seek some distraction rather than dwell on upset.

Overattentiveness to a child's negative feelings toward a sibling is quite common. Many parents feel that it is wrong to stop the expression of hostility toward a sibling as long as the hostile child is not expressing his feelings through physical aggression. Although parents often feel bothered by the extent of the hostility expressed (one little boy of 5 spent hours with his playmates drawing pictures of killing his 2-year-younger sibling) they feel guilty about censoring or suppressing the youngster. Similarly, the parents of an 8-year-old little girl were tolerant of the youngster's chronic complaints that it was unfair how much more time her younger sister had at home with mother while she was in school and even responded with frequent promises of compensatory time. No sense of this simply being a reality, or even of the fact that the older child had had her turn when *she* was 2, was conveyed. One must not dismiss reactions such as these without trying to understand more fully the family dynamics that led to such intense reactions. Yet by reacting to the child's upset in too understanding a way the parent is not providing the children with the motivation and message that some way to cope has to be found. When the parents of the 5-year-old mentioned above told him that he was no longer allowed to draw or get his friends to draw hostile pictures, the child calmed down considerably. The parent's tolerance had not enabled the child to muster the necessary defenses against aggressive impulses.

As discussed in detail in Chapters 7 and 8, interventions to help the child develop impulse control and age-appropriate defenses against anxiety best proceed on three tracks at once: (1) The child must be given some tools for self-control and anxiety reduction, (2) the parents must positively reinforce appropriate defenses and provide negative consequences for loss of control, and (3) the family and school environment must be worked with so that the stimulation that the child finds hard to handle is minimized at the same time that the child is learning coping and defense mechanisms.

THE CHILD'S DEFENSES AND THE FAMILY SYSTEM

Thus far, the focus of this chapter has been the individual aspects of the child's maladaptive defenses and has been systemic only insofar as the difficulties are understood as being sustained by a pattern of interaction between parent and child that makes the problem worse. It is important at this juncture to remind the reader that the child's problems must also be understood from the more standard systemic viewpoint. In understanding both the child's anxiety and the reinforcements the youngster is receiving, the therapist must ask herself what role the child's behavior plays in the interactions between family members. A symptomatic child, for example, may be serving a stabilizing function in the family system. As described in Chapter 3, one must look at such issues as, whether the child is echoing the anxiety of one or both parents. If so, is the anxiety openly expressed or is it an unconscious feeling which is expressed covertly? Are there difficulties in the marriage that are contributing to the child's sense of instability and danger? It is well-known that many children have an almost uncanny ability to pick up on parental tensions and often it is this anxiety that is expressed in irritability, anger, or clingy behavior. The children become symptomatic in response to tension in the home that they are unable to control.

As discussed in Chapter 1, there is consensus among a wide range of family therapists that stress between a couple is often resolved by "triangulating" in a child. The child's difficulties may be used to deflect parental conflict or, conversely, may be reflective of an alliance with one parent against another. When a child's symptoms are enacted primarily with just one parent, it is likely that the systemic dimensions of the problem are particularly important. For instance, a child with rigid and excessive bedtime rituals may be insistent on having one particular parent put him to bed and will shriek if the other attempts to substitute. Such a pattern has important systemic meanings. The child may have been enlisted, for example, in a covert expression of anger toward the excluded spouse. Or the parent who lets herself be possessed by the child to the point of feeling that she has no alternative but to deal with his anxiety by spending hours in his room while he falls asleep is also making a decision to be less available to her husband. Or a husband may go along with the child's insistence that only the mother will do as a way of keeping rigid role definitions in which he remains apart from the family.

Another important systemic factor which the therapist should keep in mind is that a child's maladaptive defense mechanisms may reflect a defensive system characteristic of the whole family. By this I mean that rather than the child's acting out denied aspects of self, the child may instead be expressing in an exaggerated form a coping or defensive posture that is generally endorsed by the parents. Children are powerfully influenced by their parents' belief systems, "myths" (Ferreira, 1963; Palazzoli, Cecchin, Prata, & Boscolo, 1978), and "realities" (Minuchin & Fishman, 1981). Family belief systems are rarely directly expressed or explicitly acknowledged, and it is this very lack of explicitness that can make them so powerful. Ideas such as "you can't trust anybody but your family," "authority figures will be harsh and critical," "your friends will be jealous of you," or "you need to have a competitive edge to get ahead in the world" powerfully shape the child's sense of reality, thereby significantly affecting the child's coping and defense mechanisms.

Similarly, there are implicit family rules that prohibit some emotions and encourage others. The excessive use of repression by a child is commonly related to a family's discomfort with particular types of feelings. What is acceptable and expectable in the way of expression of feelings differs greatly from family to family. Some families, for instance, "never fight," while others regard the overt expression of affection as "saccharine and sentimental."

In order to help the child feel more comfortable with warded-off feelings, it is essential that the family as a whole be able to tolerate what the child is being encouraged to express rather than defend against. For instance, the Roths were concerned about the toughness of their 6-year-old daughter, Sylvie. Apparently, Sylvie behaved in a cruel and callous manner with other children and never cried when reprimanded, punished, or shunned. A crucial step in helping this youngster was to understand this behavior in the context of the family's attitude toward showing vulnerability. Mr. Roth was a holocaust survivor who while hiding witnessed his parents being taken away, never to be seen again. Mrs. Roth also was schooled in invulnerability at an early age. She had hardened herself to a cycle of abandonment and reconciliation on the part of her mother who had a history of serious psychiatric difficulties. With these histories it is no wonder that the Roths inadvertly reinforced Sylvie's denial of soft and vulnerable feelings. Although they would never overtly tell the child not to cry or even actively discourage the expression of sad feelings, nonetheless they taught Sylvie to move away from hurt quite quickly. Rather than "owning" her own feelings, this youngster, by being cruel to others, induced them to feel the painful emotions that she herself repressed. Before being able to design interventions that would help Sylvie be a "pussycat" rather than a "lion" (see Chapter 7) it was important to discuss with the parents their own issues around vulnerability.

A WORD ABOUT AN INTEGRATIVE PERSPECTIVE AND SPECIFICITY

Although an understanding of the systemic dimensions of a child's difficulties is an essential component of an integrative approach, it is (as discussed in Chapter 1) rarely sufficient. Once we know how the child's difficulties fit with the system either in expressing disowned feelings, deflecting parental conflict, or manifesting family assumptions and concerns, the next step is to articulate with as much specificity as possible just *how* the systemic, behavioral, and psychodynamic dimensions intersect. Thus, for instance, in the case of Sylvie, speaking to the parents about their discomfort with vulnerability was only the first part of the process of integrating systemic understanding into the work. Next, it was important to understand exactly *how* each parent jointly and separately actually discouraged the expression of this affect and instead encouraged the child's problematic defense mechanisms. Noticing, for instance, that they would affectionately laugh at how "tough" she was and act helpless in the face of her strength led to coaching the parents on some behavioral methods that would reinforce the expression of her "soft" rather than tough side.

Just as our understanding of family dynamics is translated into observations of specifics, so too do we try to concretize and make precise our understanding of just what affects the child's intrapsychic conflicts and unconscious wishes. For instance, we notice the moments and interactions that contribute to a child's negative feelings about himself or that lead him to feel afraid of what he is feeling. Thus, once we have a psychodynamic formulation regarding a child (e.g., that he is defending against feelings of vulnerability), we try to know with as much specificity as possible what is going on in the child's life that leads to such strong feelings, and what specifically encourages the child to defend excessively against feelings. Chapter 7 discusses the use of concrete interventions to address intrapsychic issues and problematic defense mechanisms.

6

Essential Psychodynamic Concepts

This chapter presents some of the psychodynamic formulations regarding children's difficulties that enable us to design active interventions that address the intrapsychic component of the youngster's difficulties. The purpose of this chapter is to provide perspectives that complement systemic and behavioral concepts and thus, in this chapter, the explanatory theories for common symptoms in children will be, by design, temporarily one-sided. The concepts I describe here are not based on one particular psychodynamic theory exclusively but rather are a selection from a range of psychodynamic perspectives. Whereas the previous chapter discussed the importance of understanding the *defense mechanisms* utilized by children and how these defensive strategies interact with the family system, this chapter describes the types of psychodynamic *conflicts* (both conscious and unconscious) that, if troubling a child, contribute to the development of symptoms or the maladaptive use of defense mechanisms.

The reader should keep in mind that although in the child–family work being described psychodynamic formulations enhance the therapist's understanding of a troubled youngster, the therapeutic methods used are quite different from the theories of psychotherapy that derive almost exclusively from such formulations. The purpose, in the child-in-family approach, of understanding the child's symptoms from a psychodynamic point of view is not to make interpretations or to provide a therapeutic experience in individual sessions. Rather, the psychodynamic perspective is used to help craft active interventions that will address the child's unconscious conflicts.

One could in principle list dozens or perhaps even hundreds of specific formulations that derive from a psychodynamic point of view. Inevitably, however, any particular therapist is likely to emphasize some more than others. This chapter focuses only slightly on the various differences in viewpoint among psychoanalytic theorists.[1] It presents instead, whenever possible, areas of convergence that cut across the conventional distinctions between ego psychology, object relations theory, self psychology, and interpersonal theory.

FRIGHTENING OR DENIED ASPECTS OF THE SELF

Anger

There are many reasons why a child disowns and represses angry feelings rather than acknowledging them even to himself. Although, as discussed in the previous chapter, the family environment certainly contributes to a child's comfort or discomfort with anger, there are also intrapsychic dynamics at play when a child banishes anger from her sense of self. At the most obvious level, children fear their anger because to "hate," even temporarily, the person on whom you depend for love and support is to risk psychological, if not actual, abandonment. The child fears that his own extremely hostile and violent feelings will be known by the parent and that the parent, disgusted, will withdraw love. Even worse, the child may fear retaliation for his hateful, competitive, and aggressive thoughts and, if one subscribes to a classical psychoanalytic theory, the child may even imagine "castration" as a natural consequence of his destructive wishes toward the parent of the same sex.

Intense feelings of rage are terrifying too because the younger the child, the more readily do ego controls give way to emotions. The young child's capacity to anticipate, reason, control impulses, and sort out reality from fantasy is quite vulnerable to disruption. When the child is in the grip of tremendous rage, his developing sense of control is threatened. If one thinks of how terrifying it is to adults when their own rage reactions lead to impulsive and destructive acts, one can imagine how frightening loss of control can be to a child whose ego functioning is fragile and not fully developed. By repressing his angry feelings, the child protects himself from the frightening experience of regressing to a state in which he was overwhelmed by anxiety, unmodulated impulses, and fears of abandonment.

Finally, as a child gets older and his sense of right and wrong develops into an internalized conscience or superego, a youngster wards off hateful feelings because they lead to self-criticism and guilt. Object relations theory provides another useful perspective as to why a child might feel the need to repress strong negative feelings. This theory sees the central issue of development not as the control over impulses but rather as the reconciliation of good and bad images of the primary caretaker. It is through the process of internalizing feelings about objects that one's sense of self develops. According to Fairbairn (1952), for instance, the good mother (or primary caretaker) is internalized as the ideal object and the child thus carries within himself the feeling of being loved. When the child experiences hateful, bitter, and vengeful feelings toward the loved object, he internalizes these feelings as well, and thus experiences himself as unlovable. Therefore, from an object relations perspective, the child who fears his own rageful feelings fears them not only for the reasons described above but also because his own sense of self as lovable depends on his experiencing the primary caretaker in a positive way.

When the child is confronted with intensely negative feelings toward a loved object, "splitting," the process by which the child preserves the good parent by not perceiving negatives, may occur. Splitting enables the child to continue to experience and incorporate a sense of the parent as good. In its extreme forms the child alternates between seeing the parent as all good or seeing him as all bad. An integrated sense of the parent as both good and bad is not internalized and thus the child cannot accept in himself the simultaneous existence of loving and hateful feelings.

Theory aside, over the years I have seen many children for whom fear of their own intense angry feelings is a prominent dynamic in the symptoms they are exhibiting. Guilt over such feelings is often expressed in young children in the concrete form of hating their own body. Children as young as 4 years of age may talk about disliking particular parts of their body, wanting to break their bones, or wanting to die. Chapter 9 describes the treatment of Sara, a 4-year-old girl who, overwhelmed by her own rage, made statements of this sort.

Disowning angry feelings can manifest itself in many other forms as well. One can surmise that a child is disowning feelings of anger when she is overusing certain defense mechanisms. The child who compulsively and repeatedly states, "You're the best Mommy," or "I love you," is generally struggling with dreaded negative feelings. Similarly the "disowning" of intense negative feelings may manifest itself in excessive worry about the physical well-being of a parent. Some children become extremely anxious when a parent is away from home and fear imagined catastrophic events. Others may even check on a sleeping parent's breathing. Behavior of this sort reflects the magical thinking of young children and their belief that bad thoughts can cause real harm.

Of course, worry about the well-being of a parent when he is away can also reflect fears of abandonment. Fear of the destructive capacity of one's own anger and fears of abandonment are not always separable. Young children may worry that a parent will reject and leave them both because the parent omnisciently knows of the child's angry thoughts and because the child has projected his own rejecting feelings onto the parent and fears rejection in return.

As discussed in the previous chapter, although all children use projection and fear the "robbers" and "monsters" who embody their anger, when a child cannot stop obsessing about some fantasied danger, she is probably battling mightily with strong aggressive impulses.

The more intensely a latency-age child fears his angry feelings, the more he may resort to rigid obsessive compulsive rituals. When a child has become extremely rigid in wanting to follow particular prescribed routines and becomes highly distressed if the precise order of doing things is not followed, the child is probably trying to control, through external order, some internally disruptive feeling.

Other signs of guilt over "bad" feelings are accident proneness or blatantly provocative behavior which invites the unconsciously longed for punishment. When children behave in ways that invite teasing by others, they may be getting their peers to act out their own self-loathing (Sarnoff, 1987). By getting other children to behave in a punishing fashion toward themselves, they deny their *own* anger and their consequent dislike of self.

A big discrepancy between the way a child perceives himself and the way others perceive him is often an indication that the child feels guilt over unacceptable feelings. A young child who insists he is unpopular when he is clearly sought after by other children, or who describes himself as "fat" when he is unquestionably thin, may be struggling with "knowing" something about himself that he believes is unattractive and unacceptable.

Vulnerability and Dependency

Children as young as 2 or 3 may be engaged in an active denial and splitting off of feelings of vulnerability. These youngsters often are precociously independent. Tears on partings are not for them. Reunions (whether at the end of the school day or on return from a parent's extended business trip) are treated with indifference. Anxieties and fears are not acknowledged, not to others or to themselves; the youngster truly believes that he does not feel vulnerable.

When denial is at its strongest, the child will act in ways that appear fearless. He may behave recklessly—for example, wandering off from his parents on city streets or plunging headlong into physically dangerous situations (such as jumping into a pool) when he lacks the skills to cope with the situation. These behaviors do not stem from some cognitive deficiency or delayed maturation but rather reflect the child's denial of feelings of fear and vulnerability. At the less extreme end of the scale, the child, while denying to himself any fear, may simply be avoidant and rationalizing away his lack of interest in some activity.

Although many of the behaviors just described are seen in almost all children from time to time, what differentiates the kind of youngsters I am talking about from others is the *degree* to which they renounce the need for parental contact and protection. For instance, although many children (especially young ones) act indifferently to returning parents whom they have missed, the children I am describing seem indifferent to the comings and goings of one or both parents most of the time. Similarly, many young children act braver than they really feel from time to time. These children in contrast may have a long-standing pattern of engaging in inappropriate and often dangerously fearless behavior.

Parents of children who have defended against feelings of vulnerability may feel quite rejected and even unloved. The child may seem to have virtually no need for demonstrations of affection. I have seen children who never allowed themselves to be hugged or kissed by either parent (though often a babysitter or grandparent *was* allowed to express some modicum of physical affection). Although many children proclaim, "I'm not a baby," from time to time, these youngsters have an intense need to act beyond their years. They want to do as much as they can for themselves, and, as soon as they can, they start working so they have their own money. Although most parents are happy to see their children strive for independence and competence, there is a point at which the child's need to say, "I can do it," or "I don't need your help," feels more like rejection than growth. When a child not yet old enough to read never permits a parent to read to him but instead insists that he can do it himself, a line is crossed in which what might be "cute" feels instead like a wholesale rejection of the state of being a child. Some children (see the case of Sara, Chapter 9) even insist that they are older than they actually are.

Again, although all children do some of this, a child who is excessively intolerant of dependency will do it far more persistently and rigidly than a youngster for whom it is but a passing issue. Even when a child's behavior is less extreme, a parent may feel frustrated by the seeming lack of relatedness. Ethan, for instance, could only ask for a hug by assuming a robot-like posture, walking mechanically with arms extended, and stating, "Robo want hug."

Indifference to disapproval or punishment (to be discussed further) may also be a sign of denial of need for parental affection. One 6-year-old girl acted like a "bad seed." The child was experienced by her mother as sadistically trying to "torture" the mother with extremely provocative behavior. Although the mother was projecting her own relationship of a psychologically "torturing" mother onto her child, she *was* correct in perceiving that the child did not seem to care about the rage she was inducing in her mother. Once again the reader must keep in mind that this phenomenon can be observed in almost all children but not to this degree. Many children, like Pierre in Maurice Sendak's *Really Rosie,* sing the refrain "I don't care," when they are being chastised or punished for misbehavior. It is only when this stance persists and becomes chronic that one need be concerned that the child has renounced his need for warmth and approval.

DEPRIVATION, FRUSTRATION, AND ABANDONMENT

When children are experiencing emotions that overwhelm them the therapist must try to understand how they have come to have feelings so intense that they feel the emotions must be denied and split off from their sense of self. Since all children at times feel strong anger or vulnerability, the therapist must ask why a particular child's feelings fall outside expectable bounds. When one looks carefully at the family environment and family history of children who are struggling with extreme feelings of anger it usually becomes apparent that the child has in fact had to endure intense frustrations and deprivations.

It is not uncommon for children to be abandoned by parents either literally or symbolically. Often there is a period of several months just prior to and immediately following a marital separation when parents are emotionally unavailable to children. Furthermore, it is well-known that not only do many fathers not honor their financial responsibilities to their children, but contact is frequently severed or seriously diminished when they separate from the children's mother.[2]

Even in those instances in which parents eventually reconnect with their children, the child who has experienced a sudden and serious rupture in a relationship with a parent not only fears abandonment but often carries around extreme feelings of anger toward a parent who is, at the same time, greatly loved and missed. Similar feelings can occur when a child loses any caretaker to whom he is strongly attached. Strong attachments to babysitters are often unacknowledged by parents and when the caretaker leaves the child may feel extremely angry and powerless.

It is well known that children who have been severely abused physically or verbally deaden their feelings through dissociative states. Similarly, the child who feels he can do no right may develop a defensive immunity to his parents' opinions. When a child feels constantly criticized, punished, or corrected she may convert feelings of hopelessness to indifference.

The therapist must keep in mind that parents and children both may be part of a vicious circle that has developed. A child who is seen negatively (perhaps because he is unconsciously seen as the equivalent of some other person or perhaps because he is the embodiment of denied aspects of self or is simply a youngster with a "difficult" temperament) begins of course to fulfill the parent's critical vision. The more difficult the child's behavior, the more criticism he gets, and, feeling hopeless about ever getting anything else, he no longer allows himself to need his parent's approval. Without the incentive of approval the child's behavior deteriorates further and the parents become more and more angry at the child's rejection of them.

Of course, it is also important not to blame the "victim." Children may not play an equal part in this vicious circle. Unfortunately, often they are truly the victims of adult drug abuse, pathology, or just plain cruelty, and it may in fact be true that nothing they can do will result in a positive response from a parent. When children have steeled themselves against this kind of hurt they respond negatively to any signs of tenderness or affection. Sullivan (1953) has described this phenomenon as a "malevolent transformation" (p. 213) in which a child actually becomes more comfortable with hostility than with love.

Serious psychological difficulties in a parent can also leave children feeling emotionally abandoned. Even when no extreme forms of physical or emotional abuse have occurred, the children of highly volatile parents may feel assaulted by inexplicable anger and outbursts of rage. Or, a child may feel confused and angry about an emotionally disturbed parent's preoccupied and halfhearted attempts to parent. A child may experience his parent as physically present but emotionally absent. When looking for elements of the family history that may have led to extreme anger or fears of vulnerability, the therapist should inquire about depression and family stress which could dramatically change a parent's ability to relate emotionally to a youngster. Children who in their first few years of life have been primarily looked after by a depressed and emotionally unavailable mother may develop a schizoid like character defense (Chethik, 1989) (see Chapter 8). Their detached and aloof manner is thought to be a defense against a painful sense of self (called by Willock, 1983, the "disregarded self" [p. 402]); these children feel that they simply do not have what it takes to hold the interest of adults.

Often, however, the provocations in the home environment are by no means obvious. I have seen children as young as 3, from "normal" family situations, who have vowed never to show warmth to parents and who rebuff all affectionate overtures. A number of youngsters with whom

I have met (again from apparently normal homes) have resisted a good deal of social pressure to show affection to their mother on Mother's Day, and one youngster was so angry that he gave his mother a gift of cut-up worms in a box of "snot."

Common and expectable experiences can leave some children feeling powerless and angry. A child may feel abandoned when a parent returns to work or when a grandmother who has been caring for her becomes ill and the child is placed in day care instead. New romantic relationships that develop after a separation can have a profound effect on the intensity of connection between a parent and child. Frequently, children experience themselves as being displaced by a parent's lover or new spouse and consequently feel extreme feelings of powerlessness and frustration and a loss of status. And, of course, children may get attached to people who prove to be only temporary relationships in their parent's life.

Many young children find their parents' long working hours quite frustrating. They feel anger because they want more of their parents than they can have. Long hours, extended out-of-town business trips, or even frequent interruptions by business calls can leave children with a residual anger even when the parent is home. Many children whom I have seen in my practice really suffer from the lack of contact with and *control* over the amount of contact they have with a parent. When parents start spending more time with their child, the child's anger often diminishes rapidly.

And then there are youngsters who are extremely angry despite the fact that their family seems to be providing consistent love and attention. These are situations in which therapists would have to be stretching facts to fit theory to find withdrawal or deprivation sufficiently severe to account for the child's anger. One explanation for this phenomenon is simply that there is a mismatch between the child's temperament and that of the parents. Thus, a naturally strong-willed or "difficult" youngster may react with rage to what is within the normal range of "control" that parents exercise and the parents in turn may not be sensitive enough to *this particular child's* strong need for autonomy. Other children in the family may have little or no trouble with the same parenting style. This is not only because no two children in fact grow up in the same environment (Dunn & Plomin, 1991) but because one child may simply be more adaptable than another or simply better suited to the parents' style (that is, they might have fared *worse* than their troubled sibling were the parents' style and temperament different). Conversely, there are children whose disposition seems to enable them to withstand extreme deprivations and emotional assaults without becoming so angry that healthy functioning is impaired.

OVERGRATIFICATION AS A SOURCE OF RAGE AND FEELINGS OF DEPRIVATION

Ironically, a child may be vulnerable to feeling extreme anger not because she has been deprived but, rather, because she has not had to learn to cope with frustration. On occasion one sees families in which the parents have been so attentive to a child's needs and wishes that the youngster feels extreme loss and anger when the power he has is taken away or diminished by some change in the family system (Haley, 1979; Stierlin, 1977).

Parents and therapists alike tend to assume that a child who gets love and attention will be secure enough that she will readily cope with the inevitable separations and changes that come with growing up. Yet, although there is an overall validity to the notion that children who have experienced love are more secure than those who have been deprived, we have all seen children whose anxiety about separating or level of hostility toward a sibling is perplexing given how much love and attention the youngster has received. Clinical experience demonstrates that children can develop unrealistic expectations regarding the amount of attention and accommodation to their needs that they "ought" to receive, and because of this they have trouble adjusting to more demanding interpersonal situations. In my practice I have encountered a number of youngsters whose rage at being thwarted was expressed not only at home but in school as well. Well-meaning teachers and even school psychologists often relate the child's distress to lack of attention at home, but when one looks closely at the family system, one may see quite the opposite.

For instance, Jessie, age 9, was a lovely, engaging youngster who was the light of her parents' and grandmother's life. At the time I met her she had never gone to sleep alone in her bed. Some adult would lay down with her until she dozed off, and if she awakened in the night she called for someone to come in to her again. Almost any request Jessie made was granted. When Jessie complained about a babysitter, her parents would fire that person virtually no questions asked. Or, if she expressed upset that they were leaving her behind, they would take her along with them on evenings out. And on several occasions the parents either did not use expensive theater tickets (or one parent stayed home) when the youngster expressed upset that she could not come along.

Jessie's parents and grandparents held her in awe. They were charmed by her cuteness and intelligence and communicated to her just how special she was. This child, so used to unconditional admiration, was ill equipped to deal with the demands made of her at school. When a formerly admiring teacher began to express frustration and annoyance at Jessie for her lack of effort in her school work, the youngster, rather than trying harder for approval, felt extreme rage at the teacher's withdrawal of admiration. The youngster, whose sense of self-worth was very dependent on praise and admiration from others, became quite desperate about the teacher's "not liking" her and the parents sought help through family therapy. This, of course resulted in further frustrations for the youngster, because the parents were now determined to get the child out of the middle of their relationship as well as to prepare her for a world that would be less nurturing. The tantrums and extreme rage this child felt at being thus "dethroned" were terrifying both to herself and to her parents.

Some parents who are overly indulgent of children develop rather deep feelings of resentment and antipathy to their now very demanding offspring. Feeling guilty about such sentiments, they may bend over backwards to be good to the child and a vicious circle develops in which the child's neediness leads to parental resentment (and sometimes the intermittent expression of rage) and the parents' guilt about these feelings in turn leads to overindulgence, demandingness, parental resentment, and so on. When children get attention this way they sense the parents' underlying irritation. Although they are in some sense being overindulged and get more attention than most of their cohorts get, they do not in fact get what they really want—a feeling of closeness and love. Thus, despite the objective amount of attention they are receiving, they in fact feel unattended to and this leaves them with an "unexplainable" feeling of frustration and anger. Like the parents, the child is caught in a vicious circle. Even when the parent gives in to the demand, the child does not really feel satisfied; the child wants love, not time per se, privileges, or material gifts. The more she tries to get what she thinks she needs, the more resentful the parents become and the more needful the child feels. Breaking these vicious circles is of course the work of family therapy.

UNDERSTANDING HOSTILE AND AGGRESSIVE CHILDREN

Perhaps the most common complaint of parents bringing a young child to therapy is that the child is "difficult." Although sometimes parents describe a situation in which the child is blatantly defiant, more often it is simply that life feels like a constant strain with these children. They repeatedly push parents and teachers to their limits. Although many of these children specialize, so to speak, in being passively hostile and aggressive (the most effective means to express hostility and anger if you are a small child dealing with much bigger and stronger adults), some children will express hostility quite overtly. Seven-year-old Marcus, for intance, told his father he wanted to gouge his father's eyes out, and on first meeting the therapist said, "I hope you get run over by a car." A little girl of 6 describes how she "teased" another child all day by insulting her about how she looked. And another little girl said quite calmly in a family meeting that she wished her brother was dead. Although there are occasional nice moments with these children, parents and teachers tend to describe them as surly, sour, negative, controlling, and bossy. Often, though not always, the dysphoric mood and angry feeling extend to relationships with peers. Play dates are few and far between and often end in the other child's crying. Nursery school teachers often describe these children as intimidating and manipulating their peers. Sadly, at a very young age they are regarded as a "bad influence" on their more cooperative classmates and are shunned by their classmates' parents. Children as young as 4 may already have become proud (defensively, of course) of their reputation as "toughest" in the class. These children may be disturbingly comfortable with being a bully.

Frequently these children feel that their aggressive behavior is warranted as a reaction to having been *aggressed upon*. Feeling slighted and offended easily, they often misinterpret accidents as intentional assaults and retaliate covertly (e.g., by causing another child to trip) or by an explicit "defensive" assault in return.

Similarly, what to others may seem like mild and reasonable requests by parents are responded to by these children as if they were major interferences with their autonomy. Described by parents as very "strong-willed," these youngster appear to suffer a tremendous loss of pride by doing what they are asked or told to do.

Confronted with what at times appears to be a "paranoid" and "bizarre" overreaction, and dismayed by the child's failure to display any remorse, parents often wonder whether the child has inherited some serious psychopathology. The ghost of schizophrenic relatives may haunt the parents, and they fear that the youngster is destined for some enduring mental illness. If this angry child also happens to be adopted, the parents may worry that the child is genetically predisposed to psychopathic tendencies. Filled with guilt and anger, parents of hostile children vacillate between feeling that they have done something terribly wrong and, on the other hand, that the child is simply a "bad seed."

The Oppositional Child

To a degree, oppositionalism can be regarded as not only a normal but also a positive and *necessary* part of the developmental process (Levy, 1955; Redl, 1976). When the young child is "oppositional," he is demonstrating an ability to resist the influences of the environment. Crucial to the development of inner controls is this capacity to ignore and even defy external pressures.

It is by practicing saying no that the young child develops a sense of autonomy. Simultaneously, by resisting the influences of the environment, the child is strengthening her ability to steer her own course. However, oppositionalism that is so consistent that it has become part of a child's character structure has gone well beyond its developmental usefulness. Consistently oppositional behavior develops either because the child has no other way to resist truly overcontrolling and authoritarian adults or because the child, as discussed earlier, has come to believe that his dependency needs are dangerous and does what he can to ward off a wish to submit.

Strongly oppositional children evoke tremendous frustration and hostility in adults who have to deal with them. It is easy to see how a vicious circle develops. The child experiences his parents' negative feelings toward him and this experience strengthens the youngster's self-defeating character defense. Sullivan (1953) describes how a malevolent transformation of personality can take place:

> If one is led by consistent experience to expect rebuff and humiliation whenever one shows a need for tenderness, for friendly cooperation, it may become the case that one ceases to show any need for good treatment at the hands of others, but instead, when one would feel that need, acts hatefully as if to anticipate a presumedly certain rebuff. When such a deviation has occurred in developing one's potentialities for interpersonal relations, one can scarcely but become ever more firmly convinced that one is unlikable and unattractive, that one is disliked and avoided, and that others are unkind and unfriendly and chiefly interested in making life unpleasant for one another. (p. 303)

A systemic understanding of the development of a negativistic personality in a child does *not,* however, assume that the root of the problem is the parent's rebuffing of the child. As described earlier, many factors can lead a child to excessively protect himself against vulnerability, but once such a pattern develops the child is *correctly* experiencing negative feelings from the parents and further needs to protect himself from wishing to please them.

Clinicians and parents alike may forget that the negativistic, oppositional child really feels quite bad about himself. The child who is provoking strong negative responses internalizes those feelings and generally feels a good deal of self-loathing. This feeling, in turn, contributes to the vicious circle of negative interaction. Feeling unlovable, the child only feels able to have an impact and be important to adults by being provocative. Helping children learn new ways to hold the attention of adults is one of the interventions (described in Chapter 7) that can break the self-destructive pattern that has developed.

The Acting-Out, Aggressive Child

Like the oppositional child, the overly aggressive youngster is regarded by most psychoanalytic therapists as a child who at core feels highly vulnerable. Chethik (1989), describing his work with an "antisocial" youngster, notes that the child interpreted any adult control or criticism as well as the perceived "aggression" of peers as serious assaults on his self-esteem.

> Any command or request by parent, teacher, or therapist was seen by Roger as an attack on his self-esteem, an attempt to bring him to his knees. It was out of these feelings of humiliation that his defiant acts arose. (p. 146)

Chethik (1989) sees the hyperaggressive child as feeling

> massively threatened, helpless and weak. They "cope" with this threat by the mechanism of "identification with the aggressor—they transfer themselves from the person being threatened to the person making the attack." (p. 138)

Willock (1983), too, describing his work with highly aggressive children, notes that minor and imaginary threats or "slights" are readily taken to be major, real dangers. Criticism of one aspect of the child's behavior is felt to be a total condemnation of the basic self. Feeling so vulnerable, the child feels it necessary to maintain a constant readiness to call on primitive, aggressive security operations in order to defend against such "attacks" (p. 389).

Therapists can readily see the core sense of insecurity in these overly aggressive children when attempting to play even mildly competitive games with them. Their need to win is extreme, and their reactions to losing (e.g., disruption of the game, anger, or simply taking the "chips" one is supposed to win) indicate intense feelings of vulnerability and feelings of humiliation at loss.

Beyond feeling unimportant, these children also believe that there is something essentially unlovable about themselves. Willock (1983), writing on this aggressive, acting-out character style, describes what he calls the "disregarded and devalued self." "These youngsters harbor the fear that in the eyes of the world they are not merely insignificant and worthless, but utterly repulsive as well" (p. 390). It is this underlying vulnerability that is behind the rejecting, hostile attitude that serves as armor against narcissistic injury.

It is generally assumed that something happened during the first few years of life to engender such feelings; the child is seen as fixated at a developmental phase where threats to the self are relatively undifferentiated. A cyclical psychodynamic understanding of such issues is less concerned with how the pattern began than with what currently keeps such seeming "fixations" alive. As described earlier in the section on denied aspects of self, various circumstances ranging from actual abuse or neglect to the more subtle lack of availability due to a parent's emotional distress may have profoundly affected the child's sense of worth. Currently, interactions with adults, siblings, and peers are such that the child receives little feedback that counteracts these negative assumptions about himself.

One must keep in mind that there is often validity to these children's feelings that aggression is being directed *at* them. Frequently, a child who expects hostility from peers is used to being the butt of an older sibling's hostility. Not enough attention has been paid in the literature to the effects of the sometimes chronic hostility of older children toward their younger siblings. Clinical experience with families shows, however, a striking ripple effect in which children who feel helpless at home in turn act out on their classmates.

Finally, one must keep in mind that children may simply differ in the strength of their impulses. Freud (1937) posits the existence of children with excessively strong instinctual wishes who have a low threshold for frustration and tolerance for anxiety. Research has indeed shown that some children are constitutionally more aggressive, irritable, and active than others (Chess & Thomas, 1986) and that these children have a harder time than others in accepting limitations. Parents need to be more skilled than average in helping these "difficult" children adjust to conventional expectations.

A basic premise of a psychodynamic orientation to working with these highly aggressive children is that they need to be more comfortable expressing what they regard as "weak" feelings. Some of these children may engage in impulsive and dangerous behavior with the unconscious hope that, seeing the child risk bodily harm to himself, the parents will show that they, in fact, care about the youngster's well-being (Willock, 1983). These children have serious difficulty handling anxiety, fear, embarrassment, and longing, and they will often act out aggressively when these emotions arise.

OVERLY ANXIOUS AND DEPENDENT CHILDREN

This section of the chapter presents some psychodynamic theories that relate to what I will broadly term *overly dependent behavior in children.*

The children being discussed in this section are described by parents and teachers with one or more of such terms as *lacking in self-confidence, fearful, clingy, immature, school phobic, having trouble with separation, cautious, staying apart from the group, clinging to Momma's coattails,* or even *mama's boys* (an old sexist phrase still quite commonly used). Alternatively, they may be thought of as children who are "spoiled" and who want adults to cater to them rather than doing things for themselves. Perhaps the most descriptive and least pejorative of these characterizations is simply the word *immature.* By this I mean that these are children who are not comfortable with doing the things, (e.g., dressing themselves or going to sleepaway camp) that the majority of their age-mates do with relative ease. In a milder form, these are children who though functioning appropriately in some respects, seem to find age-appropriate expectations something of an imposition. These youngsters, for instance, may state that they wish they were in nursery school so they could just play instead of having to learn. One little boy with intense struggles around dependency, though functioning maturely, longingly "recalled" drinking warm milk from his mother's breast. Another little fellow, age 7, who had gone through severe separation difficulties in nursery school but who now was comfortable with overnight visits with friends, spent a good deal of time wrapped tightly around his mother and often demanded baby food. Resorting to baby talk is of course a common occurrence with young children, but some youngsters continuously speak babyishly long after they are capable of doing otherwise. In myriad ways these children exhibit reluctance to develop skills that are within their capacity.

The most extreme form of the behavior described above is seen in young children who become highly anxious, to the point of panic, when separating from one or both parents. Some of these children express fear about calamities that may occur. Others just have a terrible sense of dread when they are separated from a parent and may exhibit this by tantrums and panic attacks or withdrawal and apathy. This, of course, is a problem commonly confronted by family therapists and is usually treated by focusing on the contribution of the family to the child's anxiety (Combrinck-Graham, 1989) and, conversely, the role of the child in "solving" family difficulties. This section reviews some psychodynamic perspectives on separation anxiety and the next chapter looks at how such perspectives can be utilized to formulate family interventions.

Viewed from a traditional psychodynamic perspective, separation anxiety, sleep disturbances, and school phobia are understood as resulting from the child's use of the defense mechanism of projection and displacement. The child who is anxious about separating from a parent is anxious both because angry feelings have been projected onto the environment — making the environment feel like a hostile place — and because the child, believing that the parent knows about his hostility, fears abandonment.

The "worry" about the mother that family therapists so often observe in children who are school phobic can be understood as resulting not solely from a family system in which the child acts as the support and protector of a vulnerable parent but rather as a defense (a reaction formation) against the child's own angry feelings and destructive fantasies. Furthermore, mothers of anxious children may themselves, according to Gardner (1985), worry and be overprotective as a reaction formation against unconscious hostility about which they feel guilty. He notes:

> Interestingly, an almost identical pattern of psychopatholgy develops in the child. The child is basically angry at the mother for a number of reasons. . . . However, [the children] cannot directly express this anger. They are much too fearful of doing that. They are much too dependent on their mothers to allow such expression. After all it is she, more than anyone else in the world, who has designated herself to be their protector from the dangers that await to befall them "out there." . . . And the children too come to deal with their hostility in the same way that their mothers do. Specifically they use repression, reaction formations and fantasized gratification. Each time they envision calamity befalling the mother, they satisfy in fantasy their own hostile wishes toward her. By turning the wish into a fear they assuage their guilt. (p. 20)

Kessler (1966) points out that the child who defends against his unacceptable aggression by becoming increasingly dependent on his mother for protection against his own projected hostility may become more than ever in conflict about his aggressive feelings toward her. Fears of loss of love as a consequence of hostile thoughts are heightened by the child's excessive dependency on the very person with whom she is angry. The psychoanalytic assumption that symptoms simultaneously express and deny unconscious conflict can be seen in how "aggressively" children hold on to parents when they are anxious. Often parents feel quite angry with the child who will not let them separate because the fearful child is also experienced as extremely controlling and demanding. The force with which the child expresses his need for the parent can be understood as a derivative of the defense against aggression.

Separation anxiety and related difficulties are understood quite differently when one looks at these problems from the perspective of developments in psychoanalytic thought that, rather than emphasize, as just described, the conflict between unconscious impulses and the demands of the ego and superego, regard instead as central the internalization of the relationship with the mother. Rather than asking what might the child be defending against, these approaches look at the quality of the child's early relationship with the mother and whether the youngster has developed a sense of self which enables him to feel secure.

Winnicott (1965), who coined the term *good enough mothering* to describe a mother who, while not perfect, was attentive *enough* to the infant, believed that basic trust develops out of the child's internalization of the experience of merger with a "good mother." As the child begins to sense his separateness from mother, he transfers his dependent attachment onto a "transitional object," which maintains the sense of fusion with mother and helps the child deal with separation anxiety. The child's growing sense of separateness is accompanied by anger at not having every need met. When the infant experiences that his destructive feelings toward his mother do not in fact destroy her or lead to abandonment, he develops a sense of both self and object as separate and constant. If the mother is either not sufficiently responsive or does not provide a "holding environment" in which the child's aggression is tolerated, the child does not develop a secure sense of self.

Mahler, Pine, and Bergman (1975), like Winnicott, postulate that the infant merges with the mother in the first few months of life and feels secure and powerful in that state of merger which she calls the phase of normal symbiosis. Mother is regarded as an "auxiliary ego" in the sense that there is no differentiation between "I" and "not I." In order for the child to achieve a sense of separateness and the ability to function apart from the mother, the child needs first to have had a period in which there was a symbiotic fusion with the mother. The developmental task of the child is gradually to separate from the symbiotic bond with the mother and to develop a sense of himself as an individual with his own characteristics. During the separation–individuation phase, which lasts approximately until age 3, the child repeats over and over again a cycle of letting go and returning until security develops. The mother needs to encourage the child to explore and venture forth and at the same time to remain available for the child to return to for infusions of security. If the mother is not available for this "rappprochement" phase, the child does not adequately separate and move out of the symbiotic stage.

Slipp (1984), in his work on the relationship between object relations theory and family therapy, has given a good description of the importance of Mahler's work in understanding anxiety:

> Mahler defines individuation as equivalent to the development of intrapsychic autonomy; separation deals with differentiating the self from the object, distancing, and structuring boundaries between the self and the mother. If these processes are successful, during the rapprochement subphase the mother becomes internalized. The child can trust that the mother's love will continue even in her absence. The child is able to evoke an image of the mother in its memory that is psychologically available when needed, just as the actual mother

previously was present to supply comfort, nurturance, and love. Object constancy can now occur, as well as the development of a separate cohesive self that is relatively autonomous. The child can thus assume the equilibrium-maintaining functions of the mother within itself, providing soothing and self-regulation of narcissistic supplies to sustain self-esteem. . . . If developmental arrest occurs, so that symbiotic relatedness continues, the individual remains overly sensitive to the regulation of self- esteem by others in the environment. (pp. 50, 51)

Both the conflict theory of symptom formation and the idea that there have been some early disturbances in the mothering relationship can be useful perspectives in evaluating the source of separation difficulties. In the next chapter both these theories are used to formulate interventions that address separation problems not just as systemic events but as reflecting intrapsychic difficulties as well.

THE MORE SERIOUSLY DISTURBED CHILD

A variety of terms have evolved to describe children who exhibit more severe disturbance than the typical child patient. These terms include *narcissistically disturbed, schizoid, borderline,* and *schizotypal personality disorder,* to name but a few. I address here some ways of understanding this level of severity which can be useful in the context of a family-oriented treatment. I mention these diagnostic terms only to enable the reader to identify clearly the type of difficulties I am talking about; I will not, however, utilize these terms myself because I believe that they imply a false level of precision and a degree of pseudomedicalization that impedes rather than enhances our ability to address these children's difficulties.[3] Attempts to determine criteria for diagnosing a child as "borderline" (not a DSM-III-R category), for example, reveal that the symptoms described in articles on the subject cover an extremely wide range of behavior. Vela, Gottlieb, and Gottlieb (1980) did find a consensus on 6 out of 19 symptoms described by eight authors. These 6 symptoms, however, also met the DSM-III-R criteria for separation anxiety disorder, oppositional disorder, attention deficit disorder, and schizotypal personality disorder. Furthermore, face (or descriptive) validity in regard to classification does not necessarily provide prognostic predictive validity (Shapiro, 1983). Although there may in fact be real differences in functioning between the borderline child and the child who is described as narcissistically disturbed or between the schizotypal personality disorder and the schizoid disorder of childhood and adolescence (Kestenbaum, 1983), I have found that these classifications are not useful when working with these children in family therapy. Rather than enhancing one's understanding of the specific characteristics and difficulties of a particular child, categorizations of this sort may lead the family and the therapist to overemphasize the extent of the child's psychopathology.

The types of children I am talking about in this section, though not psychotic or schizophrenic seem "strange" and clearly different from more typically troubled youngsters. For instance, a child may be so hypersensitive to feeling that he is being aggressed upon that, although he is not delusional, he is in a loose sense of the term *paranoid*. Children like this respond with great excess to what other children might regard as a small provocation. Their aggressive response to what they perceive as hostility may be so extreme that school officials decide they cannot have such a child in a regular classroom for fear that others will get hurt when an eruption occurs. Children such as this do not merely have problems with impulse control, as described earlier in this chapter, but seem also to have difficulty with reality testing in that their interpretation of events is highly personalized.

Then there are children who, though able to function in the school environment, are nonetheless extremely socially isolated. Their "strangeness" lies in their almost total lack of relatedness to others. Ethan, for instance, made no eye contact with anyone at school, and even at home seemed to be constricted and emotionally distant. He isolated himself from the rest of the family and spent hour upon hour compulsively drawing sharks. Any attempt to interrupt this behavior was met with tremendous resistance and anger.

Withdrawn and aloof children may not even seem distressed by their lack of social relationships. Ethan had built such a wall around himself that he genuinely (at a conscious level) seemed not to care whether he had friends or not. Other severely disturbed and socially isolated children indicate a wish for social contact but behave so oddly and inappropriately that they are shunned when they approach others.

Some seriously troubled youngsters are so anxious that they cannot function without the presence of a comforting adult. Chethik (1989) for instance, describes a borderline child he worked with as becoming agitated and terrified without any apparent provocation. "All new stimuli terrified him. He appeared to be constantly traumatized and had no effective adaptive or defensive system to negotiate the daily environment" (p. 161).

Another phenomenon is drastic and often rapid fluctuations in mood. Episodes of rage or despair seem to appear out of nowhere. It is often quite bewildering to parents and teachers when a child's affective state changes so rapidly and without any obvious precipitant. Six-year-old Jared, for example, suddenly ripped to shreds a painting that to his teachers looked fine, and for the next hour he engaged in an inconsolable tantrum during which he had to be forcibly restrained from harming himself by head banging. Similarly, 4-year-old Sara (see case study in Chapter 9) would alternate between episodes of unprovoked destructiveness toward peers and heart-wrenching "fits" of self-loathing sobbing. These children may also express extreme emotions with regard to how they feel about important adults in their life. A parent or teacher once loved may become "hated" with an intensity that is chilling in its extremity.

Combrinck-Graham (1989) interestingly describes how the difficulties of borderline children can be understood in systemic terms. In my experience, however, although the systemic perspective is crucial, it is rarely sufficient. An approach that also integrates an understanding of the psychic life of these children synergistically enhances the effectiveness of family interventions. Thus, the reader is again reminded that the psychodynamic understanding offered here is utilized not to pathologize the youngster but rather to enhance the power of behavioral and systemic interventions.

Psychoanalytic clinicians describe these children as having inadequately developed ego structures. Pine (1974), for instance, writing on borderline children, describes them as exhibiting "chronic ego deviance."

> Central to the features of the more disturbed children are failures in the establishment of the reality principle, unreliability of the signal function of anxiety and fluidity of object attachment. . . . Thus, these children lack the basic *stabilizers* of functioning that other children acquire: a reliable anchor in external reality and in patterned object relationships that give the children shape, and an array of intrapsychic defenses reliably set into motion when anxiety is aroused. (p. 348)

Pine see these difficulties as arising out of a severe developmental failure that reflects problems in the realm of object relationships rather than the intrapsychic conflict and defense mechanisms that result in symptom formation in less disturbed youngsters. Paulina Kernberg (1983) too sees the source of these difficulties as problematic object relationships during the period of rapprochement and separation–individuation (described earlier). From her point of view, it is the "splitting" of the good and bad internalized objects that results in the failure to develop ego functions with which to handle anxiety and aggression. Similarly, Chethik (1979) describes the borderline child as having achieved only a partial transition out of the state of symbiotic union with the mother. Since the child does not have an internalized "good object," she may experience panic and terror when separated from the "object" who keeps her safe and may become overwhelmed by aggressive fantasies and primitive rages which her poor ego functioning does not help her repress.

It is important to note that the psychoanalytic focus on a failure in early object relationships does not necessarily imply poor parenting. Otto Kernberg (1975), for instance, believes that there may be in some children a constitutionally determined lack of tolerance for anxiety and an excessively strong aggressive drive, which he sees as a factor in the splitting that occurs.

Even if one does not accept the notion of internalized good and bad objects and splitting, it is helpful to think of these children as deficient in the development of some fundamental ego functions. Thus, these children may have poor reality testing, insufficiently developed defenses against impulses, an inability to delay gratification, and inadequate defenses again disorganizing anxiety. As a result, they resort to a variety of massive defenses that interfere with normal functioning.

Many psychoanalytically oriented child therapists, although working from a radically different model of therapeutic intervention than the one propounded in this book, nonetheless describe the goals of their work with borderline or narcissistically disturbed children in terms quite compatible with an integrative family–child model. For instance, Chethik states that a major goal of treatment is to help the child bind the primitive material and to bring it under the control of secondary processes. Similarly, Paulina Kernberg (1983), in describing her approach with these children, talks about the importance of working in the here and now. She utilizes concrete games to practice superego functions, talks realistically with children about their deficits, articulates what is happening in the therapeutic relationship for the purpose of developing empathy, and helps the child tolerate anxiety about primitive fantasies.

In Chapters 7 and 8, some specific interventions designed to strengthen the youngster's ego functioning are described.

INTERPERSONAL EXPECTANCIES

Theorists of all persuasions recognize that the images and expectancies that people have are a powerful determinant of their behavior. Among psychodynamic therapists these notions were initially embodied primarily in the idea of unconscious fantasies. In early psychoanalytic theory, the concept of fantasy was closely tied to the concept of drive, and at times fantasies seemed scarcely more than mental or visual representations of the young child's experiences of gratification. Increasingly, however, even within the drive model, the concept of fantasy began to be elaborated to include a picture of how the world works, what is to be expected, and what is worth pursuing. In more recent years, as interpersonal, object relational and self psychology perspectives have come to the fore in psychoanalytic thought, there has been increasing emphasis on internal representations of interactions between self and others that are better described as expectancies rather than fantasies. Research on infants has demonstrated that even very young infants organize experiences into memories that give rise to generalized expectations (Stern, 1985). Bowlby (1969/1982) has called these internal representations of relationships "working models." Zeanah, Anders, Seifer, and Stern (1989), in reviewing the research on infant development and its implications for psychodynamic theory and practice, described internal representations as follows:

> Essentially memory structures that re-present a version of lived experience to an individual. . . . These large networks [of internal representations] not only re-present lived experience, but also are presumed to perceive and interpret incoming information selectively, to generate anticipations, and to guide behavior in relationships. They are not merely passive filters of experience but contribute towards an individual's active recreations of relationship experiences. (p. 663)

Much empirical support for the existence and relevance of internalized constructs has come from the study of "attachment behavior" in the "strange situation," a laboratory paradigm in which babies are observed separating and reuniting with their mothers (Ainsworth, Blehar, Waters, & Wall, 1978) Babies whose behavior is classified as indicating a "secure" versus "avoidant" or "ambivalent" attachment did significantly better on subsequent measures of psychosocial adaptation (Sroufe, 1988). Although most of these predictive studies deal with children only slightly older than infants, the studies done of school-age children also show that the children who presumably have internalized a secure attachment are more competent in overall functioning (Main, Kaplan, & Cassidy, 1985) and have higher self-esteem (Cassidy, 1988) and less psychopathology (Lewis, Feiring, McGuffog, & Jasher, 1984) than those who were classified as insecurely attached.

These theoretical conceptions begin to merge or overlap with the expectancy notions that have independently been developed by cognitive and cognitive-behavioral theorists. Notions of schemas, to be discussed in Chapter 8, will be seen to have much in common with these concepts.

In the work described in this book, it is these latter, more cognitively formulated notions that are most directly applicable, because they have a more elaborated notion of the ongoing transactions that reflect and simultaneously confirm internalized expectancies and ongoing events. It will be apparent, however, that among the child's expectancies are some that lie considerably outside the conceptual framework of cognitively oriented therapists. In this, as in much else in the book, the cyclical psychodynamic perspective provides an easily crossable bridge between the insights into our deepest and most irrational thoughts provided by psychodynamic theory and the recognition of the connections between psychological structures and manifest events that have characterized cognitive-behavioral approaches.

When working with young children and their families, one can readily see both that the parents may be reinforcing certain internalized expectations and that the child brings to situations "working models" that, however they developed, seem to function relatively autonomously of current reinforcements. I say *relatively* autonomously because internalized expectancies are not static entities. Expectations influence the child's behavior, which in turn influences the patterns of interactions that develop between the child and his family. These interaction patterns in turn themselves subtly modify the child's internalized working models. This same cyclical process, of course, also holds true for the child's interactions in the extended world. Children who expect to be rejected, for instance, often behave in ways that elicit the very response they expected, thereby further "confirming" the utility of the internalized expectation. Of course, the child's expectations do not totally control the responses of the environment, and when the response does not fit with the expectation, the schema can be modified (see, e.g., P. Wachtel, 1987).

Sometimes the difficulties that brought a family to therapy reflect a discrepancy among the various environments the child encounters. Expectations that may be accurate within the family context may have little predictive value in the larger social world the child inhabits. For instance, a child's expectation that his "babyish" self will be admired and even adored may accurately reflect his accumulated experiences in the family, but this expectation may lead to serious disappointment and anger when the child utilizes this schema in more demanding environments such as camp or school. Or a child who is in some sense correct in assuming that one must be on the alert for unprovoked outbursts of hostility may have a defensive posture that is inappropriate for the nonhostile environment in which the child spends his day.

The need for combining psychodynamic, systemic, and cognitive-behavioral perspectives is perhaps nowhere as crucial as when working with a child and a family to alter "working models" that interfere with comfortable and appropriate functioning in the world. Close observation reveals that these assumptions and cognitive schemas both contribute to and are maintained by systemic interactions. Understanding (via projective methods and other means) the unconscious assumptions the child carries within himself, and understanding through careful observation of the child in his family the ways in which the parents may inadvertently contribute to maintaining those expectations, provides the foundation for a more comprehensive and fully transactional approach. The next chapters show how these varying perspectives point to a range of interventions to help the child and family resolve the dilemmas in which they are trapped.

7

Interventions Based on Psychodynamic Formulations

This chapter describes a variety of interventions with families and children that utilize psychodynamic formulations. The aim is both to address the child's concerns through specific active interventions and to incorporate psychodynamic perspectives into an overall treatment plan. Unlike psychoanalytically oriented child therapy or child psychoanalysis, the approach described here does not use the understanding gained of the child's dynamics to make *interpretations* to youngsters. Rather, psychodynamic formulations are used to better tailor systemic and behavioral interventions to the specific needs of the child.

Sharing formulations and tentative hypotheses with parents is a crucial element of this work. Most parents are eager to learn more about their children and psychodynamic understandings often function in a manner similar to the reframings of family therapists; they enable parents to see their children differently and with less anger.

Generally, parents are quite receptive to psychodynamic hypotheses regarding what might be going on for the child. Their receptiveness is in part due to the fact that they are *not* being informed just so that they can be patient and understanding. Rather, they are offered specific advice about what they can do to help the child with his problems. Furthermore, linking behavioral and systemic interventions to psychodynamic understandings seems to dramatically increase the willingness of parents to try new approaches. Many parents, for instance, who would otherwise resist attempts to get them to set firmer limits for fear of being too harsh are comfortable making such changes when they understand them in the context of the effect on the child's intrapsychic processes and his temporary need for external ego controls. Thus, psychodynamic formulations not only inform interventions but can at times significantly reduce resistance to suggestions for changing interactional patterns.

The reader must keep in mind that these examples are meant to demonstrate an approach and are not intended to be an exhaustive survey of ways to use psychodynamic conceptualizations. Such a survey would be impossible because each child and family presents unique issues and challenges. As in all good therapy, there are no formulas. One cannot say, for instance, that when a child's aggression is understood as a defense against vulnerability, one should do such and such. Rather, how exactly one utilizes this perspective is a complex matter that takes into consideration systemic, social, and behavioral factors as well. The aim of this chapter is to give the reader the tools to achieve such a synthesis and to apply psychodynamic insights appropriately and creatively.

Psychodynamic conceptualizations often inform aspects of the work even when the main focus is not psychodynamic. Thus, for example, the particular reinforcements suggested in a behavior modification plan might be based on an understanding of the unconscious needs of the child (see the case of Mathew in Chapter 9). Similarly, an analysis of what structural changes in the boundaries and alliances in the family would help the troubled youngster is aided significantly by the therapist's understanding of the unconscious needs and conflicts of the troubled youngster.

We begin by looking at two types of interventions, "Play Baby" and the "Story-Telling technique," which are particularly useful ways of addressing a child's psychodynamic conflicts.

PLAYING BABY

The Play Baby intervention involves asking parents to initiate pretend games and other activities whose aim is to let the child know that the parents are aware of, accept, and love the child's baby self. Having the parents relate, in play, to the baby that still exists under the facade of the "big" child has proven to be extremely useful both with excessively anxious or immature children and with youngsters whose surface adaptation is almost the opposite — children who have renounced dependency needs and seek neither affection nor approval from parents. It has also been helpful in dealing with resentments, both expressed and unexpressed, that an older child may feel for a younger sibling despite the parents' attempts to give the older child equal or more attention.

Play Baby is a shorthand term I will be using to cover a wide range of activities all aimed at, in one way or another, reminding the child that no matter how big she has become or how self-reliant she acts, the parent knows and accepts the unarticulated or even renounced wish to be nurtured. Parents are asked to initiate games and other activities that will let the child know that although the youngster is still expected to behave in an age-appropriate manner, in some sense "you'll always be my baby." In making a "game" of the child's needs, the parent models for the child the acceptability of regressive longings without threatening the child's growing sense of maturity and autonomy.

The Play Baby activities will vary greatly depending on the age and personality of the child and how comfortable the parents are with regressive play. For instance, some parents report having great fun wrapping their school-aged child in a "blankie," giving him a "baba," and pretending that he is a newborn infant just arrived home from the hospital. Other parents and children will be more comfortable pretending that the parent is excited to see her toddler just learning to crawl, walk, or say his first word. For others, Play Baby might simply consist of the parents' reminiscing about when the child was a baby or taking out baby pictures or dearly loved transitional objects.

Essentially, this technique attempts to address the child's longings without the youngster having to "admit" overtly to these wishes. This is particularly important with children who have repressed or renounced dependency needs. Rather than "interpret" to the child the meaning of his behavior, the therapist helps the child get in touch with and gratify largely unconscious longings through these symbolic enactments. Thus, it is the parent who suggests the game because "though I'm proud of how big you are I sometimes miss my little baby." Play Baby statements and games not only obliquely bring the child's needs to consciousness and symbolically speak to her needs but, perhaps most important, actually change the quality of the parent–child interactions. Youngsters who are receiving this kind of attention are far less likely to try to involve their parents in provocative and negative ways. Similarly, parents who indulge their child's fantasies in this way are often much less apt to "pamper" their youngsters at times that are in fact detrimental to mature development.

It is important to make clear to parents that Play Baby should be initiated by the parent only when the child is not in fact acting in a manner inappropriate for his age. Since Playing Baby is usually great fun for the child, it is important that the parent be aware of just what is being rewarded or reinforced. For this reason, it is best to Play Baby when the child is behaving in ways that are acceptable to the parent. If it follows closely on the heels of immature or negative behavior, those behaviors will be inadvertently reinforced.

Anna Freud (1965) has pointed out that backward moves occur in every child's normal development. At bedtime, for instance, "even the most reasonable and well-adapted children begin to fret, to whine, to talk nonsense, to cling and to demand the physical attentions which they used to receive at much younger ages" (p. 101). Playing Baby at times like this is not recommended, because it will teach the child to associate acceptance of regressive needs with behavior that is actually unwelcome by the parents.

Because engaging in Play Baby often results in rather quick, noticeable change, it is important to convey to parents that this activity must not be thought of as pleasant-tasting medicine that once administered cures the ailment. Rather, Play Baby is meant to communicate to the child an attitude of acceptance and love for the banished parts of himself. Reminiscing about the child as a baby, lingering over baby pictures, or taking out ancient, beloved toys are activities that parents will, it is hoped, engage in throughout the many years of fits and starts in the child's development during which there is always some battle going on between the wish to grow and the wish to stay a child.

Some parents are uncomfortable with the Play Baby method. It is important in such instances to discuss with the parents the theory behind the intervention. Thus, for instance, it might be explained that a child who is unaffectionate to parents and hostile to a younger sibling has renounced her own longings. When reassured that this is to be a "game," and that they should *not* in day-to-day life relax appropriate standards for maturity, parents are often willing to give it a try.

Frequently parents are skeptical about their "macho" or coolly independent child warming up to such a game. It is helpful to alert parents to the fact that although a child may not show any obvious enjoyment of the activity, and may even seem to reject the parents' overtures, nonetheless the child has heard and taken in the parents' symbolic communication regarding the child's needs. It is important to keep offering this to the child even when he does not accept it. The offer alone begins the process of breaking through the child's defensive armor.

When a parent is very uncomfortable with the Play Baby method, the therapist should not push or insist on its importance. As trust develops, it will become clearer why this method may be particularly difficult for the parent to accept. Once again the reader is reminded of the artificiality of separating the systemic, psychodynamic, and behavioral aspects of the work. The Play Baby method is not done in isolation. Family sessions are also used to address the issues of vulnerability and regressive longings for the family as a whole. Thus "resistance" to this approach is regarded as a clue to productive directions in family sessions.

Examples of Using Play Baby

Miranda, age 7, often seemed to be quite angry at her parents. They reported that although she complained that her younger sister got more attention than she did, she in fact, rejected most of the overtures that her parents made to engage her. A voracious reader, Miranda hardly picked her head up from her book when her parents said good morning, and her scowling expression said to them that they erred in interrupting her. Aloofness of this sort alternated, however, with clingy, whiny, and dependent behavior. When Miranda's mother left for work in the morning Miranda cried and complained that mother was not available to take her to the school bus. When the parents went out at night together Miranda interrogated them as to why they would not or could not take her. Extremely articulate and verbal, Miranda often succeeded in making her parents feel quite guilty and sometimes was effective in getting them to change their plans. Although Miranda was overt about her dependency needs, conflict about wanting nurturance from her parents was evident in the way Miranda interrupted warm and intimate interactions shortly after they began to occur. Thus, for instance, moments after joyously laughing during some playful roughhousing with her father, Miranda would get angry that he had inadvertently "hurt" her or should have stopped the wrestling earlier when she was jokingly yelling "stop." Similarly, shortly after cozying up with mother for some quiet reading time, Miranda would get miffed about some annoyance (often an interruption caused by her younger brother) and would reject offers to resume even when mother had remedied the difficulty and made herself completely available.

The reader should keep in mind that the problem being described was only one part of the difficulties that brought the family to therapy. Both the parents and school were concerned about how upset Miranda got with herself when she did not do extremely well on some new academic challenge. This exceedingly bright youngster could not accept anything less than near perfection from herself and would become withdrawn and teary if she failed to live up to what seemed to be her own expectations. There was also great concern about Miranda's lack of appetite and her preoccupation with not eating fattening foods. Last, and perhaps most disturbing to Miranda's parents, was the intense hostility she showed toward her younger brother.

After meeting with Miranda and her family it was hypothesized that Miranda's intense need to succeed and her resentment at her brother stemmed from some core feeling that she did not have what it takes to hold her parents' love. She vacillated between trying to get their love by demanding it (behavior that annoyed her parents and further confirmed her feelings of rejection) and renouncing any need for them. When the parents initiated Play Baby, Miranda was at first reluctant to participate. Only when they persisted in telling her stories about how cute she was as a baby (and conveyed to her that it was *they* who wanted to relive through play those wonderful baby years) did she relax and enjoy the gratification of a need that she was not required to "own" as her own. A great deal of warmth developed between Miranda and her parents just from this simple intervention. Miranda quickly became noticeably less rejecting and demanding. Her parents felt much better about their interactions with her and were more able to say "no" when it was appropriate to do so.

Obviously, there was much more to Miranda's difficulties than her conflicts around vulnerability and dependency. Family sessions dealt with marital conflict, alliances between a parent and child against the other parent, the family ethos of seriousness and hard work, and the high and self-critical standards by which the parents judged themselves. It is my belief, however, that the Play Baby intervention made all the other work go much more smoothly, because it rapidly addressed the child's underlying need, which, in turn, led to positive systemic changes.

According to his parents and babysitter, Adam, age 10, had always been "difficult." In fact, without quite saying it overtly, everyone indicated that Adam was often quite nasty and had the knack of saying things that really cut to the quick. He especially went after his younger brother, Benjamin, who, though often disobedient and impulsive, had according to the parents a much sweeter nature than Adam. Teachers, relatives, and especially his father were disturbed by the rudeness and arrogance with which Adam addressed them. Thus, although Adam was basically "good" in that he did his school work and conformed to rules at home, he simply was not likable. Particularly disturbing was the lack of empathy Adam seemed to have for the suffering of others. When his father showed upset at the illness of his elderly father, Adam's response was on the order of "he's old anyway." To add insult to injury, Adam had no qualms about being extremely demanding in regard to material goods. He "needed" expensive sneakers and sports equipment and the only time he seemed to truly enjoy his time with either parent was when they took him shopping for things he "needed."

In this family, the parents had clearly "pegged" each child and the discrepancy between the warmth they felt for their younger son and the obligatory parenting they did for Adam, was sensed by Adam and increased both his hostility and his need to demand signs of love through a preoccupation with material objects. Of course, his parents' feelings in turn derived from how hurtful and difficult Adam had become. Furthermore, both parents felt terribly guilty about the fact that they had separated and subsequently divorced when Adam was 6 years old. To make up for the injury they had caused him (and also for the injury done to him by having a second, adorable child) each parent gave in to his demands and overlooked his hostility as understandable given the loss he had suffered. Both parents, to varying degrees, allowed Adam to dictate their social life. Although Adam said he could not have cared less about whether his parents remarried, he stayed completely aloof from his parents' new romantic interests. He spoke of his mother's new boyfriend as "an asshole" and the string of women in his father's life as "airheads" to whom he would not bother talking.

The same guilt noted earlier also led both parents to treat Benjamin quite permissively. Both agreed that Benjamin was "babied" quite a bit and that Adam had been much more mature when he was that age. It was clear that each parent in some sense enjoyed Benjamin's vulnerability and got tremendous pleasure from being able to comfort this warm and cuddly youngster.

Although Adam's parents superficially were cooperative with one another and were able, with only intermittent difficulty, to handle a joint custody arrangement, there was in reality a good deal of hostility between the two parents. Adam's mother clearly experienced Adam's arrogance and demandingness as something he had learned from his father. The father understood Adam's hostility as a reaction to his mother's excessive need to control him and the fact that she put a great deal of pressure on Adam to succeed.

Clearly, addressing the systemic aspects of Adam's "nastiness" was crucial. It was also important, however, to find ways to help Adam alter his negative view of himself. In a meeting alone with Adam in which childhood memories were invited, it became clear that he had no "cute" stories or memories from his childhood. Instead, Adam said with an air of some pride that he had learned to walk and talk very early, was told he was very independent, and had a really bad temper. He was told how he would kick and scream if made to leave someplace he did not want to leave.

Family sessions were used in part to remind both Adam and each parent of the tender moments in their history together. The Play Baby technique was explained to each parent in separate meetings and they were encouraged to engage in a variety of Play Baby activities with the aim of helping Adam know his softer side and his wish for affection from his parents. The mother decided to Play Baby by undertaking some "spring cleaning" in which she discovered some of the items that had been saved from Adam's childhood. She asked whether Adam remembered playing, for instance, with his trucks and would say almost incidentally something about how cute he was when he was little. Another variation of Play Baby used by Adam's father involved taking out some photographs of Adam as a young child and jokingly asking at bed time if he would allow a favorite story to be read to him just for old time's sake.

Combined with many other interventions, including the noticing and positive response to the slightest bit of warmth or niceness on his part, Adam began to be less hostile and clearly enjoyed this reminiscing. When his mother brought home a cuddly little bear for him one day and had the bear say in a squeaky, high-pitched voice, "I'm little and I'm scared. Can't I sleep under your arm tonight?" Adam's coolness totally melted and he softly replied, "Sure you can."

THE STORY-TELLING TECHNIQUE

The "Story-Telling technique" (E. Wachtel, 1987) involves asking parents to tell stories that embody the feelings the child has banished. The stories incorporate not only feelings the child may feel guilty about but also his unspoken fears and unconscious concerns. Young children are usually enchanted with animal stories and easily identify with the baby elephant or school-age tiger whose feelings and thoughts closely resemble those that the child has disavowed.

Parents often express concern that their children are too sophisticated to fall for this ploy and thus this method will not work for their youngster. It seems, however, that even when a child does catch on (and certainly to some degree most do), the fact that it is *just* a story, and that the issues are being addressed obliquely rather than frontally, allows the child to listen and enjoy vicariously the pleasure of having his darkest side known.

Children (and adults as well for that matter) are enchanted by tales. When these tales are tailor made to fit closely with the youngster's issues, children often love them so much that they ask to hear the same story over and over again. Many parents feel concern that they do not have the creativity to invent interesting stories. Parents need to be reassured that children love stories that speak to their unconscious concerns even when the story is not elaborated on with fanciful and creative detail. Most children are so happy they are being told the story that they are very forgiving of inconsistencies and lackluster plots. Some children eagerly join in and provide detail and subplots which further reflect their concerns, but most youngsters are content to passively listen.

It is important to provide parents with some detailed instruction as to what they might include in the story. Sample plots which they can build on should be offered. Thus, for example, a child who unconsciously fears that he will not be as lovable once he grows up and is no longer "babyish" could be told a story about a little elephant who refused to go to Elephant School to learn circus tricks because he thought that once he was big, Mommy and Daddy elephant would no longer find him cute and funny and would not give him rides and squirt him with water anymore. Or a child who is horrified by and tries to repress hateful feelings toward a younger sibling could be told a story about a lion cub who would wrestle and nip the younger cub in fun but who sometimes felt so angry that he hoped his brother cub would step in the trap set by hunters. The stories can end with the animal confessing his feelings to someone (a kind aunt, a fairy godmother, a teacher, a friend) and with reassurances that these types of feelings have been heard before. Although the stories can incorporate the child's ambivalences (e.g., the baby bear also *wants* to learn to do circus trick and the lion cub also *has fun* with the baby cub sometimes), the main thrust of the story should be the feeling about which the child is most uncomfortable.

Gardner (1971) has written extensively on the usefulness of story telling in child therapy. Gardner's technique differs from what I have been describing in several respects. First, stories are told to the child by the therapist, not the parents, and are told in response to a story the child has related. Second, the purpose of the therapist's story is to provide the child with a lesson in a more adaptive solution to his difficulties rather than, as with the stories I am describing, simply to model for the child that opening up about his hidden self will make him feel better.

In the work I am describing, the purpose of having the parents tell these stories is to reassure the child that his hidden self need not be so frightening. For this reason parents must be made to understand that it is important that these stories do not cover up or have happy but unrealistic endings. In helping parents prepare to tell stories, the therapist should make sure that the parents understand the basic feeling and unconscious conflict that is to be the theme of the story. If possible, the parents should tell the child a few different stories which incorporate the same basic conflict. Throughout the work with the child and the family, new issues may arise which, with the help of the therapist, the parents can incorporate into new stories.

REAL-LIFE STORIES

It is helpful to ask parents to search for incidents in their own life that demonstrate the types of conflicts about which the child is concerned. For instance, do the parents remember any time they felt guilty about intense anger toward somebody they were supposed to love? Do they remember any instances of trying to feel more independent and less needy than they actually felt? Can they think of current occasions when the same or similar feelings were at play? Are there times in their day-to-day interactions with colleagues, friends, family, or even salesclerks when they have feelings that in some way parallel those of the child? They may, for example, have been afraid to say something critical to a colleague for fear it would sound too harsh. Or perhaps they tried to push away feeling hurt that a friend seemingly became distant, or had to push themselves to act maturely rather than give in to what felt like a childish impulse.

Most children love to hear anecdotes about their parents' lives, at least when these anecdotes are not told to them as object lessons or for the purpose of emphasizing how easy the child's life is by comparison). When parents tell stories that reveal authentic feelings and conflicts, children are tremendously engaged. Especially with older children, for whom childish animal tales may no longer be appropriate, real-life stories that embody the child's repressed or forbidden feelings are extremely effective. Although these stories can be about events in the past, incorporating into one's conversation *current* instances of conflictual feelings can be even more meaningful. Sharing with a youngster one's feelings about current experiences and relationships lets the child know that conflictual feelings are not something the parents *once* felt (and then, in the child's mind, presumably outgrew) but rather that they are something adults still have to deal with from time to time.

TELLING STORIES AS EXPOSURE TO BOTH PARENT AND CHILD

Parallel anxieties are often found in parent and child. Frequently, the very feelings about which the child feels conflicted or guilty are also anxiety producing for one or both parents. By asking the parent to actively make the child more comfortable with these feelings (through modeling or story telling) the therapist is also communicating to the adult that these taboo feelings are natural and acceptable. Not only is the therapist giving the parent permission to feel these feelings, she is also providing a rationale and a method that allow the adult to work indirectly on his own issues without having to consciously "own" the problem as his own. Thus, by telling the child stories in which the disowned feeling is of central importance, the parent inevitably is exposing himself to the feeling that he too has been uncomfortable acknowledging or expressing. There is much evidence that exposure to what has been fearfully avoided is an effective means of anxiety reduction (Marks, 1969; P. Wachtel, 1977; Wilson & Davison, 1971).

TELLING STORIES AND THE ALTERATION
OF THE FAMILY STRUCTURE

When a parent tells a story to a child as a way of changing problem behaviors, the activity itself involves certain structural changes in the family. The child is now getting attention in a new and unaccustomed way.
Perhaps the parent tells the story early in the morning or at a meal, and
thus changes the pattern of interactions in the family at those times.

When parents talk about their own experiences they are frequently
surprised and gratified by the child's obvious interest. Often parents resent
(but do not see their contribution to) the self-centeredness of children and
a shift from focusing on the child to focusing on the parent is a major
structural change.

Furthermore, by giving the parent this task, the therapist provides
the parent with something to do, and is thereby alleviating feelings of
powerlessness and frustration. Like any task, telling stories gives the parent
a new solution to substitute for old ones that have been largely unproductive.

Brief Examples

Laura, age 7, avoided challenges. Her teachers were concerned that she
needed an inordinate amount of attention and reassurance to get her to
work at something that was difficult. She was particularly resistant to
working on new material when in a group. She avoided being asked to
"guess" at something she did not already know and would avoid possible failures by such maneuvers as wandering off, feeling sick, losing
her place in the book, or simply saying "I know this already." Laura's
projective stories contained themes of humiliation and taunting for inadequate performance.

The Story-Telling technique was used with Laura to help her deal
with the fear of humiliation, which lay behind her avoidances. Animal
stories about kittens and baby birds who avoided learning how to hunt
and fly for fear of doing these things foolishly were intriguing to her.
Although she never related these stories directly to herself, she did begin
to talk about how difficult some things were for her and bit by bit dropped
the bravado with which she had announced how "great" she was at things
that in reality were difficult for her.

In addition, Laura's mother (but not her father) was able to relate
current instances in which she felt foolish even though she knew she really
should not feel that way. For instance, Laura's mother told Laura how
silly she felt when she did not know how to unlock the gas tank cap on
a rented car and had to ask the garage attendant to figure it out for her.

Or, she related feeling silly about not knowing how to fill out some bank forms and having to ask a bank officer for assistance for something quite simple. Laura was very interested in these events and asked her mother whether people had actually laughed at her. This of course led to a discussion of how when one does something that is potentially embarrassing one usually (but not always) learns that people will not in fact laugh.

Once again the reader should keep in mind that Laura's problems were approached from the systemic and behavioral perspective as well. Surely, one must ask what in the child's interactions with family, babysitters, teachers, and peers might be contributing to this anxiety. One wonders, too, what the child has observed in regard to competition between the parents, particularly in light of the fact that Laura's father had a great deal of difficulty relating real-life stories.

Ethan (described briefly in Chapter 6) was a severely disturbed youngster who kept himself at a great emotional distance from peers as well as family. In school he would engage with children only when absolutely necessary. At recess he preferred to be by himself and would play one-person electronic games. His parents felt concerned that he did not seem to want to participate in family life and would spend hours at a time compulsively drawing sharks.

Ethan's need to withdraw was understood as a result of a fear of intense rage. This rage manifested itself both in the stories he invented in response to projective material and in occasional eruptions of almost bizarrely hostile verbalizations (e.g., "I hope you are run over by a truck and that it breaks all your bones slowly"). Generally Ethan was well behaved, but his good behavior felt much more like compliance than true cooperation. Subtle passive aggressive struggles left adults with a bad feeling about interactions with Ethan: He evoked feelings of anger even when he was in fact doing what was asked of him.

On two occasions between the ages of 3 and 5, Ethan, in fighting with his younger brother, got so mad that he lost control. Once, he threw a heavy firetruck at his brother's head which resulted in a bloody gash requiring stitches. A year later, a shove resulted in a head injury which, though it turned out to be inconsequential, at first caused great alarm because of accompanying vomiting.

Both Ethan's father and his stepfather had a powerful temper which his timid and excessively sweet mother had to cope with. Ethan had not only witnessed a great deal of fighting in his home but had also been on the receiving end of each man's volatile temper. Again, the reader is reminded that the full work on this case involved many different types of interventions with both sets of families as well as direct behavioral work with Ethan to help him modulate anger and develop appropriate ways to assert himself and to express anger. One piece of the work, however, was telling Ethan stories to help him acknowledge his fear of his own anger. He would become completely absorbed by stories about cubs with bad tempers that could be very dangerous. Freddy the Ferocious Lion, for instance, did not even want to play with other cubs for fear that he might get so mad when scratched that he would bite off another cub's paw. Ethan's interest in the content of these stories was so great that it overcame the youngster's defense against the wish to be passively dependent on his mother. Thus the Story-Telling technique not only addressed an important issue in terms of content, but the very act of having these stories told to him addressed the split-off need to be babied.

UTILIZING PREWRITTEN STORIES

Some parents feel very intimidated at the prospect of telling a child stories and ask whether there are any books that they can read to their child instead. Although there are some books that do attempt to help children accept their fears, worries, and angers, such books do not generally incorporate themes of unconscious conflict, anxiety about abandonment, or retribution for angry thoughts. Furthermore, a story invented by a parent is a much more powerful communication to the child that the parent accepts these emotions than merely choosing a book to read that has these themes. Nonetheless, reading stories that invite the child to express his feelings on sensitive topics is certainly of value and should be encouraged as an adjunct to the Story Telling technique or as an alternative to it when the parents feel unable to create stories tailor-made to the concerns of the child.

In trying to create their own stories, some parents might find it useful to look at *Annie Stories* (Brett, 1986), a book on creating therapeutic stories for children. Although the book is useful in providing concrete advice on how to incorporate the child's concerns into stories, the stories Brett describes are much more elaborate than what I am suggesting and incorporate modeling and desensitization into the narrative. Nonetheless, if a parent takes the time to read this book and to create intricate plots and fantasies, the child is sure to benefit.

NEGATIVE REMINISCING

In an effort to help children adjust, many parents avoid talking about events that may be painful reminders of hurts, losses, and fears. By avoiding topics that evoke disturbing feelings, parents often inadvertently reinforce the child's own maladaptive defense mechanisms. It is not uncommon for children simply to banish disturbing memories from their thoughts. In order to keep memories and the troubling feelings associated with them repressed, the child may avoid situations that in any way evoke the excised emotions. A child who has experienced terrible feelings of abandonment, for instance, may be excessively independent and reject attempts at closeness. Or a youngster who has been terrified by the angry scenes she has witnessed at home may prefer to play by herself at recess rather than to engage in games at which fights might erupt.

Negative Reminiscing is used to help a child remember the repressed events (and associated feelings) that are limiting the child's repertoire of behaviors. It is also used in working with children who, even if they have not repressed their memories of a traumatic event, have not thoroughly worked them through.

It is important to prepare parents for Negative Reminiscing sessions. Sometimes children feel a need not to talk about memories they feel will be painful to the parent. Thus, work with each parent is necessary to ensure that each is in fact comfortable talking about the disturbing events. By explaining to the parents exactly how the need to "forget" the feelings associated with upsetting incidents has affected the child's functioning, parents are helped to overcome their own discomfort at the prospect of dredging up feelings they believed were better left buried.

When the parents are ready to talk about these painful subjects a meeting is held with the child and the parents in which the child is encouraged to recall the painful episodes in her life. If the parents are divorced or separated and the child would find it stressful to be with them together, two separate sessions are held. At this meeting, the parent prompts the child (saying, for instance, "Do you remember the time when you were 5 years old that Mommy and I had a big fight and threw things at each other?") It is important that the Negative Reminiscing be as specific as possible. If, for instance, a child is repressing memories of abandonment, it is not enough for a parent to say, "Remember the day Mommy left home?" Instead, the therapist should encourage the parent to describe the event as vividly as possible. The father might say, "Do you remember the day when you got off the bus in second grade and Mommy had a suitcase packed and said she was leaving? Do you remember how I was grabbing Mommy and telling her not to go and that I would kill myself if she left?"

It is the therapist's role to encourage the child to actively add to the recounting of the events rather than passively listening to the descriptions proffered by the parents. This can be facilitated by such questions as: "Do you remember what Dad is describing?" "Do you remember anything at all like that?" "Where were you?" "What did the room look like?" "Can you close your eyes and picture yourself at that age?" "In that place?"

"Can your body feel what you felt then?" "Do you remember any thoughts you had at that time?" "Where were the other people in your family when this was happening?"

Very young children, instead of being asked verbal questions alone, can be encouraged to draw pictures of the frightening event. As they draw, they are asked to describe what happened so that a parent can write down for them an accompanying text. Older children can be encouraged to keep a journal of any memories they have of their childhood, using the Negative Reminiscing session as the start of the journal.

Brief Example

Mrs. Lang consulted me about the extremely aggressive behavior of her 5-year-old daughter Kaitlin. A few months prior to the session, Kaitlin's father had been hospitalized for depression, and although he was now at home, he remained seriously depressed. In a session with Kaitlin and her mother (Mr. Lang refused to come to sessions), Mrs. Lang was asked to describe some of the upsetting things that Kaitlin had witnessed and was still continuing to witness. With family puppets, Kaitlin and her mother acted out the scene in which, at the urging of her mother, Kaitlin ran to a neighbor to get help in removing a knife from her father's hand. They enacted the father's screaming that he would kill himself someday and the subsequent arrival of police and ambulance workers. Kaitlin then quietly and calmly drew pictures (which her mother would later help her make into a book) that showed the different scenes the child remembered. She also drew pictures of how her father seemed now and of her mother crying because she was "mad at Daddy."

POSITIVE REMINISCING

It is not only negative memories that children repress. Not infrequently children repress memories of positive events which, nonetheless, can evoke feelings of loss, vulnerability, anger, or even guilt. Parents, wishing to spare their children any more pain, may contribute to the child's loss of important positive memories by simply never talking about the person or event whose complex implications include significant elements of loss or hurt. A loved babysitter or parent, for example, who has abandoned the child may never be mentioned.

When the occurrence of such omissions becomes clear in the course of the work with a family, it is helpful for the parents to begin to mention (at first casually) the excised event or person. With a child who is not dealing with feelings regarding a divorce, for instance, it is helpful to ask the parents to incorporate into routine conversation mention of places and occurrences that took place when the parents were together. Or, as in the case of Sara (see full-length case study in Chapter 9) a parent may begin to bring up the painful memory of a figure who represents loss to the child by such simple statements as, "Oh, that's the kind of car your father drove when he lived with us," or "That color was the favorite of so and so when she used to babysit for you."

After some preparation of this sort at home, a session similar to the Negative Reminiscing sessions described above can be held. The adults who remember the positive memories that the child has repressed are asked to share their memories with the child. This, of course, can be quite difficult for a parent who may prefer, for his own reasons, to remember only negative things about the spouse who has left. When, however, parents understand the psychological repercussions to the child of not dealing with feelings of loss, they can often overcome their own reluctance to participate in such reminiscing.

A session in which Positive Reminiscing is the focus can also be very useful when a parent and child are so locked in a hostile interaction that they are defending against conscious awareness of close and warm times they have had together. Anger at a parent often serves as a defense against feelings of loss and vulnerability. Similarly, when a parent feels chronically angry at a youngster, he too may be keeping from consciousness memories and images that would evoke the more complex emotions of loss, regret, and rejection. Often, an individual session with the parents enables them to recover positive memories. Once this has been achieved, a family meeting strictly devoted to reminiscing can be very helpful in starting a process in which the child is helped to experience a fuller range of emotions.

USING PSYCHODYNAMIC UNDERSTANDING TO INFORM SYSTEMIC AND BEHAVIORAL INTERVENTIONS

Psychodynamic formulations inform my work with families and young children in myriad ways that are not as discretely describable or as broadly and generally applicable as the methods described thus far. The uniqueness of each family and child frequently requires the therapist to be inventive in thinking about how an understanding of the child's needs and unconscious conflicts can be applied in pointing the parents and child toward new behaviors and patterns of interactions. Although some family therapists eschew discussion of the child's individual psychodynamics, or prefer altogether to intervene in the family's patterns with minimal explanation, it has been my experience that parents are vastly more cooperative and consistent in trying out new ways of interacting with their children when they have an understanding of how such changes relate to the child's fears and anxieties. Thus, I regularly give feedback regarding my understanding of their child's conflicts and defense mechanisms and make clear how specific suggestions I offer are based on such an understanding. Of course, any changes the parents make on behalf of the child are systemic changes as well, and one must strive to keep both perspectives in mind simultaneously.

LIMIT SETTING TO ADDRESS THE CHILD'S FEAR OF HIS OWN ANGER

When a psychodynamic understanding of the child's conflicts and anxieties is offered, parents are often able to change their own behaviors in ways that previously may have seemed to them wrong, unsupportive, insensitive, or harsh. When parents understand, for example, that their child is actually feeling quite afraid that she will hurt someone with her uncontrolled aggression, they often find the wherewithal to set the protective and reassuring limits that the child needs. Parents need not be highly sophisticated or well educated to understand that a child feels bad about his "dark side" or fears that he will hurt someone with his anger or that his parents can read his mind and will retaliate even for bad thoughts much less actions.

It is important in enlisting the help of parents to provide them not just with the therapist's conclusions regarding the psychodynamic issues but with a report on some of the behaviors and information obtained in sessions alone with the child that support the interpretations being offered. This is one of the advantages of supplementing the more obviously systemic work with sessions with the individual child. Such sessions are not an alternative to work on the systemic patterns of interaction but are often a crucial factor in implementing such systemic work successfully.

To illustrate the considerations just put forth, let us consider the Walker family. Mr. and Mrs. Walker were quite alarmed by how upset their 7-year-old son, Mickey, could become. When frustrated with himself for his own inability to do something (e.g., stay up on skis or bowl) or when another child teased him or even accidentally pushed him, Mickey generally became quite withdrawn for the next hour or 2. With a brooding, somewhat fierce expression on his face, this well-built muscular boy would sit hunched over in self-imposed isolation and would be totally unresponsive to attempts by either adults or children to interact with or comfort him.

Ever since Mickey was a toddler he had been known to have an explosive temper which led him at times to do things that were truly physically dangerous. In family sessions as well as in meetings alone with Mickey it became clear that he felt quite vulnerable and reacted to this feeling with rage. His withdrawal was seen as an attempt to control his violent temper, for he felt frightened of the harm he could do to people when he was mad. Frustration at not being able to accomplish what he wanted to do was dangerous too, because although Mickey was angry at himself, he felt that he was so mad he might hurt somebody.

For a variety of systemic and individual reasons, which will be explained in the full-length case study of Mickey and his family in Chapter 9, each of Mickey's parents had been rather lax about setting limits on how aggressively the youngster could behave. Only when they understood how painful and frightening it was to Mickey to feel out of control were his parents amenable to being much firmer with him about temper tantrums. In addition to the limit setting, Mickey's parents, based on their new understanding that this child felt tremendously vulnerable and that self-control would enhance his sense of security, cooperated in *rewarding* Mickey for his attempts to control and redirect aggressive responses. They were also encouraged to protect Mickey during this learning period so that his attempts to use some cognitive and behavioral methods to feel better would be successful. This meant that family time needed temporarily to be restructured so that Mickey would not be exposed to situations that stimulated aggressive impulses or to challenges that some children his age ordinarily do with ease but which Mickey could not participate in without feeling overwhelmed by anger. Play wrestling, socializing with his elder brother's friends, and participating in team sports were all activities that were *temporarily* curtailed while Mickey and his family worked on helping him get his aggressive impulses under control.

LIMITING THE EXPRESSION OF NEGATIVE FEELINGS

Many parents feel that it is important to let children express hostile feelings openly. Often, this is a good policy in that it communicates to the child that his aggressive emotions are natural and that he is still loved despite how angry he may sometimes get. There are two situations, however, when the freedom to express negative feelings can become excessive. First, children who are given too much license to express hateful feelings can become quite frightened by the primitiveness of their rage. Young children are unclear about questions of personal power and causation, and when they are allowed repetitively to make statements such as, "I want to kill my sister," "I'm going to rip his heart out," or "I hope he gets run over by a truck," or, as in the case of one little boy I worked with, the child is allowed to write and enlist his friends in writing hate letters to his younger sibling (who fortunately could not yet read), they can become quite frightened by the power of their emotions.

Although it is clear to an adult that words cannot actually harm someone physically, children are often quite unclear about how much harm such expressions can cause. Furthermore, when the parents allow the child over and over again to express hostile feelings, the child is, in a sense being overstimulated by his own verbalizations and is not being given sufficient help in taming her aggressive urges.

It is also useful to note that children generally feel *ambivalent* about a sibling, not just negative. Excessive focus on hostile feelings can interfere with the child's awareness of the full range of her emotions. When this occurs the child's functioning is disrupted by surges of anger and she has trouble achieving the calm necessary for concentration and age-appropriate mastery. Parents are often quite relieved when I spell out for them reasons it is not good to allow so much expression of hostility; indeed, often they have been *wanting* to say "enough" but did not feel it was acceptable parenting to do so. It is helpful to give parents some concrete examples of how the child is feeling afraid of the impulses stirred up by so much freedom of expression. When parents understand that children sometimes need external support to develop ego controls and can be quite overwhelmed by primitive feelings without help from parents, they can experience this sort of limit setting not as repressive but rather as a way to assist the child in becoming more mature.

The second reason for limiting the expression of negative feelings is that at times parents are so responsive to complaints, criticisms, and negative perceptions that children are being inadvertently taught to be "grievance collectors." Trying to be responsive to the dysphoric feelings of youngsters is, of course, extremely important. Too often, children learn to put on a happy facade and feel that they must hide sadness and negative feelings from their parents. Yet, at times, parents can go too far in listening and responding to unhappiness. The child not only learns that this is a way to engage the parent, but more important, the parent is not helping the child to develop a more philosophic or relaxed attitude toward things that are not always to one's liking.

AVOIDING OVERSTIMULATION OF REGRESSIVE URGES

Although it is often helpful for parents to attend to the regressive needs of their child through such means as the Play Baby technique described earlier, an understanding of the psychodynamic issues of a particular child can also at times lead to the suggestion to be *less* encouraging of regression. When a child is having a particularly difficult time, for instance, with separations and is struggling to develop ego strengths that will quell anxieties, it can be important for parents not to stimulate the child's more regressive longings. Just as sleepaway camps discourage parents from calling during the period when children are conquering homesickness, for fear that the sound of the parent's voice will upset the youngster, so too, it is helpful for parents to understand that some perfectly normal activities may be ill-advised during periods when their child is struggling to develop more mature behavior.

Sometimes a simple change in routine is enormously helpful in making it easier for a child to mobilize the ego strengths he needs to cope with emotionally taxing situations. For example, in the case of Todd, age 6, a change in his bedtime routine helped him master rather severe separation anxieties which often led to vomiting as he was being put to bed. By suggesting to the parents that right before turning out the lights they play some games with Todd that utilized his cognitive capacities (checkers, word games, puzzles), and that they no longer read to him books that put him into a regressive loll, the child was given a little extra support for his developing ego strengths. It is easier to be mature when you have just felt "smart" than it is to be mature when you have been metaphorically rocked like a baby.

Again, the reader is reminded that this is only one small intervention among many. This child's difficulties with separations not only served a function in the system but were in part due to the covertly negative feelings of his mother, which were themselves a result of systemic interactions in which she was overly permissive. Without systemic interventions, the strategy of changing the bedtime routine would have been unlikely to be helpful. By understanding, however, that activities that connected to the child's more regressive self made it all the more difficult for the youngster to separate, the therapist was able to give the child the extra help he needed to overcome anxieties that were increasingly less relevant to his actual family situation.

A similar approach was used with a 2½-year-old whose half hour cuddle time with his mother had begun to be ruined by his crying over not wanting her to go to work. A change in routine, in which playing and watching television with mother in her bed prior to her getting ready for work was replaced with more active play in the family room, made the toddler's separation from his mother go much more smoothly. Even with a child that young, one should keep in mind that is may not be helpful to relate to the child's "younger," more regressive self.

Some families are so protective, nurturant, and willing to accommodate to their child's upsets that they not only hinder the development of the child's ego capacities but set up expectations regarding the responsiveness of adults that do not accord with reality. Paul, age 7, was the youngest of three children. Very much the baby of the family, Paul often cried and had tantrums. Both parents regarded him as extremely sensitive and felt that he had always had a hard time handling the playful (and sometimes not so playful) aggression of his older siblings. He was insulted easily and would sob in sadness and in rage at being teased. When playing board games he would disrupt the game or pout as soon as he felt he was losing. Each of Paul's parents was extremely responsive to his upset. Paul's mother would cuddle him and stroke his hair, all the while assuring him that everything would be all right. Similarly, Paul's father would sweep him up in a bear hug and allow him to snuggle up for as long as he needed until he felt calm.

Both parents, felt that Paul had always been a very sensitive and sweet boy who was having a particularly difficult time adjusting to his parent's separation which had occurred when he was 5. For this reason they were not only very comforting to him when he was upset—even if his upset took the form of an angry tantrum—but also tried to grant almost all his requests. Moreover, the parents were competing with each other to be the more responsive parent and at a moment's notice would drop what they were doing in order to meet the youngster's needs. This included playing games and sports with him, helping with school work, and letting him sleep in their beds whenever he felt like it.

Although there were times when each parent's patience wore thin and explosions of rage would occur, by and large Paul almost never heard the phrase "please wait a minute," "later," or "cut it out." When Paul was upset about losing a game or cried about something being unfair, the comforting response of each parent gave the unintended message that he, in fact, truly had something to be upset about. This reflected each parent's feeling that in fact Paul *did* have something to be upset about, namely, the divorce. Yet by responding to their son's crying with heartfelt concern, Paul's parents were reinforcing emotional collapse rather than helping him develop the ego capacities that would enable him to be heartier. Furthermore, Paul, who had spent his first years of school in a small and highly nurturant private school, was having a very difficult time adjusting to the public school he now attended. He had learned to think of himself as "cute and sensitive" and of adults as almost limitlessly supportive and comforting. Only when his parents began to understand how they were contributing to Paul's difficulties were they able to shift from blaming the school for a lack of support to helping Paul develop better coping mechanisms.

THE CHILD'S FEARS

A psychodynamic perspective on children's fearfulness often leads to some rather nonobvious behavioral and systemic interventions. Nine-year-old Olivia hated to be alone even for a few moments. She became highly anxious and sometimes quite hysterical if her mother (Ms. Brown) stepped out of their extremely secure apartment just for the few moments it took to put laundry in the basement washer. Even when her mother took a shower, Olivia became quite anxious and insisted on the door's being open; sometimes Olivia could not even tolerate the shower curtain's being fully drawn. And if her mother, despite the child's protestations, dared to leave the building to do 10 to 15 minutes of shopping at the market across the street, Olivia, whose fear resulted in stomachaches and occasional nausea, would stayed glued to the window until her mother returned.

Olivia's mother was an ambitious woman who found her work gratifying though stressful. As a computer problem solver and systems coordinator for a large corporation, Ms. Brown was "always on call." Although she found it difficult to juggle her career and her responsibilities as a single parent, she felt that changing jobs was not something she wished to do. She got no financial support from Olivia's father and felt that a less demanding job would not only be less challenging but would not provide the kind of income that she felt she and her daughter needed to live comfortably.

Ms. Brown did not have a predictable work schedule. Although she was in a position of authority and could set her own hours, she often worked rather late when there was an important job that she felt had to get done immediately. She frequently went on business trips and often these were arranged on just a day or two's notice. An elderly neighbor would babysit for Olivia whenever Ms. Brown was not able to be home.

Olivia was quite vocal about her resentment of her mother's schedule. She regularly reproached her mother about the business calls that her mother believed were a "necessary" part of her work. Olivia felt that her mother spent "hours" on the telephone each night. Although Ms. Brown denied that it was "hours," she did acknowledge that a typical evening often included five or six important business calls from home.

Ms. Brown experienced Olivia as extremely controlling and was often irritated by her behavior. Olivia was a very "picky" eater and not infrequently, after Ms. Brown prepared something that Olivia had requested, Olivia would state that it did not taste good and would demand something else in its place. Olivia, who bitterly complained about her mother's absences due to business trips and late hours, would often, when her mother *was* home, beg, much to her mother's dismay, to be allowed to have an overnight play date at a friend's house. These behaviors were understood both as an expression of anger at her mother and as a manifestation of Olivia's need to control emotional "supplies."

Given Olivia's life experiences, her fearfulness about being left alone when her mother was in fact technically "home" was understood as an expression of the feeling that even when her mother was home she was not really there for Olivia. Olivia could be described as a child who was not securely attached and who felt that her emotional hold on her mother (as well as, of course, on her father) was rather weak.

Most important, however, Olivia's fears were understood as stemming from her own anger. Olivia often behaved in a way that was so "difficult" that given her underlying feelings of insecurity, she could easily feel that her irritating behavior would lead mother to abandon her. Furthermore, her anger could lead to retribution in the form of injury to herself or her mother.

Interestingly, Olivia was not terribly anxious when her mother flew on business trips or when mother had to work late. She seemed most anxious at those times when she "had" mother but temporarily had to let her go. The anger this child felt when her mother was home but not available (for example, when mother was on the telephone or doing chores) was far greater than she felt when her mother *had* to be at work. The fact that mother seemed to be *choosing* not to be with her was what provoked extreme anger, and the terror the child felt at these times was understood as a direct consequence of this anger.

The psychodynamic understanding of Olivia's fears was helpful in devising systemic interventions that would work synergistically to increase the effectiveness of behavioral methods (e.g., relaxation training, cognitive strategies, and gradual desensitization) aimed at helping Olivia feel less anxious. First, instead of offering reassurances about how soon she would be back or about how nothing could possibly happen when she was in the shower, Ms. Brown would simply state that she knew how angry Olivia felt sometimes and that this anger could not cause anything to happen. Second, since the source of Olivia's fear was understood to be her angry feelings, it was important for her to have some nice time with her mother right before these short separations. Both mother and daughter had to do their part in making some pleasant times possible. In contrast, the anger both parent and child felt when Olivia had tantrums to prevent her mother from leaving or taking a shower, served as fuel for the fear. By having some "close" time immediately before the feared event, Olivia's anxiety was reduced and with less anxiety to overcome, the behavioral strategies had a better chance to work.

Once again, I wish to remind the reader that, for the purpose of demonstrating the usefulness of psychodynamic understanding I am describing just one small piece of the work with this family. Olivia was seen with both her father (who had recently been discharged from a drug rehabilitation center) and stepmother as well as with her mother and babysitter. The work included giving Olivia more control over time, helping Ms. Brown sort out the ways she saw Olivia as like her ex-husband, helping her be there more when she was actually home and working with Olivia to deal more directly with Olivia's disappointments and anger about her father.

PSYCHODYNAMICALLY BASED REASSURANCES

As discussed in Chapter 4, in the method of working described in this volume, the therapist seldom makes direct interpretations to children. It has proven very helpful, however, to explain to *parents* the possible meaning of certain behaviors and to devise with them a set of statements that address the child's underlying concerns. We have already discussed the usefulness of parents saying to children who have conflicts over giving up regressive needs, "You'll always be my baby." In such instances, without ever "interpreting" to the child his conflicts over growing up, the parent speaks to the child's concern. Similarly, in the case of Olivia just described, Ms. Brown was advised to address the child's anger rather than her fears. She did not state directly, "You are afraid because you are angry," but rather offered reassurances regarding the underlying anxiety.

By speaking to the child's unconscious rather than interpreting it, one bypasses defense mechanisms. The idea of addressing the unconscious in a noninterpretive manner has been used by a wide range of therapists— from the psychoanalyst Winnicott (who dialogued with children by answering their unconsciously created squiggle drawings with those of his own) to the hypnotherapist Milton Erikson whose stories indirectly spoke to the patients fears and anxieties.

When suggesting to parents that they utilize what I think of as psychodynamically based "nonsequiturs," it is important to rehearse with them the exact statement they should make and the specific circumstances during which the comment should be offered to the child. These statements should be short and simple. If parents deviate too much from terse declarative statements, their comments begin to be received in the same way as interpretations and thus lose their impact. Once again, the reader is asked to keep in mind that this type of intervention is only effective because it occurs in the context of a complex mix of systemic, behavioral, and psychodynamic work.

Brief Example

The parents of 5-year-old Ivan were concerned because this youngster was behaving very aggressively, was extremely resistant to authority, and would become compulsively demanding about doing things in a particular way. Though many children of Ivan's age are fascinated by the concept of "policemen" who punish for wrongdoing, this youngster's interest in guilt, arrest, and punishment was extreme. Preoccupied with this theme, Ivan told numerous stories about thefts, misdeeds, capture, and punishment, and though these themes are common ones at this age, the intensity of Ivan's concerns were such that he often could not shift attention back to the immediate task at hand. Explaining to the parents that Ivan was struggling with the feared consequences of his challenging attitude enabled the parents to set firmer limits so that Ivan would be less fearful of the consequences of his aggression. In addition, it was suggested that when Ivan became cranky and upset for no apparent reason, they should say to him, "Don't worry, we won't let you be bad and nobody will arrest you."

Crucial to this statement is the idea that nobody will arrest the child because he will not be allowed to behave in ways that warrant it. If the parents had simply said, "Don't worry, we won't *let* anybody arrest you or punish you," the child would not have been reassured, because central to his concern was his worry about the consequences of his own "bad" behavior.

Ivan's parents followed this suggestion closely and reported an almost immediate decrease in their son's upsets. This decrease occurred even before the youngster's behavior had actually changed. From a systemic viewpoint, giving the parents something specific to say in itself alters the systemic interaction and helps them feel more able to cope with the child's upset in a nurturant way.

An example of the use of a psychodynamic nonsequitur in the context of a whole case can be found in the full-length case study of Sara in Chapter 9.

RECOGNIZING A CHILD'S UNARTICULATED NEED FOR MORE ATTENTION

Often the problematic or difficult behavior exhibited by a child can be understood as an expression of the youngster's unstated and often unconscious need for more parental attention. For instance, Doug, age 8, the second oldest of four children, the youngest of whom was just 6 months old, had been stealing money from his mother's pocketbook. One instance occurred the night of his return from camp just as he and his older brother (the two younger children were half-siblings) were once again to leave their mother, this time for a 2-week vacation with their father (see Chapter 4). It became clear in meetings alone with Doug as well as with the whole family that he felt his mother was overwhelmed with responsibilities and upset by her stormy and sometimes violent relationship with Doug's stepfather.

Doug took pride in being particularly mature and able to handle things for himself. Understanding Doug's stealing both as a statement of his need and a statement regarding his belief that he should not overtly *ask* for attention led to interventions that would address both issues. Thus, family sessions focused both on how the mother could get more support for all she had to handle so that she would have more time for the older children and on the importance of Doug's, as well as his older brother's, feeling freer to ask for what he needed.

Understanding the meaning of Doug's stealing also led to the suggestion that despite the parents' need for a "mature" children in the house, they refuse Doug's offers to make their life easier by being more self-sufficient. It was noted that a new episode of stealing had followed a recent decision to accede to Doug's request to be allowed to walk to school by himself. When family sessions focused on the reversal of that decision, Doug uttered not a word of protest. Individual meetings with the youngster focused on helping him be more comfortable asking for what he wanted even if it might be refused.

RELAXING WITH CHILDREN

It is important to make clear to parents that they do not have to do special activities with children to give them the attention they are craving. Most children love to have a parent simply hang out with them without being distracted by other things. Parents these days are often so harried by the demands of earning a living and running a household that they groan at the thought of now having one more thing to worry about (i.e., giving the needy child yet more attention). It is essential therefore to structure this additional attention in a way that is actually feasible and that the parents will themselves enjoy. Sometimes, for instance, just relaxing in a child's room, perhaps glancing at a magazine while the youngster plays, is all that the child needs.

Parents are often perplexed by a child's feeling that she is not getting enough of a parent's attention. Often, hours spent helping the child with homework or even on fun family outings are not experienced by the child as the parents' *really* being there for them. This is because what the child is longing for can be thought of as something akin to the nondemanding parental presence offered to babies and toddlers as they explore and parental to home base. Thus, the main ingredients for spending time with a child are that it be nonstressful and as uninterrupted as is realistically possible. Playing a board game or watching a favorite television show together, uninterrupted by the telephone or perhaps on some occasions even by the demands of younger siblings, is often just what an older child desires.

Parents' attempts to provide stimulating and enriching experiences to children on weekends, though loved by some children, are experienced by others as the parents' *still* not being available. When a child is experiencing the pace of activities as too much, he will often dawdle and become whiny and difficult. Parents who are trying so hard to provide their children with something enjoyable feel hurt, angry, and resentful at the lack of gratitude, much less pleasure, the child is exhibiting. Thus, family outings can become fraught with tension and evoke negative rather than positive associations. Memories of negative experiences often lead to more dawdling and whining when future activities are proposed and what is intended as a way to pay attention to a child becomes something that involves disappointment, coercion, and power struggles.

As so often happens, parents and children keep trying to solve a problem and get what they desire by more of the same. Thus a child craving attention often whines, misbehaves, and *demands* parental involvement and of course is not satisfied with what she is able to wheedle out of the parent. And parents who *want* to give to their children often give what the children does not actually want. Breaking this cycle and helping a child get what he needs is often quite simple. Parents are amazed by how much calmer everybody is when part of a weekend is devoted to doing nothing but hanging out. By explaining to parents that by not providing as much they may in fact be providing more, one empowers them simply to relax and be there for their youngsters.

UNDERSTANDING THE CHILD'S NEED TO HAVE SOME CONTROL OVER THE PARENT'S AVAILABILITY

Children are often frustrated by the fact that they have little control over just when a parent will be available to them. When a child feels angry at not having enough of a parent or frustrated by a parent's leaving at times when the child wishes the parent would stay, the youngster may cope with these feelings by, in turn, finding ways to control his *own* availability.

There are many arenas in which these issues are often acted out. One fairly common way in which children reject parental offerings of nurturance is through food. A child may reject outright a parent's cooking or may ask the parent to prepare something the youngster then decides is not desired after all. Similarly, some children complain about a gift a parent has brought, focusing on how it is not exactly what had been desired. It is not uncommon for parents to complain that they leave work early only to find that they cannot wrench their child away from the television. Or perhaps, as in the case of Olivia, described earlier, the child insists on having a sleepover with a friend on the very night the parent has returned from a business trip.

There are several separate but related aspects to this sort of behavior. In "rejecting" the parent this way, a child simultaneously expresses anger, expresses a wish to have more control over when and where dependency needs will be met, and tests out the strength of the parent's commitment and devotion to him. Unfortunately, the indirectness of this communication does not allow the child's feelings to be addressed or his needs to be met. Instead, many parents become angry and frustrated and withdraw themselves. Furthermore, the child who acts like he does not care whether the parent is home provides some parents with easy rationalizations for putting other commitments and needs ahead of those of the child.

When a dynamic of this sort exists it is helpful to start by working with the child and the parents on ways that the child might be able to have more of a say in *when* and *how* he gets attention. The child needs to be helped to express feeling more directly so that he does not act them out in ways that deprive both himself and his parents of the closeness that they all want. Often behavior of this sort diminishes when the child feels that when the parent *is* home she is not distracted by business or other concerns and is really there for the youngster. The parent might decide to give the child the option of deciding when in the evening he would like undivided attention and how he would like to spend that time. Or perhaps the parent can arrange his work schedule so that he is home at times that are particularly important to the youngster. The specifics will vary with each case. The point is that when parents understand the child's behavior in the terms just described, they are less apt to withdraw and more willing to find ways to give the youngster a greater sense of control over emotional "supplies."

A WORD ABOUT THE CHILD'S NEEDS FOR AUTONOMY AND MASTERY

Throughout this book there has been frequent discussion of the need to meet children's dependency needs. In today's fast-paced society, we more frequently find children who are growing up too fast (Shelov & Kelly, 1991) than children whose need for mastery and competence is not being acknowledged. Despite the general tendency to encourage children to grow up rapidly, however, there are many instances in which a child in a family continues to be dealt with as a "baby" well into childhood. As described earlier, some families stimulate regressive needs or are overly responsive to the less mature behavior of the youngster. Children who have not been encouraged to develop age-appropriate ego controls often have also been discouraged from expressing their need for autonomy, mastery, and independence. Thus, along with not being so "comforting" that children have no need to develop *self*-comforting mechanisms, it is also important for parents to actively encourage the development of skills and competencies of all sorts. The thrill that children derive from becoming competent at activities that just a short time ago seemed beyond their capacity goes a long way toward compensating for the loss of parental coddling.

In family sessions and with the parents alone, it is helpful to continually explore the boundaries between what the parents are comfortable with and what a child might like to try. Instead of coaxing or rewarding a child to do things the parent wants him to do (e.g., dress himself or clean up his toys), it is best to move a child from babyish behavior to maturity by gradually giving the child *permission* to do some of the things the child actually *wants* to do. If the child is *rewarded* for behaving maturely she can experience it as something that is for the *parent* and is not inherently pleasurable. Instead, the therapist can help the parents and child discover together some of the things that the child wishes to be able to do.

Of course, there is an element of paradox here. When behaving in a self-sufficient and competent manner is treated like a *privilege* rather than a demand, most children are far more eager to engage in activities that are at first difficult and challenging.

It is helpful for the therapist to "brainstorm" with the parents what new activities the child might be allowed to try. By using her understanding of the individual and systemic dynamics, the therapist can suggest things that may meet multiple needs of the family and child. Thus, in a family that is uncomfortable with aggression, a child may be allowed to use a sharp knife to cut or slice vegetables. Or in a family that tends to lock children into rather narrow gender roles, a girl might be allowed to try repairing a toy while a boy could be allowed to make his own sandwiches for school.

Thus far we are describing children whose wish for mastery has been dampened by too much encouragement in the other direction. There are many children, however, whose oppositional or difficult behavior results from a direct clash of wills with a parent around issues of autonomy.

Even very young children can feel a good deal of resentment about what they experience as too much intrusion in their life. Sometimes the degree of limit setting that was easily accepted by one child in a family is experienced by another child, with a different temperament, as excessive. Just how much freedom to give a child is a complex issue. As described in the case of Doug (discussed earlier) a child's wish to do something himself (e.g., walk to school) may be a defense against other needs that the child has renounced. By understanding both the psychodynamic and family systems dimensions of the youngster's difficulties, the therapist provides important input as to whether the family should accede to a youngster's desire for increased independence. One must determine whether there is a true wish for more autonomy and mastery, which should be respected, or whether the child's desires reflect a rejection of age-appropriate dependency.

For instance, Kenneth, age 7, insisted that he could stay alone in his apartment when his mother went shopping and demonstrated to his mother that he knew how to telephone a neighbor if something was wrong. This same child would wander off in stores and on one occasion, when staying with his mother at a hotel, left the room while she was still asleep and attempted to order his own breakfast at the hotel restaurant. Knowing the dynamics of the child and the family well it was clear in this case that the child's wish for even more independence stemmed from a feeling that he could not really rely on his mother.

Kenneth, was an angry little boy (the reasons for which would take us far afield at this point) whose extreme oppositionalism resulted in a good deal of rejection by the important adults in his life. He was caught up in a cycle in which his anger led to further rejections. His wish to be independent was both an acting out of *his* rejection of those he felt rejected him and an expression that he had better take care of himself since nobody would be there to take care of him.

In contrast, when Jessica, age 10, protested about her parents being too protective and not letting her do things she felt fully capable of doing—like going by herself to local stores or taking a city bus to a friend's house—it was understood as a genuine wish for growth. Jessica's parents had stated privately to the therapist that they stayed together only for the sake of the children. Jessica, the youngest of three, had not been permitted to do things that her older sisters had done at the same age, ostensibly because the city had become "bad." Jessica, who sensed that her parents needed her to remain dependent, had, until the family work addressed some of the couple's difficulties, been rather content to be a sweet homebody. As she began to feel it might be safe to grow away, Jessica became extremely sociable, wanted to stay overnight at friends' houses, and became increasingly insistent on expanding her repertoire of independent behavior. Although it was up to the parents to assess what they felt was safe for her to do, the therapist was able not only to point out the family dynamics but also to reassure the parents that the youngster's wishes were genuine and were not simply a result of peer pressure.

WORKING COLLABORATIVELY WITH TEACHERS

Whenever possible it is extremely helpful to enlist the support of the child's teacher. Not only can the teacher provide us with much needed information, but he can also be advised on ways to act with the child that are consistent with and reinforce some of the changes that have been suggested to the family. I have found that even when teachers have large classrooms to handle, they generally are quite cooperative and welcome the opportunity to be involved with the child in a way that enhances the therapeutic work.

By means of frequent telephone conversations with the teacher I am able not only to monitor the child's progress but also to ask the teacher to do specific things that will carry the psychodynamic and behavioral analysis of the child's difficulties into the classroom. Teachers are often at a loss as to how to handle a troubled child and welcome the chance to discuss the difficulties they are having. As do parents, teachers respond positively when they feel they are being worked with respectfully and collaboratively. It is not enough, however, to ask them simply to be understanding while the problems are being worked on in therapy. Difficult children frequently evoke strong negative reactions from their teachers. A child's sense of self is very much affected by how he is regarded in school. Immeasurable harm is caused to a child when he is disliked by a teacher. Yet, both teacher and child may be caught in a system of repetitive interactions in which each feels frustrated, thwarted, and disregarded by the other. For this reason it is essential to work with both the child and the teacher on new ways of interacting with one another. It is difficult, however, to tell teachers with whom one has only a telephone relationship to stop doing what they have been doing, even if it has not worked, and in fact only exacerbates the difficulties they experience. By making specific suggestion for positive things the teacher can do that will be therapeutic, problematic patterns of interaction change without the teacher's feeling criticized.

As described earlier, suggested interventions derive from the specifics of each child and the system in which he lives. Just as with the suggestions made to parents, there are few interventions that can be applied in completely unmodified fashion from case to case. Instead, one must craft interventions that reflect the particular child's issues and that are feasible and appropriate to the way the teacher runs his classroom. For instance, in the case of 10-year-old Mathew, a parentified child who was mature beyond his years (see detailed case study in Chapter 9) it was important for the teacher to temporarily encourage him to sometimes choose *less* challenging options for assignments rather than ones that would be an intellectual stretch. Thus, when the class, which was of mixed ages, was divided into groups for a particular activity it was suggested that the teacher resist Mathew's requests for more responsibility and instead say something like "even though you could probably do the work that the older kids are doing, I think doing what the other children your age are doing today might be a nice change for you." In order for a teacher to be comfortable with doing something like this, it is important that she understand how the suggestion fits into the therapeutic work as a whole. When teachers understand the reasoning behind the therapist's advice, they are not only more apt to follow it but they themselves come up with suggestions that fit with the general principles involved. For example, when Ms. Alport understood that 7-year-old Joshua's "silliness" reflected his inability to handle the anxiety he felt when presented with challenging work, *she* suggested that she would teach the whole class some deep-breathing exercises that a child could do before beginning new work. She then also easily accepted the therapist's suggestion that she no longer coax Joshua to do his work since it was important for this youngster to learn self-calming mechanisms. Together we planned how she might use a simple chart that would reward Joshua for efforts to stay with a task despite the anxiety that was generated.

As are parents, sympathetic and supportive teachers are sometimes greatly relieved by suggestions to be firmer with a child. When they understand the firmness as a way of helping the child feel secure or as a means of helping the youngster consolidate his struggle for mastery over impulsivity, they are able to be stricter without feeling that they are being harsh to an obviously upset and troubled youngster. There are times when it is even important to treat tears and upset as "misbehavior," but for a teacher to be able to do this, a sensible rationale must be presented.

Teachers can also sometimes assist in helping a child become more comfortable with disowned feelings. Some teachers are willing to read stories to the whole class that deal with issues of concern to this particular child. Many teachers are quite receptive to the idea of suggesting to a youngster that he write on themes that relate to the psychodynamic issues the therapist suggests. For instance, with one child it might be helpful for the teacher to suggest that she write about "a time you missed somebody," whereas another youngster might be encouraged to write about "a time he got so mad that he was scared."

A Note of Caution about Working with Teachers

Before speaking with a child's teacher, it is absolutely essential not only to get the parents' consent but also to discuss with them just what they feel comfortable sharing. There are times when parents do not want teachers or school psychologists to be aware of marital tensions or other stresses in the family. One must be careful in working with school personnel to reveal no more than what one has prior approval to disclose. Because of the collaborative and collegial tone used in working with teachers, they often do ask questions about the family that one must deflect as tactfully as possible so as not to jeopardize the working relationship.

There are times when parents wish to keep the very fact of the therapy secret and thus do not want the therapist to have *any* contact with the school. Though ultimately the parents' wishes must be honored, it is important to discuss with them the implications of the child having to keep a "secret," as well as the effects on the child of problematic interactions with a teacher. Of course, when a child's difficulties are not being manifested in school, contact with a teacher is less crucial. Often as parents become more comfortable with the therapy process and see that concrete interventions can be helpful, they become somewhat more willing to allow the school to be part of the therapeutic team.

USING PSYCHODYNAMIC FORMULATIONS IN INDIVIDUAL SESSIONS WITH A CHILD

The line between information gathering and actual intervention is a blurry one. As described in Chapter 4, in order to get to know the child's concerns the therapist engages the youngster in story telling and emotion-revealing board games. The therapist tailors his answers to a game's questions in a way that encourages the child to speak more openly about himself. Although the primary purpose of this interaction is to better understand the child's worries and needs so that they can be addressed by the parents, revealing feelings to the therapist is in itself therapeutic. Despite the therapeutic value of sessions of this sort, it is important to distinguish between individual meetings in which the primary purpose is to get to know the youngster's concerns and those meetings intended to offer direct therapeutic assistance.

When I first started to do integrative work with young children and families, I used individual meetings with children *only* to get to know them better so as to integrate psychodynamic perspectives into the systemic work. I was concerned that to work therapeutically with the youngster myself would usurp the parents' role and that the individual sessions might be perceived as the central focus of the work. Furthermore, if my contact with the child individually was going to be limited, I did not know what I could possibly do in just a few sessions that could make a real difference. In time, however, as I continued to explore new ways of working with children and families, these concerns no longer seemed to have the weight they had once had. I discovered that it is quite possible to have individual meetings with a child without the work with the family becoming peripheral. By working collaboratively with parents to plan the direction of my individual meetings with the child and then describing the sessions to them, a family focus is maintained.

Generally, meetings alone with the child are interspersed with family and parent meetings, and if for some reason it is important to see the child for two or three consecutive meetings, the parents are informed as to why this format seems appropriate. Because the children know that the individual meetings are part of the family work and generally are not confidential, they do not react to me in a way that displaces their parents. Most children, although they are happy to see me alone, also enjoy the family sessions and would be disappointed if the individual meetings began to dominate the work. Parents too want the family sessions and rarely want to convert the work to individual therapy for the child.

There are exceptions to every rule, of course, and some parents *will* try hard to make me the *child's* therapist. Similarly, there are children who *prefer* to have me to themselves and resent sharing me with siblings and parents. Firmness in not acceding to these pressures is, of course, extremely important, because often the wish for individual therapy for the child reflects a parent's (or child's) feeling that the family cannot provide what the child needs.

Although children do not tend to develop very strong transference reactions to me, and because of the way I work with them do not think of me as a substitute "good parent," often some do become quite attached. I no longer fear that this attachment may have negative consequences for the family system. Instead the attachment is used in the child's service as leverage to get him to try some things that will make interactions with parents more gratifying. When children are attached to me, they are more willing to try out some of my suggestions regarding new behaviors with family members and teachers.

I have also found that my concern that just a few individual therapy sessions with a child could not accomplish very much no longer seems warranted. I have come instead to believe that with careful planning and a clear sense of what one hopes to accomplish, even a few individual sessions with a child can be of significant therapeutic value. Once again the reader is reminded that for the sake of clarity I am artificially separating in the discussions in this chapter the psychodynamic component of the individual work. Behavioral and systemic considerations inform the work of individual sessions every bit as much as psychodynamic ones, and in practice all three perspectives coexist and are often part and parcel of the same session. This will be apparent as the reader proceeds through the book.

NEUTRALIZING THE DISCUSSION OF FORBIDDEN MATERIAL

Expressive Play

Individual sessions with a child can be used to help the youngster integrate into his sense of self feelings that he has split off and disowned. This work supplements and enhances some of the work being done by the parents through the Story-Telling technique and Play Baby. Helping a child feel comfortable with disowned feelings can be done in a variety of ways. With young children, puppet play, in which the therapist has a puppet say "forbidden" things, often leads to gleeful, relieved laughing and is the beginning of increased self-acceptance. Five-year-old Tanya, for instance, giggled with glee when she heard the baby bear puppet say to Mommy, "I'm so mad I'm going to bite you, chew you up and throw you in the river." Later in the session, this withdrawn, passively oppositional child began to talk about something that had made her angry earlier that day.

When a youngster is extremely frightened by his feelings, he may at first turn away from play that touches too closely on the taboo feelings. If this occurs, the therapist knows to proceed more gradually. The message can be softened somewhat by a statement which, although expressing the feeling, also takes it back. Thus in the example just given the puppet bear might add "and then I'll dry you off and put you back together again because I really love you."

As part of the process of helping the child "own" his feelings, it is helpful to ask the child what the puppet should say next. The more the child is able to have the puppets use *his* words rather than the therapist's, the closer he becomes to accepting his feelings. When a child has become more comfortable with the emotionally loaded script the therapist has provided for the puppet, it is often possible to get the child to switch puppets and become the voice of the puppet who is expressing the heretofore outlawed feelings. One can then ask whether the child has ever felt anything like what the puppet character feels or whether the story reminds her of anything in her own life.

Art materials, such as clay or finger paints, can also be of great use in sessions aimed at helping a child feel more comfortable with banished feelings. There seems to be something inherently relaxing about playing with these media (though some children do feel anxious about the messiness of the process) and it is good to start a clay or painting session by briefly letting a child use the material without any specific aim or direction. Poking, squeezing, rolling, banging, and smushing moist clay (rather than plasticine or play dough) is extremely pleasurable to most children (and therapists as well if truth be told). Often, without any direction, a child, through his running commentary about what he is making, will begin to present relevant themes. When the child seems relaxed and somewhat open, the therapist begins to have her own artistic creations "state" forbidden themes. For example, with a child struggling around regressive urges, the therapist might mold a dog and have him defecating in the house instead of outdoors. Or, with a youngster who feels humiliated by his smallness and lack of competence, the therapist might do a finger painting of a baby bird who is embarrassed by learning to fly. If the child responds positively to this suggestive material, a transition can be made to acting out in clay or with paints some of the child's own feelings.

It is important for the therapist to model the expression of disavowed feelings in a playful, nonthreatening way. For example, one might have the child make a clay figure that represents his little sister. "Let's tell this little clay sister how mad she makes you feel." The therapist then demonstrates by saying in a caricatured, exaggerated voice, "You stupid little sister, you make me *so so so so* mad! I'm going to squash you into a pancake!"

Encouraging the child to express "dangerous" feelings in a playful way not only helps the child own the full range of his emotions but makes it clear that even intense feelings do not have to be so threatening. When working with a child in this way one goes back and forth between the somewhat wild fantasy play and a straightforward discussion of what is actually going on in the child's life in relation to these people. Eight-year-old Ned, for instance, a little boy who was brought to therapy because of his intense tantrums, stubbornness, and fear, was exhilarated by my encouragement to really smash the clay figure of his stepfather. Soon he was talking in great detail about power struggles he and his stepdad had and the fear he felt when this powerful man forcefully grabbed and twisted his arm. He was able to describe not only his rage but how terrified he felt during these episodes. Finally, exhausted from his "assaults" on his clay stepfather, Ned spontaneously brought up his stepfather's good qualities and stated quite authentically that he really liked him.

This type of progression is not uncommon. When children have been invited to fully express their feelings in this playful way they reach a point when they seem to be satisfied and make very genuine statements that express positive feelings toward those they have been demolishing. Sometimes they simply indicate that they have had enough by asking whether we can play checkers or other emotionally neutral games.[1]

Many of the methods described in Chapter 4 for getting to know the child better can also be used to help the child accept banished feelings. In playing board games like Feeling Checkers or the Talking, Feeling, and Doing Game, the therapist can respond to a child's glib, minimizing answer with an answer of his own that in effect tells the child tha *all* sorts of intense feelings are acceptable. For instance, if a child, when asked as part of the game to talk about a time she felt scared, says something such as, "I don't get scared," the therapist might say, "I do! I'm sometimes scared that people will be angry at me." Most children will be very curious about such a response, and a meaningful conversation often ensues.

Similarly, personality inventories or sentence completion questionnaires can be made into a game in which therapist and child take turns answering questions and the therapist answers in a way that invites a discussion of the issues relevant to the child. In many ways what the therapist is doing in these conversations is essentially the same as what the parents are being advised to do when they are coached in the Story-Telling technique. What differentiates the therapist's story telling from that of the parents is largely that the therapist, as a trained clinician and as an adult who is outside the system, is less likely to avoid or back away from troubling questions and responses on the part of the child. The therapist is less threatened by the feelings the child has been warding off and thus is less likely to communicate anxiety about what is being revealed.

The reader is advised to read Oaklander's (1988) book *Windows to Our Children* for an excellent compendium of activities designed to facilitate greater expressiveness in children. Oaklander ingeniously uses art materials, sand trays, story telling, and projective tests in ways that enable the child to talk directly and openly about his concerns and feelings. Although Oaklander writes as a Gestalt therapist and sees greater expressiveness as almost the sole therapeutic factor, much of what she does with children is easily adaptable to the occasional therapy session that is part of the integrative work being described in this volume.

James (1989), in *Treating Traumatized Children,* also has numerous fascinating suggestions for fostering expressiveness through structured activities such as psychodrama, poster making, and the creation of clay families.

List Making

Latency-age children like to make lists. Paradoxically, list making, which taps the child's intellect, can be used to help children get more in touch with what they are feeling. For example, when children are projecting all their negative feelings about a parent onto another authority figure, they can be asked to make a list of "five things you like about your Dad and five things that annoy you about him." As noted in Chapter 4, children answer all sorts of questions when they are framed as part of a game. So too with lists. A child who is guarded and who does not easily talk about himself can be more revealing when asked, for instance, to "name four things that are good about yourself and two or three things that you think are not so good."

When a child begins to talk about negative feelings about himself, it is important to do some work that can help him see himself different-ly. One could, for example, ask the child what a fairy godmother might say about him if she heard him say such mean things about himself (Oak-lander, 1986). This question enables the child to counter his own self-criticisms in a way that is apt to "stick" better than reassurances coming directly from the therapist. The child can also be asked to think of things he could do that would make him like himself better, and this can lead to the creation of another list, this time of things he might try to do differently.

Lists can also be used to help foster self-insight. Eight-year-old Isaac had little understanding of what he did that made children get annoyed with him. Together we made a list of all the boys in his class and instead of talking about himself, Isaac was asked to name each boy in his class and to state whether he liked the boy or not, and why. Further elabora-tions as to what the "liked" boys did that he thought was good, and what the disliked boys did that was annoying, easily led to a more realistic discussion of his own way of being with other children.

ADDRESSING UNCONSCIOUS CONFLICTS AND ANXIETIES THROUGH METAPHORIC STORIES

By using metaphoric stories, the therapist is sometimes able to speak direct-ly to the child's unconscious. Mills and Crowley's (1986) excellent book, *Therapeutic Metaphors for Children and the Child Within*, provides use-ful guidelines for constructing a story that describes the child's problem in metaphorical terms and incorporates therapeutic suggestions that the child can hear at an unconscious level. A story line is developed that presents a conflict that the child can identify with, yet is different enough that the child does not feel embarrassed or become resistant. The authors suggest that different characters in the story represent the conflict between the child's negative beliefs and fears (villains) and his abilities and resources (heros). The story culminates in a metaphorical crisis in which the protagonist overcomes or resolves his problem. Mills and Crowley spell out in great detail just how to construct a story line that will engage the child and address his concerns. In my work with children and families, I have found it useful to incorporate into these metaphorical stories attention to the intrapsychic conflict, ambivalences, and family dynamics that are not on the surface as an obvious part of the child's problem. Thus, for example, when working with a child who is very fearful, the metaphorical story would include not only symbolic references to his fear and models for mastery but also the struggle the child is having with his anger which, projected, is the actual source of his fear. For instance, one might tell a story about Benny the Bear Cub who was so afraid of an evil pack of wolves attacking him that he would not go out to play with the other cubs his age. In order to address the child's fear of the anger he is experiencing toward a younger sibling, the story might include something about just how hard Benny tried to be nice to the new Baby Cub who had just been born. Sometimes this was very difficult for Benny to do because the Baby Cub was annoying and Mommy Cub spent so much time taking care of him. Whenever Benny the Bear Cub had mean thoughts about Baby Cub he felt very bad about it. He knew how much Mommy Bear wanted him to love his new baby sister and he was worried about why he often found her annoying.

It is important to address the child's *ambivalent* feelings and not just the negative aspects of his unconscious concerns. In this story, for instance, one would want to include something about the positive feelings Benny felt when his baby sister smiled at him or reached out to pull his nose. Adapting the format suggested by Mills and Crowley, the story would include references to former successful attempts at mastery. In this case, for instance, the mastery component not only would focus on successful prior attempts to overcome fears but would also refer to times in his life when speaking about something that was bothering him seemed to help. Benny might remember, for instance, when he told Mommy Bear that he had broken her favorite plate and instead of being angry she said she was glad he had been honest. Of course, the story must conform to what is realistic to expect of the child's family. If a youngster lives in a family in which there is real reason to fear the consequences of emotional openness, perhaps the story would involve Benny the Bear Cub confiding in some supportive trusted adult.

These stories are particularly helpful as a way to address not only the child's intrapsychic conflicts but also the systemic issues that contribute to the child's difficulties. Seven-year-old Roy, for instance, acted much of the time like he preferred nothing more than staying cuddled on his mother's lap. He longed for the days of nursery school when nothing but play was expected of him and rejected his mother's attempts to get him to engage in age-appropriate self-care like dressing independently and taking care of his own toileting. Roy was told a story that tapped into the part of him that wished to become more mature and separate from his mother. The story also included a reference to his concern that his mother would be unhappy if she was no longer needed so much. Roy's mother was, in fact, a single parent who was having quite a hard time and felt isolated in the community in which she lived. Thus, Roy was told a story about Bobby the Baby Bird, who lived all alone with his mother. Bobby liked living alone with his mother. He liked the way his mother chewed his food for him and thought there was nothing more wonderful than sleeping under his Mommy Bird's wing. Bobby felt he would like to stay a baby bird forever. He noticed how happy Mommy Bird was when she did things for him. As Bobby got bigger, he began to notice that some other baby birds who lived in the same tree were beginning to learn to fly. Baby Bird said, "I'll *never* learn to fly. Besides, I don't need to. Mommy will get me everything I need."

As the story progresses, Baby Bird begins to notice how much fun the other little birds seem to be having. He notices how they play tag and do stunts and he begins to think that maybe it would be fun to do just that one thing. He would still have Mommy feed him though. And he would still have Mommy Bird give him a bath. Soon, however, Baby Bird wants to try more and more things but worries that Mommy Bird will be lonely if Baby Bird is out playing all day.

Stories such as this can be thought of as a way, without making direct interpretations, of helping the child notice not only aspects of his own feelings that may be changing, but also some of the systemic changes that therapy is bringing about. Thus, the resolution of this story involves talking to his mother about his worries and noticing that Mommy Bird (with the help of her therapist) is beginning to make some friends herself and sometimes seems to wish that Baby Bird would feed himself so that she could have more time to do Big Bird things with her friends.

With older children, one can tell metaphorical stories that revolve around people rather than animals. The fact that a child may recognize that the story has something to do with himself is not generally a problem. Some children happily state, "Oh, that's like me!" while others quietly suspend disbelief and let themselves enjoy the world of fantasy.

It is best to do this type of story telling at a point at which some systemic changes have already been instituted. When the child and the family are just beginning to change but have ambivalent feelings about it, these stories help reinforce the wish for growth. Another relevant factor for determining when to use this method is the child's degree of comfort with the therapist. Some children do not feel comfortable passively listening. They cannot relax and do not like the feeling of loss of control that they experience when asked to lie down, breathe deeply, and relax. I have found it useful to give children a big floppy bunny to hold while they lie down and to ask them if they can make their body as relaxed as Floppy's. With tense children, I suggest some deep breathing and muscle relaxation exercises before the story begins. I have learned that many young children do not like to close their eyes when hearing these stories. This is not a problem and does not seem to interfere with the absorption required for these stories to be effective. I do ask children to try to listen quietly rather than interacting with me while the story is being told. Restless or anxious children may be able to quietly listen if allowed to draw or play with clay while they listen.

This chapter has described some ways that an understanding of *psychodynamic* issues can inform our use of active interventions with parents, teachers, and the individual child. The next chapter reviews some of the basic *behavioral* principles utilized in working with families and children.

8

Interventions Based on Behavioral Formulations

T his chapter discusses the ways in which interventions based on cognitive and behavioral formulations can supplement the systemic and psychodynamic perspectives already described. As I have discussed in previous chapters, parents of troubled children are eager for concrete suggestions regarding what they can *do* to help children overcome their problems. Seeing the child's symptom as a reflection of problematic family interactions, most family therapists address the parents' wish for help in dealing with a troubled child by working on the broader context within which the child's symptoms are occurring. Thus, though family therapists are often meticulous observers of sequences of actions and reactions in families (e.g., Scheflen, 1978), what is noticed tends to be put to use in guiding the overall systemic work rather than in giving specific feedback based on learning and behavioral principles.

For example, Minuchin and Fishman (1981), in one of the most useful and widely works on techniques in family therapy describe in detail a sequence of behavior that occurs after the therapist "instructs the parents to talk without letting Ronny (age 4) intrude" (p. 70). They observe that the youngster "begins to whimper, then cry, jumping up and down in his chair and scratching furiously. . . . Mark, obviously the parental child, tosses a toy to Ronny, engaging him in a playful, slightly aggressive transaction. Soon Ronny throws the toy at Mark and runs to his mother" (p. 70).

These observations are made not for the purpose of instructing the parents in specific behavioral interventions but rather with the broader aim of pointing out to the parents the need to create a boundary around their own relationship. Giving "expert" advice on behavioral principles that could be useful in dealing with a child is studiously avoided. The goal, rather, is to empower the parents and to enhance their confidence in their ability to come up with their own solutions.

For instance, in talking with parents about a difficult-to-handle child, Minuchin and Fishman might say the following: "When a four-year-old is taller than her mother, maybe she is sitting on the shoulders of her father," or, "You two must be doing something wrong. I don't know what it could be, but I am sure if you think together, you will find out what it is, and moreover, you will find out the solution," or, "As things go you are defeating each other, and in some way you are hurting and exploiting a child that both of you love very much, so we will need to find a way in which you help each other so you can help your child" (p. 148).

Underlying this approach is a welcome respect for parents as well as a possibly unjustified assumption that most parents really know what to do if they are given support for exercising their parental authority. Often, of course, parents *do* know what to do and need nothing but encouragement to put into effect what they already know. When Mariano Barragan, supervised by Jay Haley, in one of the classic cases of family therapy (described in a chapter entitled "A Modern Little Hans" in Haley, 1976), encourages the father of a phobic boy to teach his son what he knows about dogs, and to go with him to adopt a fearful puppy, he of course not only strengthens the father–son dyad but sets in motion a highly effective desensitization procedure.[1] And he does so without ever needing to tell the parents about the importance of gradual exposure under safe and reassuring circumstances.

We know from experience, and from the groundbreaking research of Minuchin, Rosman, and Baker (1978), that children's symptoms reflect the level of stress in the marital dyad. Thus, in many cases a child's symptoms *are* alleviated when parents work on their own difficulties and the child's role as protector of his parents is addressed. Comments that let the family know what the youngster is up to—for example, "You are a nice, protective, and obedient child by misbehaving . . . having a headache . . . failing in school, whenever your parents feel uncomfortable with each other" (Minuchin & Fishman, 1981, p. 148)—can, and often do, result in a noticeable diminution of symptomatic behavior in children when they are combined with direct work on marital problems. Paradoxical techniques that directly address the protective function of the child's symptomatic behavior (Madanes, 1980) also seem to be effective with some children.

However, although these methods are undoubtedly effective with many families, in my experience, children and parents can often benefit greatly from more specific suggestions regarding behavior change. Some

difficulties that children exhibit reflect years of being reinforced for dysfunctional behavior. As described in Chapter 5, children may never have
developed adaptive coping mechanisms or age-appropriate social skills
(Rosman, 1986; P. Wachtel, 1977). Furthermore, influencing some
problematic behaviors may require more sophisticated and creative efforts than are in the normal repertoire of most parents. Behavioral principles can be quite useful, for instance, in helping a child who has learned
to avoid what is difficult, who will not risk failure, who has trouble with
impulse control, or who is overly anxious about performance. Although
I share the concern of family therapists regarding the importance of respect-
ing the competence of parents, I have found that rather than experiencing me as "expert" and themselves as "inadequate," parents' sense of
competence and empowerment actually *increases* when I work with them
on concrete and specific ways they can influence their children in more
positive directions. Children, too, are empowered by some direct behavioral work. A child, for instance, who is given some cognitive strategies for impulse control or who rehearses better social skills ultimately
feels stronger and more in control of his own life.

As described in Chapter 2, many family therapists have become uncomfortable with the directives, tasks, and overall acting-upon stance that
was characteristic of much family therapy. Some readers may be similarly uncomfortable with behavioral methods because they are concerned
that such direct attempts to influence a child may be manipulative and
entail acting *upon* rather than *for* the youngster. Others, reared in the
psychodynamic tradition, may be concerned that by using behavioral
methods to encourage and discourage particular behaviors, the parents
will crush the child's individuality and autonomy and he will develop a
false, unauthentic self. To be sure, therapists must use good judgment
when coaching parents on effective methods of behavior modification;
only when a determination is made that the child's way of dealing with
others or his way of handling anxiety is actually maladaptive for the child
and not simply a matter of parental preference should the therapist suggest behavioral interventions aimed at modifying the youngster's behavior.
However, conclusions about what *is* maladaptive cannot be entirely separated from the personality style of the parents and the milieu in which
the child lives. Children and their parents are always involved in a process
of mutual accommodation to one another, and a chronic grinding of gears,
even if each gear is individually sound, yields unfortunate results. Sometimes this may mean that a child must adapt at least to some degree to
the parents' needs if the child himself is to have a nurturant environment
in which to grow, but by no means does it imply that the lion's share
of the accommodating will necessarily fall to the child. In any particular
case, the therapist may feel that the child's patterns of behavior will stand

him in good stead as he grows up and that the parents need help in accepting the child as he is.

In deciding whether one is comfortable utilizing the methods of behavior modification, one should keep in mind that regardless of whether the therapist actively assists the parents in this endeavor, family members inevitably are engaged in shaping and modifying one another's actions. Once we permit ourselves to include in our thinking about family interactions the question of what is being reinforced and what kind of learning is consequently taking place, it becomes incontrovertibly clear that, like it or not, parents and children are *always* engaged in a process of mutual behavior modification. Unfortunately, however, often the learning that is taking place in the family is not in fact what any of the family members wishes or intends. Helping parents as well as children more *consciously* choose actions and consequences does not seem to me to be at odds with an attitude of respect for autonomy and individuality.

Contrary to what one might expect, helping parents plan behavior modification methods actually seems to *increase* their receptiveness to psychodynamic and systemic interventions as well. In my experience, family members are less defensive and more open to interpretations and suggestions for structural change when the level of anxiety and tension in the family is reduced. The predictable and rational nature of behavioral interventions can be a balm to family members worn out by high-intensity emotional struggles. Not infrequently, both the children and the parents feel greatly relieved by having a plan for how to deal with behavioral difficulties, and the atmosphere at home may improve quite rapidly. This, in turn, leads to an increased ability to hear one another and to make changes of a more profound sort.

Of course, there are also many times when it is by no means easy for family members to follow through on behavioral interventions. Thus, for instance, if a parent's *need* to have a child act out aggression is not dealt with immediately, the parent, though consciously cooperative, may sabotage efforts to teach the child better impulse control. Moreover, not infrequently, unresolved parental conflict can (though not always) interfere with the consistent application of behavioral interventions. And, apart from intrapsychic or interpersonal conflict, many parents would recoil from the idea of simply modifying a child's behavior without also addressing the child's underlying feelings and concerns.

The reader should keep in mind, however, that the approach described in this book proceeds on the psychodynamic, systemic, and behavioral phases simultaneously. We do not wait until all systemic issues are resolved before attending to the psychodynamic aspects of the problem, nor do we attempt to fully resolve psychodynamic or systemic issues before introducing behavioral interventions. Instead, psychodynamic and systemic understandings of the problem go hand in hand with behavioral methods targeted at the symptomatic behavior. From the very beginning of contact with the family, the therapist works simultaneously on helping the parents understand the child's concerns and encouraging them to address the symptom with behavioral methods.

In taking such an approach it is often the case that the behavioral methods used in this integrative approach are far less formal than those used by behavior therapists. For one thing, since they are just one piece of the work, discussion of these procedures, though important, often takes up only a small portion of the therapy time. Just as one does not have to subscribe to standard psychoanalytic practice to utilize psychodynamic perspectives, so too can we employ behavioral principles without embarking on a full-fledged program of operant conditioning, desensitization, or cognitive restructuring.

UNDERSTANDING WHAT IS BEING TAUGHT AND LEARNED IN THE FAMILY: AN ANALYSIS OF REINFORCEMENT CONTINGENCIES

The first step in planning any behavioral intervention is to get detailed information about what is being reinforced by parents in their interactions with children, as well as what the *children* may be reinforcing in their parents (Gordon & Davidson, 1981). This information can be obtained in several different ways: through direct observation, through plays or puppet shows in which scenes from family life are enacted, and through detailed questioning of both parents and children in separate meetings.

Detailed Questioning

As described in Chapter 2, the work with families and children begins by meeting with the parents privately. Distressed parents often have numerous generalized worries about their child. The first step is to help them describe their concerns in more observable terms. One must work with parents to convert statements such as, "She's hostile," or "He's very withdrawn," into statements about specific things the child says or does that lead them to these conclusions. It is often helpful to ask parents to describe the most recent occasion on which they felt the child was exhibiting the behavior or attitude under discussion. Often, they end up citing something that occurred earlier that very day. When the event discussed is very recent, it is possible to get a clearer picture of the antecedent events and of how both the parents and the child behaved afterwards.

For instance, a detailed description of the events of the morning clarified both what Mrs. Rose meant when she described her 8-year-old daughter as "socially isolated and withdrawn" and some of the inadvertent reinforcements that played a role in the problem. As Carla and her mother approached the school building, Carla was greeted by one or two children. She responded to their "Hello" with a faintly spoken "Hi." After a very brief good-bye to her mother, Carla quietly walked with the children she knew into the gymnasium where they waited until it was time to go up to the classroom. When Mrs. Rose went into the building a few minutes later to give Carla her forgotten lunch box, she noticed that many of the children in the room were running around and laughing while Carla sat quietly reading a book.

Questioned as to how things had been at home before leaving for school, Mrs. Rose said she was feeling very harried and somewhat annoyed that Carla had not wanted to go to school with some other children and their mother as had been planned and had insisted that Mrs. Rose take her instead. On the way to school, Mrs. Rose tried to discuss Carla's shyness and said something to her such as, "I think if you made more of an effort to smile and say hello you would have more friends in school." She recalls that the attempt to talk went nowhere in that Carla simply replied, "I do have friends." In relating what happened, Mrs. Rose herself pointed out that her statement was somewhat critical, as she felt that it was because of Carla's shyness that she had refused to go to school with the other children. When Mrs. Rose saw Carla sitting alone, she once again tried to talk to the child about being friendly but was met only with silence.

A detailed description of this sort points the way to new interactions. For instance, we know from this that Carla's mother is protective of the youngster and allows her to avoid the very situation that, though stressful, could also provide an opportunity to overcome her inhibitions—for example, going to school with a few other children. Furthermore, Mrs. Rose's encouragement and advice, probably because they are paired with anger, have the opposite effect from what is intended—the child become more guarded and anxious, rather than less so, in the presence of other children. We know, too, that there is some gain to the child in remaining withdrawn and socially anxious since this problem results in her mother's making time for her even if she is angry about doing so. The specificity of this type of information is crucial in helping parents change ways of interacting that inadvertently may be contributing to the child's difficulties.

In addition to the information obtained from parents, whenever possible it is important to get a description of the child's behavior from other significant adults in the youngster's life. Thus, in the case just described, we would want to know directly from the teacher what she has observed about Carla's social relationships. Perhaps the teacher has some idea as to when Carla seems most relaxed or when she is more withdrawn. Moreover, it is helpful to know just how the teacher handles her withdrawal or social isolation, because the teacher too is a potent source of reinforcement and guide to social behavior.

Interestingly, detailed descriptions of this sort often also provide clues to important psychodynamic factors as well as the more obvious behavioral and systemic forces at play (cf. P. Wachtel, 1977). For instance, Mrs. Hirsh found the behavior of her 6-year-old son Robby quite inexplicable. She attributed his extremely oppositional behavior to the fact that Mr. Hirsh worked overseas and thus only spent time with his wife and son for 10 days every 6 weeks. Alone most of the time, Mrs. Hirsh enjoyed her son's company but was increasingly worn out by his incomprehensible destructive behavior. When asked to give a recent example of this behavior, Mrs. Hirsh described something that had happened that very morning. Everything had been going along quite well. Robby had been in a good mood and was behaving quite sweetly while Mrs. Hirsh was getting dressed and ready to drop Robby off at school on her way to work. Suddenly, when asked to stop throwing a ball, his mood shifted and he intentionally threw the ball at a lamp, causing it to break.

Mrs. Hirsh was asked to describe exactly what had preceded this occurrence, how she asked Robby to stop throwing the ball, how she knew his action was intentional, and exactly what consequences followed this behavior. From this inquiry emerged some useful clues to pertinent psychodynamic issues implicated in what transpired. Apparently, shortly before this incident Robby had been cuddled on his mother's lap and in his sweet mood he threw his arms around her, gave her a big kiss on the mouth, and said, "I love you Mommy." When Mrs. Hirsh got up to get dressed, Robby stayed in the room watching television. As she put on her makeup, Robby told her how beautiful she was. Right after that, he got a ball and the event described took place. Afterwards, Mrs. Hirsh was very angry at him and banished him from her room.

Knowing these details suggested, at least speculatively, that Robby, alone with his mother so much of the time, was being overstimulated sexually. Perhaps his "bad" behavior was the result of displaced "excitement" and a need to break the unconsciously frightening closeness with his mother.

The Child's Perspective

In sessions alone with children, the therapist can supplement the information she gets from the parents with a detailed description of *the child's* perception of what happens when there are unpleasant, negative interactions at home or at school. As described in Chapter 4, young children often have difficulty telling clear narratives. By asking them to draw a series of pictures that shows the sequence of events, or by having the child role-play what has happened through puppets or dolls, we often get a fascinating picture of events from a perspective quite different from that of the parents. Not surprisingly, what the child has registered as an antecedent event is often quite different from what the parent focused on as central. Here again we see the importance of multiple perspectives and the "subjective" elements at work even in behavioral approaches. The same holds true for the child's description of the negative consequences that follow from problem behavior. Children may feel that their parents "did nothing" when the parents think that they punished the child by sending him to his room. Or when asked to describe or draw what they feel when their parents are angry, children may reveal that the parents' anger and punishment are experienced either as less powerful than intended or far harsher than the parents realized.

Family Dramatizations

Much can be learned about reinforcement contingencies by asking the family to role-play some of their difficult interactions. As described in Chapter 3, role playing can be accomplished either by using family puppets or simply by using props and pretending that the office is a room at home. Pretending that a bowl of rubber bands is the family's spaghetti dinner or putting a mat on the floor to represent the bathtub really tickles most children, and they plunge into their roles with great enthusiasm. Even shy, withdrawn youngsters or those who have angrily vowed not to participate usually eventually join in, if only to correct or comment on mistakes in the way the scene is being played. Both the action in the dramatization and the discussion that ensues about its accuracy provide the therapist with a wealth of information about the reinforcement contingencies and modeling at work in the family.

One of the concerns of the Porter family, for example, was that their youngest child, Sandy, age 7, was very difficult to handle. Extremely defiant, Sandy had terrible tantrums whenever she did not get her way. In an enactment of what happened when Mr. Porter tells Sandy that it is time to get ready for bed, it became clear that both her parents, as well as her older sister, age 10, enjoyed tremendously the zestful spunky way in which Sandy refused to comply with her father's request. The dramatization highlighted that Mr. Porter was set for a fight and signaled, by his challenging tone, that he expected Sandy to resist his request. As soon as she did resist, however, his tone changed and there was a pretend quality to his "anger." Like a cartoon chase scene, there was a sense of excitement and anticipation as Dad chased Sandy around the house. And although not infrequently the pursuit ended in tears, anger, and hitting, there was a positive affect associated with the whole scene — as if the wild steer had finally been lassoed.

In addition to this overall sense of the emotional tone of this repetitive bedtime scene, several important details emerged in the enactment. Sandy would first run to Yvette's room for protection from her father, and Yvette, who generally expressed little but contempt for her younger sister, would at that time try to protect Sandy from being captured and dragged off. Second, after finally taking her coerced bath, Sandy was comforted by both Mom and Dad, who reassured her of their love. This reconciliation with her parents was followed by some time in which she and Yvette played peacefully together — one of the *only* times they played well together — before going to bed and being read to by her mother.

High spirits and laughter accompany most dramatizations when young children are involved. For this reason it is important to ascertain whether this is what it is really like at home or whether the laughter is an artifact of the fact that the family is play acting. The therapist asks throughout, "Is this what it's really like? What would make it more realistic?" With the Porters, questions of this sort settled everyone down and it became clearer that as Sandy continued to be defiant, Mr. Porter became *genuinely* angry and Sandy revealed that she was sometimes afraid her Dad would pull her so hard that her arm would rip off.

An analysis of this role play in behavioral terms makes it clear that the child is not only being given a signal that a fight is expected, but that she is also reinforced in her resistance: The tone of the "You can't catch me" . . . "Yes I can" . . . "No you can't" is at first playful and teasing. Furthermore, although she is eventually hurt and real anger ensues, there are also some powerful positive reinforcements for engaging in this fight. Sandy's parents reassure her of their love and affection and even her sister, who is normally rejecting, comforts her. Mr. and Mrs. Porter, who are frequently upset by Yvette's "nastiness" to Sandy, are themselves reinforced in their behavior by being "rewarded" with the pleasure of seeing the two girls relate warmly toward one another.

Direct Observation

Much can be learned about reinforcement contingencies in the family simply by observing how parents and children interact in the therapy office. Family therapists are of course accustomed to looking carefully at patterns of interactions in the family. Much of the classic literature in family therapy demonstrates the value of closely noting sequences of behavior. A behavioral analysis of the interactions in the family builds on, and does

not replace, the standard systemic analyses. In order to integrate the behavioral component into the work, one attends to exactly *how* family
members reinforce one another and thus keep the behaviors going that
are part and parcel of the family structure. If parents are allowing their
conflicts to be dissipated by the frequent interruptions of a child, for instance, the therapist must try to notice exactly what cues the child is being given that discourage him from getting engaged in his own activity
and encourage him to interact with the parents. Perhaps, for example,
a parent incorporates something into the conversation with the spouse
that will inevitably capture a child's attention. Or perhaps, when talking
together, the parents simultaneously keep an eye on the child's play, and
the youngster, sensing he has an audience, shows the parent what he is
doing.

In planning behavioral interventions, it is essential to pay close attention to voice quality, facial expressions, gaze, body language, and nonverbal reinforcements. Moreover, one must observe not only what is
responded to but what is ignored. Thus, for example, when 5-year-old
Ingrid sat for the entire session snuggled under her mother's arm, thumb
in mouth, speaking in a whispery, teary voice, I mentally noted that neither
parent was encouraging her to participate in the family discussion in a
more mature manner. And when Tricia, the older child in the family,
kept her back to her father when speaking to him, he responded as if
she had been talking directly to him. These observations were important
because the parents in this case had expressed a good deal of worry both
about Ingrid's vulnerability and Tricia's poor social skills and inability
to relate normally to her peers. Clearly they were reinforcing behaviors
that contributed to the children's acting the very way the parents were
unhappy about.

To be sure, the behavior of both these children could not be understood as simply the result of not having learned more adaptive ways of
behaving. There were systemic issues in the family as well as individual
conflicts for both children that played a highly significant role in the development and maintenance of these behaviors. Nonetheless, feedback
as to the exact way the parents reinforced behavior that kept each child
in her role was extremely helpful. Knowing some of the specific ways
they had actually been reinforcing "vulnerability" in Ingrid and "unrelat-
edness" in Tricia enabled them to plan new ways of responding and thereby
to communicate effectively to the children that they really wanted to see
new behavior.

A behavioral analysis also looks carefully at the maladaptive patterns that are maintained because they bring short-run symptom relief
but at the price of long-run maladaptation. Thus, for example, parents
who tolerate a child's rudeness until the point that they shout at him and

demand an apology may feel that shouting has been effective. Yet the child may have learned that a good deal of rudeness is acceptable as long as he does not go too far and that a pro forma apology is all that is needed to make things allright.

Or a parent may deal with a withdrawn, distracted, or nonengaged youngster by coaxing the child to participate with an implicit offer of a lot of attention. Although this may be very effective in the short run, the child may come to believe that passivity and withdrawal are effective routes to rewards and engagement.

When doing a behavioral analysis of family interactions, one must carefully note what other family members do when one parent is trying to effect a change in a child's behavior. This information is generally best obtained from direct observation rather than by questioning, as more often than not, undermining takes place subtly and unconsciously and thus is not amenable to self-report or even to the report of others in the family.

By carefully observing the nondisciplining parent in a session, the therapist may observe, for example, a pained expression when a child is being scolded or that a chastised child is spoken to by one parent more quietly and gently than he normally would be after he has been reprimanded by the other parent. As with criticism, so too with praise we can observe how one parent may diminish the meaningfulness of positive feedback that has been offered by the other parent.

Other *children* in the family may also be reinforcing undesirable behavior. Arthur, for instance, was always craving the attention of his older brother, who most often had no use for him. Only when Arthur had an uncontrollable fit of anger did his older brother seem to regard him with respect. Although Arthur's parents were clearly disapproving and would sometimes punish Arthur for his outbursts, his brother's subsequent warmth more than made up for the negative consequences imposed by the parents.

One must also not forget that reinforcement goes in both directions. Studies have shown that even infants have an important influence on caretakers (Bell, 1974) in that they "train" their parents to respond to their rhythms. It is important to be alert in family sessions to the ways children positively or negatively reinforce their parents. Some children, for instance, will "reward" a parent for playing with them by being very cheerful and enthusiastic during the interaction. Others, though they have succeeded in getting a parent to play a game, may seem so competitive and frustrated with losing that the parent associates playing with the child with negative affect.

It is especially important to notice whether parents who lose their temper are being rewarded for doing so by their children. Some children when yelled at get angry back and parents often feel that it just is not worth it to get into an argument with the youngster. At the other extreme are children who try to make amends by being unusually "good" or who reassure themselves of the parent's love by being especially loving and sweet after an argument. Parents of children who behave this way are of course being reinforced for getting mad.

The therapist can get an opportunity to observe a broader range of interactions, and is more likely to see patterns which are closely related to what takes place at home, if she varies the format of family sessions. For instance, sessions in which the family plays games or enacts family scenes with puppets will elicit different behavioral sequences than sessions in which the family just sits and talks. Still other material is elicited if the therapist asks a parent to teach a child something in a session; for example, to work with a youngster on learning how to tie his shoelace or to teach a child a new game.

Observations made when a family enters and exits the therapy room can also be very useful. Some parents act helpless when a child refuses to enter the office. Others get "tough" instantly while still others engage in long negotiations rather than communicating expectations with authority. Similarly, some parents are clear that they expect children to help in putting things away when the session is over, while others will communicate such a wish in a much more ambivalent fashion. Not surprisingly children of these latter parents are more resistant to helping.

Sharing Observations

In contrast to the methods of most family therapists, I have found that it is best not to comment on family interactions while they are occurring but rather to give feedback to the parents privately. As is true in all psychotherapy (see P. Wachtel, 1993), comments on what one has observed can easily be perceived as critical and thus must be carefully worded. Although parents are eager for feedback and suggestions, they will become defensive if what they hear is that they have been parenting incorrectly. It is absolutely crucial, therefore, that feedback include comments that empathize with each parent's feelings as well as, whenever possible, the good intentions and strengths that are also part of the picture. In giving feedback to parents, we must notice and support the parenting behaviors that are effective while at the same time pointing out what needs to be changed. Although it might be possible to do this spontaneously, the wording of the therapist's comments in response to family meetings (particularly the first one) is so important that it is generally best to delay giving feedback until the therapist has had an opportunity to carefully think through what should be said.

Another reason for speaking to parents in private about what one has noticed is that it is important to avoid situations in which family members feel humiliated in front of one another. Many parents would feel diminished in the eyes of their children if an authority figure were to "critique" them in the child's presence. And, of course, when people feel embarrassed they are prone to be angry and defensive.

The same considerations are true for feedback to children. Children's vulnerability may lead them to be very defensive. For this reason, it is important that observations made to a child about counterproductive behavior be made in a positive, productive way so that the youngster experiences the therapist as helping him get what he wants rather than scolding or criticizing him. Again, it is best to do this in private sessions to minimize defensiveness.

UTILIZING PRINCIPLES OF BEHAVIOR MODIFICATION

Choosing Target Behaviors

Just as interventions based on psychodynamic considerations had to be individually crafted, so too must behavior modification methods be devised that are appropriate to the particular characteristics of both the child and family. The first step is to help each parent clarify what behavior they would like to try to change. Often, parents lose their effectiveness because they attempt to correct too many behaviors at once. The child does not therefore learn to differentiate between what is *really* important and what is only mildly desired. Working with the parents on a focus for the behavioral efforts not only helps parents pick target behaviors but highlights areas of agreement and disagreement between the parents. Even when there is serious marital conflict, parents are usually able to reach some agreement as to at least some things they *both* wish would change. When they are unable to reach *any* agreed-on goals, it is best not to embark on behavioral programs. Behavioral interventions in such cases are unlikely to be effective, not only because one parent may sabotage the other's efforts but because the systemic factors involved in the child's difficulties are likely to be far more central than the behavioral ones.

When parents are separated or divorced and the child lives in two separate households, it is possible to institute two separate behavioral programs which reflect the different concerns of each parent. Of course, when feasible it is best if divorced parents work on the *same* behaviors, and not infrequently divorced parents can reach agreements on target behaviors in joint sessions or in separate meetings with the therapist.

It is important to define with great specificity exactly what constitutes the target behavior. A crucial element in behavior modification is that the individual know exactly what is expected. Thus, for instance, if a parent states that he wants Johnny to be more cooperative, it is the job of the therapist to help the parent clarify and define precisely what behaviors would constitute "cooperativeness." Often it is best to start by having the parents carefully *observe* the child's behavior: They should note not only the specific conduct that they would like to see diminish but also the actions and behaviors of the child that please them. A valuable side effect of this initial task is that careful observation of both positives and negatives often enables parents to see their children more realistically. Statements such as, "He's got a chip on his shoulder," "He's always negative," or "He's clingy and overly dependent," often give way, under the gaze of careful observation, to more moderate and qualified statements.

It is also useful to note that many parents are unaware of how seldom they praise or show pleasure in a child's behavior. When parents are asked to keep track for 24 hours of how often they use social reinforcers (smiles, hugs, praise, etc.), they are often surprised by how rarely they interact with their child in these positive ways (Patterson, 1975).

Rewarding Desired Behavior

Many parents are much more comfortable with a behavioral plan that emphasizes positive reinforcements rather than negative consequences. Frequently, however, they are pessimistic about the effectiveness of rewards since they feel that attempts to use positive reinforcement and promises of gifts to the child have never seemed to do any good. It is helpful, therefore, to review with parents some basic behavioral principles that can make positive reinforcements much more effective. First, when trying to encourage more positive ways of acting, parents must make sure that they are not *also* inadvertently reinforcing the ways of acting that they want to discourage. If a parent is generous with approval when a child is playing cooperatively but also gives a lot of attention to the child when she is whining and argumentative, the power of the "reward" for approved behavior is tremendously diminished. Thus, conscious effort to respond positively to desired behavior must be combined with efforts to eliminate reinforcement for ways of acting that are not acceptable.

Second, it is important to explain to parents the effectiveness of rewarding small steps in the right direction—what is called by behaviorists, shaping. In order to shape behavior, one must first learn to *notice* the variations in the way an individual acts (P. Wachtel, 1993). The parent must look carefully for those periods, even if they are very brief, in which the child is behaving somewhat better, and try to consistently reinforce those behaviors until they become more routine and are the foundation for a somewhat larger step.[2] Shaping involves being attentive to steps in the right direction and consistently reinforcing those behaviors. For example, if an "uncooperative" 5-year-old picks up and puts away even one item of a pile of toys he has left on the floor, one would notice and respond positively to this small piece of cooperative behavior. This approach involves simply noticing what occurs spontaneously and strengthening that response by reinforcement (this is called operant conditioning by behavior therapists).

Some parents are uncomfortable with rewarding behavior that they feel the child should do automatically. They do not like the idea of giving rewards for behavior that seems ordinary and expectable. Giving rewards for what should be normal cooperativeness, for instance, seems like "bribing" the child and parents feel annoyed at the child for "blackmailing" them in this way. When parents have concerns such as this, it is best to recommend that they use a positive reinforcement system only for naturally occurring behaviors. Rather than setting up any formal program of objectives and rewards, parents would simply "reward" the child with positive statements and affectionate gestures whenever the child takes steps in the right direction. Doing this consistently can be extremely effective when parents are careful not to also reinforce undesirable behavior. Many parents who are uncomfortable with making "contracts" for rewards do like the suggestion that they occasionally surprise the child with a treat or a present as a gift to show appreciation for how nicely the youngster has been acting.

A more direct method of reinforcing positive behavior is to set up a reward system for the child based on the desired conduct. Children seem to enjoy having a chart with a list of behaviors that can earn them points (in the form of stickers, checks, etc.), which can be redeemed for rewards. When this method is chosen, it is important for the child to be part of the process and to select some of the things he wants to work on. This should be done in a family session with all the children present. Charts with target behaviors should be made for the other children as well, because it will seem unfair to them if the "problem" child is rewarded for behavior that they exhibit regularly without any promise of a reward.

When setting target behaviors, it is extremely important that only one or two be put on the chart at once and that at least one item is easy enough that the child is assured of some success. Usually it is helpful to divide the day into three parts: before school, after school but before dinner, and after dinner until bedtime. The child should be able to earn points in each of these three periods, and the behaviors being rewarded should be clearly defined in the family session so that there are no arguments as to whether a sticker was legitimately earned. For example, if a child is to get a sticker for doing what he is asked to do in a timely fashion rather than dawdling, it is important for parents and children to talk about what is meant by "dawdling" and what constitutes doing something soon after being asked to do it.

With young children, it is often helpful to have the parent prompt the child as a way of evoking the behavior. Saying something like, "OK, Now, I'm asking you to get ready promptly," rather than just asking the child to get ready, gives a signal to the youngster that this is an opportunity to earn points.

Latency-age children often are intensely engaged by the detailed discussion of rules and the subsequent refinement and definition of categories. Often, in fact, setting up the chart is as therapeutic as the chart itself in that children and parents are collaborating on ways to solve problems in the family.

Parents often ask whether the chart plan should also include the *loss* of points for misbehavior or failure to do what has been asked. Although some behavioral approaches do include penalties, I advise against this for two reasons. First, I think it is important for the child to have entirely positive associations to the chart, and deducting points makes the chart a mixed experience and possibly quite a negative one. Second, and more important, I think adding and subtracting points can turn what should be in essence a matter of self and parental approval into an exercise in "bookkeeping." Instead of mixing rewards and punishments in this one modality, it is better for parents to punish misbehavior separately and to use the chart only for rewarding desired behavior.

Rewarding Children for Working at Overcoming Their Symptoms

Reward systems can be used not merely to help children change behavior that is annoying or disruptive, but also to encourage the child to try to overcome anxieties or other difficulties on which his motivation to work is limited. Anna Freud (1965) notes that many pathological manifestations in children "successfullly serve the avoidance of pain and unpleasure rather than causing it, while the resulting restrictions and intefereces with ordinary life are resented by the family, not, as with adults, by the patient himself" (p. 120). Even when children *are* feeling very distressed, as is the case with severe anxiety, they are almost always reluctant to engage in a program of gradual exposure to help them overcome their fears. They are not as conscious as adults of the long-term negative effects of using avoidance and, thus, are often quite reluctant to engage in therapeutic tasks that will feel uncomfortable at first. Thus, in order to gain the child's cooperation in a behavioral plan, one can use rewards to motivate the child to participate in something for which he does not really feel a need.

In the case of 8-year-old Penny, who had developed a fear of being in the upstairs of her house when the adults were downstairs, a sticker was placed on her chart every time she took a step to overcome her anxiety. In collaboration with Penny, a plan was devised in which she got a sticker for playing upstairs for 15 minutes when an adult was at the base of the stairs, then another for staying longer, then for playing for 15 minutes when an adult was not in sight but was in a nearby room, and so on.

Similarly, if a child has developed the maladaptive habit of "tuning out" whenever he has difficulty comprehending something, a chart could be used for rewarding him whenever he carefully listens to discussions. Items on the chart might include such things as listening and contributing to dinner-time discussions or demonstrating that he has been attentive during a television documentary or church sermon. Or, children who become frustrated easily could be rewarded for "working hard at things that are difficult" or doing their homework without assistance.

Often individual sessions with the child can be helpful in enlisting the child's active participation in the behavioral plan. The therapist can work out with the child a day-by-day plan for gradually overcoming an anxiety which together they propose to the parents. Children seem to like this approach and are often quite specific in their instructions to their parents. Seven-year-old Jennifer, for instance, in planning a way to get over her school phobia, told her mother that for 3 days she wanted her to sit right outside the classroom, for 1 week in the cafeteria, and for 3 days at home by the telephone so she could be called at any time. The fact that the child is "dictating" the terms of her therapy seems to shift the child's attention away from her fear and replaces it with feelings of power and mastery. The child is also reinforced for his efforts by charting and rewarding each step in the process.

Of course, before setting up such a reward system it is important to discuss and alleviate the environmental circumstances that might be contributing to the child's difficulties. Sometimes, for instance, when a child "tunes out" it is because a highly verbal sibling is being allowed to dominate. Or the child's comments may be being mocked or laughed at by older family members. Or the conversation at the dinner table may be one that is not appropriate for young children, giving the child the message that he is not expected to participate. Similarly, before rewarding a child for working hard at homework without assistance, one must make sure that the work he is being given is appropriate for his capacities and that he is in fact capable of doing the assignment.

When devising a program that targets behaviors such as these it is often useful to supplement the naturally occurring events with planned opportunities for the child to earn points. This is helpful because it provides more frequent and rapid reinforcement for behaviors that otherwise might be rewarded only once every day or two. Thus, for instance, "stick-to-itiveness" when confronted with difficulty in learning a new skill might be a highly desired behavior, yet the opportunities for reinforcement of this trait may be so infrequent that learning the importance of this trait will be very slow unless the child encounters some additional occasions that call for persistence. Together parents, therapist and even the child can plan some situations that will enable the child to win points for persistence. Depending on the child's age, for instance, he could be give an opportunity to peel a potato, set the table correctly, learn to cut with a knife, tie a shoelace, memorize a telephone number, or learn to calculate the number of calories in a meal. Again, the very process of thinking about the chart dramatically changes the family dynamics and makes overcoming individual and interpersonal difficulties a family project.

Working with Teachers

When using reinforcement charts to encourage new behaviors it is helpful to enlist the support of the child's teacher. Often it is in the school setting that a child's maladaptive behavior patterns are most apparent. Avoidance behavior, for instance, occurs most frequently in school where the child is being challenged intellectually and socially. The effectiveness of behavioral interventions is considerably enhanced when teachers are included in the plan to reward the youngster for overcoming habitual defensive patterns.

Many teachers are happy to cooperate in helping a child earn points for new behavior as long as what they are being asked to observe is clear, simple, and does not become obvious to the other children. Thus, for instance, one might ask a teacher to put a check in a page in the child's assignment book whenever she observes that the child is sitting still and working on something that is somewhat difficult for her without getting up to ask questions, go to the bathroom, or otherwise remove herself from the situation. Or the teacher might be asked to evaluate the child in the morning and the afternoon and give one check for each period if the child met the goal for a majority of the time. The child brings the book home every day and the check is entered on his chart. The teacher is not asked to directly reward the child (except by showing approval) because singling out one child for rewards is not appropriate in the classroom situation. I have found that when teachers realize that I am genuinely interested in their observations and input, they are quite happy to participate in this way. Often they welcome a new way to understand what is going on with the child and the very act of collaboration with the therapist results in the teacher's feeling more positively about the youngster.

The Use of Rewards

A concern of both parents and therapists is that rewarding children can lead to a lack of genuineness and a diminution of intrinsic motivation. In fact, some research indicates that rewarding people for doing what they already enjoy doing *can* lead them to attribute their actions to the reward, thus undermining a perception of intrinsic motivation. For instance, people who were paid for playing with enjoyable puzzles subsequently played with the puzzles less than people who played with the puzzles without being paid (Deci & Ryan, 1985; Boggiano, 1985). This phenomenon is called the overjustification effect. With this in mind, I encourage parents to give small rewards that have symbolic value rather than money or material objects which are more likely to lead the child to believe that he is doing the required behavior only for the prize. When children receive small rewards they are more likely to realize that they are not *really* doing what is asked merely for the reward but rather because they are in fact motivated to overcome their difficulties. Whenever possible I encourage giving rewards that involve interaction with the parent.

Parents and children are generally very enthusiastic about the suggestion to make a grab bag with folded-up slips of paper stating the "reward" the child has picked. Although some small material objects can be included (e.g., "Johnny wins a pack of gum"), generally the grab bag should contain nonmaterial prizes that include parental participation. For instance, the grab bag could contain a slip that says, "Mom watches a television show that I choose," "Dad takes me with him to buy ice cream," "Mom plays cards with me for 15 minutes," or "I get to choose what video we will watch" (etc.). If parents want to offer bigger rewards for the accumulation of numerous stickers or weeks of desired behavior, these too should, ideally, involve interaction with parents. Perhaps when a child earns enough points a parent might schedule an extra trip to someplace the child really enjoys, take the child to an additional movie, or play video games with the child at a mall.

Although most parents feel much happier using a reward system of this sort rather than one that offers real material incentives, some parents propose (or give in to their child's demand for) rather big material inducements instead of the relationship rewards just described. When this type of arrangement is offered, it often reflects an assumption on the part of the parents that the child does not really *care* about engaging with them and that an opportunity to accumulate *things* will be far more motivating than time with a parent.

Having grown up in a culture that inculcates in children an emphasis on the pleasures of accumulation (see P. Wachtel, 1989), most youngsters do, of course, enjoy material possessions. Nonetheless, almost all young children enjoy opportunities to do something with a parent. When a child does not, it is likely a reflection of some problematic interactions in the family and/or defense mechanisms that parent, child, or both may be using to avoid hurt. In instances of this sort, it is best to go along with whatever type of reward the parents and children agree on while continuing to work with the family on the underlying issues that lie behind these feelings.

The younger the child, the more necessary it is that some small reward be given *daily* for points accumulated that day. An extra 10 minutes of play time in the bathtub, an extra story at bedtime, or a special dessert, all let the young child know that the efforts he made that day are appreciated. Even with older children who are saving for some bigger reward (it is hoped one involving interaction with the parent), it is important to set up some smaller goals along the way. Often, both parents and children underestimate the child's need for some immediate positive reinforcement and it is failure to include these interim rewards that often accounts for the prior lack of success with agreements and promises. A promise of a reward for a good report card, for instance, is too distant and removed from daily behavior to effectively motivate a young child. If possible, it is helpful to have the interim rewards relate to or be part of the larger goal. One little boy of 7 was working toward getting a hamster. As he accumulated stickers he was able to get a book on hamsters, some toys for the hamster's cage, the cage itself, and eventually the hamster.

A frequently encountered problem with the utilization of formal behavioral systems of reinforcement is that families often get off to a good start and then prematurely let the program drop. Ironically, it is often the rapid success of the plan that results in its being forgotten about. As noted above, the very act of devising a plan itself changes patterns of interactions in the family. That, plus the good feelings generated by the children's efforts to cooperate and win stickers, sometimes leads to a lack of attention to the plan after just a week or two because it just does not feel necessary anymore. Children as well as parents are often so much happier that they too forget about earning stickers for the sake of a reward. Of course, in one sense this state of affairs is ideal; this is what we are aiming for. However, since families can become discouraged when old behaviors reappear, it is best to urge them to continue with the plan conscientiously for a while longer. As part of this routine, children are also asked to remind parents of the sticker system if they forget to use it.

Few families can, or would want to sustain such a system indefinitely. As the family and child continue to change and new ways of acting become the norm rather than something that has to be worked at, a reward system should no longer be necessary. The child's new behaviors will most likely have become self-rewarding. It is important, however, to remind the parents that even at this stage they should continue to positively reinforce the child's efforts, albeit in a less formal and more intermittent manner.

USE OF NEGATIVE CONSEQUENCES
OR PUNISHMENT VERSUS THE NATURAL
EXTINCTION OF UNDESIRABLE BEHAVIOR

Most parents really do not like to punish. They are much more comfortable reinforcing positive steps than punishing behavior they wish to weaken or eliminate. Popular advice on parenting often suggests to parents that they try their best simply to ignore negative behavior such as whining or tantrums and that these behaviors, when not reinforced, will gradually disappear. Although in theory this approach might work, try as they might most parents simply cannot ignore behavior that leaves them feeling angry and helpless. Not uncommonly, attempts to ignore children's disturbing behavior end in a sudden loss of temper accompanied by hitting, shouting, and threats of extreme punishment. Even when parents do not explode, the effort exerted in not responding to a child's unpleasant behavior leaves parents feeling tense and frequently there is a critical, irritated edge to their interactions with a child who is taxing their patience.

Although the undesirable behavior may, in fact, slowly lessen as the child is reinforced for more positive ways of interacting, the process can be a slow one. In addition, there is a price to be paid for simply ignoring annoying behavior; sensing the parent's general state of irritation, the youngster may attribute the parent's feelings to a general feeling of dislike rather than displeasure with something specific the child is doing.

For these reasons, as well as the ones discussed in the last chapter regarding the need of some children to have their internal struggles with impulse control fortified by external controls, it is important to help parents develop appropriate responses to the behaviors they really cannot ignore. With young children, one of the most effective ways of dealing with negative behavior is by using the Time Out method.

TIME OUT

Time Out is a method based on the idea that one can diminish the frequency of undesirable behavior on the part of a child by designing a Time Out from reinforcement, rewards, and attention at the time the unacceptable behavior is occurring. It is more than "active ignoring" (Clark, 1985): It is also a mild form of punishment that not only ensures that undesirable behavior is not reinforced but actually links that behavior to a negative and mildly aversive consequence.

Time Out can be used for a wide spectrum of behavior ranging from the more serious displays of aggression or impulsivity to behaviors that fall more in the category of bad manners and minor irritants. Research indicates that it is maximally effective when it is used very consistently and when the actual period of Time Out is of relatively short duration (Ollendick & Cerny, 1981). Time Out works best by targeting just one or two very specific behaviors and responding to those behaviors as soon as they occur by placing the child in a quiet, boring area which is not reinforcing or enjoyable.

Many parents have tried using Time Out and have found it to be ineffective. They report that either the child really does not mind it or, conversely, her objection to it is so great that the parent feels that enforcing Time Out is virtually impossible to do. As simple as the technique sounds, there are a number of complexities to using Time Out which, if neglected, are likely to lead to failure.

Often, when Time Out has failed, it is because certain basics of the method have not been followed. For instance, if parents wait too long before responding to the troubling behavior, the child is getting reinforcement for his ability to anger and upset his parents. Time Out must be done calmly and this usually requires that the parent respond to the target behavior at the first sign of its occurrence. By giving a child a chance or two before using even this mild form of punishment, the child is deprived of the clear criteria he needs regarding what is or is not acceptable. Furthermore, when parents wait a while before using Time Out, the child is more likely to be out of control, and that makes it all the more difficult for him to settle down when sent to Time Out.

Another common error is that parents will talk to the child about why they are upset and sending him to Time Out, and this very talking may itself be reinforcing and thus undermine the method.

Parents who send a child to his room for Time Out are violating the core requirement of the method which is that the youngster be in a place that is not reinforcing. Most children find their rooms quite comforting and have a lot to play with and distract them when they are supposedly suffering the consequences of misbehaving. Instead, they should be sent to sit on a chair in the most boring place possible, and other family members should be instructed not to speak with them during their detention.

Another common error is that Time Out is not used consistently. Perhaps this is because parents do not realize that the Time Out should be rather short, and thus that consistent use, however frequent, need not ruin the whole day or evening. Clark (1985) recommends that Time Out be done in 10 words and 10 seconds and that the child be placed in a not overly comfortable chair in a boring room for just 1 minute for each year of his age. If the child delays going to Time Out or is disruptive while there, the time should be extended to no more than 15 minutes. If the child refuses to go to Time Out, he is not allowed to engage in some enjoyable activity until he actually does the Time Out. Clark's (1985) book, *S.O.S. for Parents*[3] covers such topics as how to use Time Out in situations away from home, what to say to a child after Time Out, and how this method can be used in conjunction with other behavioral methods designed to reinforce desirable behavior.

PENALTIES, PUNISHMENT, AND DISAPPROVAL

Aware of the growing consensus that global criticism of the child — "You never look what you're doing," or "Once again you've been thoughtless" — is destructive and counterproductive, many parents end up avoiding criticizing the child's behavior altogether. Instead, the child's misbehavior or failure to do what has been requested "costs" the child something like a loss of allowance or time watching television. Although it is a vast improvement for the parents to focus on the child's behavior rather than his character, there are also some problems with this cost approach. For many children the loss of privileges is just not that important if there is no real feeling of parental disapproval behind it. And for children who do care about losing privileges, the cost approach can foster a very mechanistic attitude toward misconduct, so that the child learns to behave well not because it is *right* and really matters to his parents but because he will be punished if he does not. By making the consequences of problematic conduct simply a matter of incurring penalties, the child is less likely to internalize expectations and generalize them to other situations.

Furthermore, when penalties are frequently used, many children become quite inured to the loss of privileges or allowance and *mean* it when they defiantly say, "Who cares?" For these reasons it is important to help parents rethink their use of punishments. If a child no longer seems to care about penalties, it does no good to increase the cost by, for instance, depriving the youngster of television for a week rather than one evening. One reason that some children become immune to penalties is that they get so little *approval* that they are hardened to the censure implied in the punishment and are highly defended against the wish to please. This almost total loss of hope for approval is expressed both in the misbehavior and in the indifference to the negative consequences the parents impose. Many children who behave this way feel powerless, hurt, and angry and find strength in the stoical acceptance of punishment.

When one sees an attitude of this sort in a child, it is a reflection of serious problems in the parent–child relationship. One of the first steps in resolving this impasse is to have parents stop *their* side of the power struggle. New ways of interacting with the child need to be pursued. Helping the parents shift to shaping through praise rather than utilizing punishment is a necessary first step.

It is important to discuss with parents the limited and controlled use of disapproval as an alternative to depriving children of privileges. Particularly when a child has become inured to punishments, it can be helpful for parents to simply state in a mildly disapproving manner, something like "I'm not going to punish you but I want you to know that it really upsets me when you behave that way." Similarly, instead of depriving a child of some privilege, a parent might want to show his disapproval by saying to a child who has misbehaved, "I'm not feeling like playing (or chatting) with you just now because I feel angry and upset about how you just acted." Of course, withdrawal of this sort should be used very selectively, and the parents should make it clear that the emotional detachment is temporary and in response to something the child *did* rather than the kind of person the youngster *is*.

And most important, the power of a parent's disapproval is directly related to the bond of *affection* that exists between parent and child. This approach should never be suggested without simultaneously working on helping both parent and child become closer to one another.

COGNITIVE-BEHAVIORAL APPROACHES AND SOCIAL SKILLS TRAINING

In recent years, behavior therapy has relied increasingly on cognitive interventions to complement more traditional behavioral methods. The central tenet of this approach is that emotions and behavior are mediated by thought and that an individual's emotional problems can be ameliorated by focusing on the maladaptive thinking and distorted cognitive processes that are contributing to the person's difficulties. By focusing on an individual's beliefs, attributions, self-statements, expectations, and underlying schemata, the therapist helps restructure the thought processes that are inadvertently supporting behavioral and emotional problems.

When working with impulsive, overly aggressive children, for instance, cognitive behavior therapists may teach the child self-instruction procedures (Braswell & Kendall, 1987; Meichenbaum & Goodman,

1971) in which the child is trained to define problems, think about various solutions, evaluate the probable consequences of each choice, and finally either to reward himself with a congratulatory self statement (e.g., "I did it right!") or, if he chose incorrectly, to use a coping statement (such as, "On the next problem I'll slow down and concentrate."). Children who are too quick to get angry may also be taught to "identify physiological and affective cues of anger arousal" (Lochman, White, & Wayland, 1991, p. 42) as well as to notice anger-augmenting and anger-reducing cognitions.

When working with depressed and anxious children, cognitive approaches focus on the distorted information processing that results in emotional distress. Interventions are designed to reduce both the negative self-critical style of thinking which is characteristic of these youngsters and the maladaptive underlying beliefs that lead the child to overgeneralize from negative experiences. Children are taught to more accurately evaluate the extent to which their own efforts, actions, and abilities can influence the outcome of events (Reynolds, 1988).

Cognitive approaches with children are often used in group settings and are almost always combined with other behavioral interventions such as social skills training, relaxation training, desensitization procedures, and programs of contingent reinforcement. Thus, for a child who suffers from depression or dysthymia, the treatment plan might include role playing geared to helping the youngster make friends as well as setting up rewards for efforts to engage in positive social interactions. (Reynolds, 1988; Frame, Johnston, & Gibliln, 1988).

Social skills training is an umbrella term for a conglomerate of methods which, taken together, aim at improving a child's interpersonal skills. Social skills programs are multifaceted and generally include the use of modeling, positive reinforcement, coaching, behavior rehearsal, and cognitive strategies for better problem solving. Modeling consists of demonstrating to the child, either in real life or on film, the behaviors that need to be learned. Through role taking, a child practices what has been modeled while the therapist acts as his coach. Progressive approximations to the desired behavior are reinforced while the child is given some feedback as to what he might do just a little differently.

Michelson, Sugai, Wood, & Kazdin (1983) describe well the delicate process of using reinforcement to shape and correct a child's role-played performance:

> The child may be requested to pretend he is approaching and asking a friend to play with him. The child may correctly walk over to the playmate (played by the trainer) and ask whether she wants to play. The child may actually walk up to the role-played peer and ask a question, in an almost inaudible

voice, while staring at the floor. The trainer might then praise both the approach and the request. Rather than punishing poor eye contact and inappropriate intonation, the trainer would provide corrective feedback, rewarding what was done correctly and emphasizing what the child should concentrate on during the next practice segment. (p. 43)

Social skills training can be used with a wide variety of behaviors ranging from helping withdrawn youngsters to make better social contact to teaching overly aggressive children to be appropriately assertive verbally rather than acting out physically.

UTILIZING COGNITIVE METHODS, MODELING, AND ROLE PLAYING

Impulse Control

In working with children and parents in the model described in this volume, one can readily incorporate into the work some aspects of cognitive therapy. Depending on the particulars of the case, one might utilize these methods in sessions alone with the child or one might coach the parents and children on how to employ some of these procedures together. For instance, sessions alone with Suzanne, age 7, who was brought to therapy by her parents because of her extreme temper tantrums and inappropriate behavior with peers, focused on helping her develop better frustration tolerance. Together, we made a list of times that it is hard for her to be patient. By focusing on the bodily sensations the child experienced as she began to get frustrated, Suzanne learned to identify the situations where work on cognitive strategies was needed.[4]

The youngster was then asked to think of some things she could say or do that would help her stay calm. With her mother's help, she decided to pick one or two toys that would be kept in a special place and that would be reserved for use when she was becoming impatient. She called these toys her "waiting toys." When outside the house the child was to carry a "Magic Slate" drawing pad so that she would have something to focus on when feelings of frustration and impatience arose.

In individual sessions, Suzanne learned to engage in "self-talk" and used the slogan "slowly and carefully" when she was becoming frustrated in learning a new skill. When she got upset she would often say, "Stay cool."

Suzanne's parents agreed to put a sticker on her reward chart whenever she utilized one of these methods in frustrating situations. Parts of sessions alone with Suzanne were used to help her practice these strategies. It was explained to the youngster that we would do an "experiment" to see whether she could use some of her self-control methods. At some point in the session I would interrupt her play and remove a toy that she had been enjoying playing with; that would be a time that she would need to find a way to wait patiently until I allowed the activity to be resumed. Even though the interruption had something of the quality of a "game," Suzanne did in fact experience it as frustrating and did have to utilize self-talk to stay calm. In future sessions she was given further opportunities to practice: She worked, for instance, at learning to tie her shoelace as well as staying calm when receiving instructions on how to play a new game.[5]

Children enjoy having a system or method for self-control. I have found them to be quite receptive to learning Kendall's (1992) Stop and Think method in which the child learns to follow a set procedure consisting of five distinct steps. I have found this to be a particularly useful method with children who have poor self-control in the classroom or who do not do as well as they could academically because they answer impulsively rather than really thinking about what they have been asked. In an individual session with the child I rehearse with him the elements of Stop and Think (Kendall, 1992). The child is taught five steps to use to help him slow down. Step one consists of the child's evaluating "What am I supposed to do?". The second step is to "Look at all the possibilities." Step three is to "Pick an answer." Next the child "Checks the answer," and finally, if the answer was correct the child gives himself positive feedback ("I did a good job") or if incorrect reminds himself to "Be more careful or go more slowly next time" (p. 3). Once the child has learned the steps involved in the method, we spend some time practicing. To make the practice resemble the school situation, I might give the child some math problems to do, or might read a page or two from a book and ask him some questions about what he has heard. I make clear to the youngster that the purpose of this is not to tutor him but merely to help him develop a method of slowing down and thinking before he answers. Practice can also easily be integrated into the playing of the "feeling" games described in Chapter 4. The child is given extra chips when he demonstrates that he has really thought about his choice of answer. Once the child and I have worked on Stop and Think, we tell the parents about the method. Parents can help the child make the method habitual, by setting up a chart to record and eventually reward demonstration of the Stop and Think approach. Young children enjoy the Stop and Relax and Think (1990) board game which some parents want to purchase to play with the child at home.

In vivo rehearsal of strategies for self-control can also take place in family sessions. For instance, in order to help 7-year-old Mickey practice impulse control, his older brother, Kevin, was asked to intentionally behave provocatively. Kevin happily accommodated by threatening to grab away the marker Mickey was using and by taunting him about the inadequacy of his drawing. Although there was, of course, a "pretend" quality to the interaction, because it had been prescribed, the scene was so close to what spontaneously happens between them that Mickey really did have to work at not losing control. He had practiced using words rather than reacting physically, and successfully spoke to himself about not letting Kevin get to him.

Balloon play can be a particularly good way to have a child practice self-control. Hitting a balloon back and forth, an activity that usually starts out as great fun, can easily turn into an experience that stimulates impulsive acting out and emotional volatility. It is this very potential that makes playing this game such a good vehicle for practicing impulse control. Spontaneous or planned "provocations" can be used to observe and coach the child in better ways to handle his reactions. We can observe, for instance, how the child responds when a balloon is hit to him badly or perhaps even pops in his face. When the therapist or family member "bops" the youngster with a balloon, the child can practice "self-talk," which helps him not respond as if the playful or even mildly aggressive "assault" were an act of major aggression.

Coping with Anxiety

When a child is extremely anxious and worries over events that others take in stride, the youngster can be taught problem-solving strategies. Parents often respond to a child's anxiety by offering reassurances and solutions. The very act of asking a child what he could say to himself so that he will be less worried, or inquiring about what solutions to his problems he can think of, shifts responsibility for handling his anxiety onto himself rather than the parents.

In individual sessions with the child the therapist can help the youngster anticipate the situations that cause apprehension and then work with the him to plan some things the child can do to help himself feel less afraid. Eight-year-old Tricia, for instance, was very fearful of burglars entering her apartment. She would worry that her parents forgot to lock the door or that, thinking she would not wake up, they would decide to go out. Although these fears were worked with psychodynamically and systemically (addressing the youngster's worries about not getting the protection she needed), it was also quite helpful to work with the child on ways that she could counteract these worries, which a part of her knew were not realistic. Thus, for instance, we discussed what Tricia could say to herself if, in bed, she started to worry that the door was not locked, and what she could do to prevent herself from compulsively checking the door or calling her parents. Tricia's parents were taught how to provide the cues that would get their daughter to engage in self-talk and more rational thinking, and instead of reassuring her when she was worried, they learned to ask how she could think about her concerns differently.

Perfectionism

Many parents are concerned that their children seem to be overly perfectionistic. The child may destroy drawings or other things he has produced because they do not to live up to his expectations. Or the child may get frustrated with himself easily and refuse to continue trying to master a new skill. In addition to using rewards to encourage children to stick with tasks they would otherwise withdraw from (as described earlier in the chapter), parents can help perfectionistic children by modeling more tolerant attitudes toward oneself. They might, for example, model congratulating themselves for *effort* rather than accomplishment or labeling an activity as "just for fun" rather than something one has to do one's best at.

A game like Pictionary, in which drawings must be made quickly simply to communicate, provides good practice in being able to do something without perfectionistic standards. The parent models being able to enjoy something of that sort by saying things like "I know I'm not much of an artist, but it's OK because I'm having fun." Modeling can also be used with activities that one *is,* in fact, trying to do well. A family task might be for everyone to do something that is difficult for them to do and to stick with it even if they are at first disappointed with the results. Points could be given for whomever sticks with his activity. While working on difficult problems, the parents model for the children tolerant and accepting self-talk, saying, for instance, "I know if I keep at it I'll get it," or "Even if it didn't come out that great, at least I tried."

Often parents of perfectionistic children are puzzled because they feel they are supportive and accepting of the child's efforts. The child may, however, be picking up on a parent's *self*-criticism and intolerant attitude toward his *own* efforts. By making this a family task, the parents also confront their own attitudes and a discussion of this in a family meeting can contribute significantly to relieving the child from his own excessive demands.

Modeling can also be done through story telling. Just as parents can tell children stories that model for them greater acceptance of denied affects (see Chapter 7), so too can stories be used to teach children cognitive strategies and problem-solving skills. The rapt look on the face of a child (or an adult for that matter) who has become engrossed in a story indicates that in some sense he is in an altered, trancelike state of consciousness. When the plight of the protagonist of the story resonates with the child's struggles, he identifies with the character and "vicariously" tries out behaviors that were not previously in his behavioral repertoire. A child who is avoidant, for instance, might be told a story about a little girl who always pretended she did not like things that she was too embarrassed to try. When the same little girl in the story decides, say, to ask for help in overcoming her embarrassment, or talks to herself about how it does not matter if she does it well because it will still be fun, the listening youngster is exposed to new solutions and is more likely to try some of these techniques himself. *Annie Stories,* by Brett (1986) provides guidelines for parents on how to tell stories to children that model adaptive solutions to their difficulties.

Learning the Consequences of Interpersonal Behavior

A cognitive perspective is also extremely useful in helping children develop appropriate expectations regarding how their actions influence the way others will react to them. As obvious as it may be to the adults who deal with them, many young children have only a hazy sense of the connection between their behavior and the effect it has on others. Thus, it is useful to ask children to articulate how they understand the reasons for good as well as bad reactions on the part of adults and peers. For example, when a child gets a check from a teacher for good behavior, it is important to ask the child to name some of the things she did that pleased the teacher.

Making a list with the child of some of the things he does or can do that are likely to be pleasing to others is a way of using the child's cognitive abilities to plan for new interpersonal behavior. This method can be used even with young children by being very concrete and by drawing pictures next to the written statements on the list that will remind the child of what we have talked about. Five-year-old Andrew was intrigued by the idea of making a list of things he could do that would make his Mom and Dad smile. He decided to place his picture list in a secret spot where he could look at it whenever his parents seemed to be getting annoyed at him.

It is also helpful to work with children on articulating some of the *don'ts* in interpersonal relationships. Seven-year-old Brad often got into fights with children at school and at home. Children initially found him quite appealing but budding friendships dissipated quickly. Brad not only seemed to have no idea what his side of the difficulties were but was very resistant to discussing it. He was, however, happy to make a list of all the boys in his class and to state which ones he liked and which he did not. By evaluating with him in a slow and careful way how each of these children acted in various circumstances (e.g., when they were angry, when their team lost, or when they won a game) this youngster was led to reflect on his own behavior. When asked to compare himself to some of the children he described, he was able to recognize that he was more like the boys who got mad and frustrated easily than those who laughed a lot. This beginning of self-reflection became the foundation for some role playing and rehearsal of cognitive strategies.

Translating cognitive understanding into action needs practice. Both sessions alone with a child and family sessions can be used to rehearse and try out new ways of interacting. Rehearsal is particularly useful when the interpersonal skills that need to be developed are in relation to parents. Many children benefit from some coaching on ways to interact with parents that will not only please the parent but will result in the children's getting more of what they want. They may be asking for things in a manner that is accusatory (e.g., "You never let me get comics!") or in a manner that pushes exactly the wrong buttons in parents who hate to be compared to others (e.g., "*Jimmy's* mother lets him watch R-rated movies").

Many children automatically respond to limit setting by "negotiating" (e.g., "one more story," "10 more minutes," or "just one more show"). Often they have been doing this their whole life and have only a vague sense of alternative ways of responding. Furthermore, they frequently do not distinguish the immediate success of having the parent finally give in to their demands from the more distant consequence, that is, that the parent is annoyed with them. When working with a child on how to ask for things from her parents in a way that is not only more likely to get a positive result but also creates a better overall mood, the therapist can first model the behavior for the child and then role play the parent in a typical situation. It is important too to role play the situation where no matter how nicely the child asks, the parent still says no. Children need to have realistic expectations regarding their changed behavior and not think that simply putting "please" before all requests ensures that the requests will be granted.

Even with more severely disturbed children, role playing interactions with parents can be quite helpful. Ethan defended against the need for his mother by having his "robot" self ask for the nurturance he craved. Ethan and his mother spent a session practicing a better way to ask for what he needed. She explained to him that she would no longer respond to him positively when his robot self grabbed her but would be happy to hug and kiss him whenever he wanted it if he asked in a more direct and real way.

When Ethan was first learning this new behavior, his mother gave him a prompting cue, saying, "Let me have a good hug and kiss," and each time he did it as himself rather than in a mechanical fashion she gave him a warm hug and a kiss and a pat on the back for trying hard to break a bad habit. Other sessions were spent with his mother giving him feedback about his grimacing and the monologues that he would tend to go into that made it difficult for her to listen to him. The problems of this very troubled youngster and his family were quite complex, and the behavioral methods were just one small but extremely helpful aspect of the treatment. With practice, this child did learn to behave in ways that were more socially appropriate, both at home and at school.

Another problem of great concern to many parents is the difficulty a child may be having with his peers. They worry that other children do not like to come to visit or that play dates end in fights and tears. In my experience it is the issue of social rejection that, perhaps more than any other, stirs the most projection and consequent loss of differentiation between the parent and child. Painful experiences in their own childhood color perceptions of their child's social interactions, resulting in excessive concern and hypervigilance for signs of social rejection.

When a parent worries that a child is having social difficulties, it is important to ask questions that can lead to a more realistic assessment of the situation. What a parent may regard as excessive fighting or aggression may, for instance, be counterbalanced by other behaviors that children find attractive. A parent's admonishments that "other children won't like you if you behave that way" may not resonate with the actual experience of the child who correctly perceives that his peers are more tolerant than his parents believe. When parents are excessively sensitive to the quality of a child's social interactions, they tend to intervene too much in his conflicts with visiting friends and thus may be inadvertently interfering with the development of social problem-solving skills.

Generally, teachers are a particularly good source of information regarding the quality of a child's social interactions. If a child is lacking in expectable social skills, it is almost always noticed by the teacher. One should try to obtain as much detail as possible regarding the child's behavior and how she is regarded by classmates. For instance, some children who do not socialize are obviously *keeping* themselves apart. Teachers sometimes report that a child is exactly the type of youngster that other children are attracted to but that when approached, the child remains aloof. Or a teacher may observe that a child is "overeager" to make friends and that the "gifts" he gives are experienced by the other children as an attempt to buy friendship.

It should be noted, however, that although teachers may know that a child is not well liked and that, for instance, murmurs and giggles accompany his contributions in class, they frequently do *not* know the extent and nature of the teasing that might be taking place outside earshot.

When a child has severe difficulties with peers, he is most often best helped by participating in a social skills training group. Unfortunately, in many areas of the country these groups are hard to find. If no group is available, some social skills can be taught in individual sessions with the child.

Social rejection is so painful that many children develop rather strong defense mechanisms to ward off feeling terrible. Because of this, they may have trouble acknowledging or experiencing a need to learn new social skills. Often the child's guardedness is further increased by advice from parents which can be experienced (not incorrectly) as veiled "criticism." Because children can easily feel humiliated by a discussion of their social difficulties I have found it best not to talk about this topic in sessions that include other family members. When the topic is raised by a parent in a family session, I usually state that I know a number of ways to teach children how to have a better time with other kids but it is something that would be best for the child and I to talk about in an individual meeting. This statement, while ostensibly made to the parent, communicates to the child that there are solutions and things that he can learn that will help solve his problem. Having heard this, many children begin to open up about their problems, as it now seems worthwhile to do so.

Social skills can be taught both by role playing and by interacting with the child in a way that the very behavior his peers find negative. The latter method was used with Robby, age 6, who, through the course of therapy had become less oppositional but who still remained socially isolated. This little boy, who once had been highly defended, would now cry about children not liking him and having nobody with whom to play.

Robby, who suffered acutely from the fact that he had very little contact with his father, seemed to want to compensate for his feelings of deprivation by "winning" at everything he did. He turned noncompetitive activities into contests and had no interest in playing or doing anything with me that would not have a clear winner or loser. Thus, Robby and I played his favorite game, Chutes and Ladders, and he would squeal with glee when misfortune befell his opponent (me). Conversely, when he was winning he would be ecstatic with joy. Robby, so intent on winning, would cheat whenever possible. Although many children that age "cheat" and have an intense desire to win, Robby's behavior was excessive; his gloating felt cruel.

In approaching this pattern with Robby, I relied on a principle emphasized earlier in this chapter—that nobody behaves absolutely consistently and positive reinforcement of variations in the right direction can often result in the gradual shaping of more consistently positive behavior. Thus, after brief periods when Robby *was* playing in a more low-key way, I shared with him how much I liked playing with him when he acted that way. It also gave him—at times when he was *not* doing it—feedback regarding how it felt when he gloated, cheated, or seemed excessively pleased by his good fortune. To make the social skills training somewhat more comparable to actual play with peers, puppets were used in which my puppet initiated a competitive game and feedback (via my puppet) was given to Robby's puppet regarding how playing with him felt. This method can be effective when the child is motivated to change and, most important, when some of the underlying systemic and psychodynamic issues in which the behavior is rooted are also addressed.

Even when a child will not openly admit to having social difficulties, the therapist can use information he has obtained from parents and teachers to initiate difficult scenarios in puppet plays. Hannah, age 6, was frequently teased by her classmates. The teacher reported that Hannah's social behavior was quite inappropriate. She grimaced, did not look at children when she spoke, and touched and hovered too much when she wanted to interact. In puppet play with Hannah, it was possible to have puppets tell her what they found annoying. It was also possible to rehearse with her effective ways of responding if she was teased. As Hannah became more comfortable with talking about what happened in school, direct discussions about and role playing of social skills became possible.

Whenever possible, it is helpful to enlist parents in role-playing situations. This can be done, however, only when parents have achieved some emotional "objectivity" and can be helpful without feeling too pained or angered by the youngster's difficulties. Often, after some individual work with parents on what the child's behavior is evoking in them, they are able to assist the youngster in practicing social skills. Parents can also assist the child by arranging for the youngster to interact in a variety of social situations. When children are perceived negatively by their classmates, it can be difficult to change these perceptions even when the child is behaving differently. For this reason, it is important for the child to have a variety of social experiences in which to try out new skills. Enrolling the child in a class, sports league, or day camp with children who do not have preformed negative impressions enables the child to have some new experiences that can enhance his self-esteem and that in turn will change how he interacts with his classmates.

Relaxation Training

Often I supplement the more cognitive and interpersonal work with progressive relaxation. The child is taught to relax by paying attention to his breathing and progressively tightening, holding, and ultimately relaxing each muscle group. Young children enjoy trying to make themselves as relaxed as a floppy bunny or a Raggedy Ann doll. It is helpful for the child to have a quiet place and perhaps a special mat on which he routinely does relaxation exercises. The child can then use this technique when he is having trouble falling asleep, is overly excited, or is feeling anxious and unable to calm down. Teaching the child this method not only gives him a skill but communicates to the youngster that he can manage his own emotional states. Generally I introduce this technique in an individual session. This helps the child experience it as something that is his to use (or not use) when he wants rather than as a method of parental control.

SUMMARY

This chapter has described a variety of traditional behavioral approaches and some of the ways that they can be adapted to work with families and young children. It is hoped that readers will familiarize themselves further with the behavioral literature and find their own creative ways to utilize active problem-focused methods. Although I have described a variety of particular techniques, even more important for effective clinical functioning is the simple appreciation of the centrality of learning and behavioral change in work with families and children. As both children's and adults' ongoing interactions with other people play a crucial role in maintaining both psychodynamic and systemic structures and patterns (E. Wachtel & P. Wachtel, 1986), the behavioral dimension, far from being an alternative to psychodynamic or systemic work, is an inextricable feature *of* such work. It is not a matter of being behavioral *instead* of systemic but, rather, being behavioral *to be* systemic. When the reciprocal relationships among dynamic, behavioral, and systemic perspectives are appreciated, the therapist's ability to intervene creatively and comprehensively is greatly enhanced.

9

Pulling It All Together: Five Illustrative Case Studies

T hrough a detailed description of the work with five families, this chapter pulls together, summarizes, and reiterates the various points made in separate chapters of the book. In practice, the work with families proceeds along systemic, psychodynamic, and behavioral tracks simultaneously and these case studies are intended to illustrate how the strands are woven together.

As described in Chapter 1, the guiding principle behind the work is the belief that children's difficulties are multidetermined and that no one perspective sufficiently addresses the complexities of the child's difficulties. However, the cases described in this chapter vary in the weight given to any particular perspective. Thus, though in all cases the psychodynamic, systemic, and behavioral perspectives are used, a consideration in the selection of these particular cases was that they demonstrate how the relative balance given to any one of these outlooks will vary from situation to situation. In the case of Sara, for instance, interventions based on a psychodynamic understanding of her difficulties were most salient. On the other hand, with Mickey and his family the work centered primarily on cognitive-behavioral interventions. And with Mathew and his family, the primary interventions were systemic ones.

While the emphasis varies from case to case, the overall therapeutic strategy remains the same. As described in Chapter 1, the work proceeds on three fronts simultaneously. First, regardless of the reasons for the symptomatic behavior, the parent is encouraged to be clear with the youngster that certain ways of acting are acceptable and others are not. Behavioral interventions are used to encourage new behaviors and to discourage symptomatic ones. Often the child is given some individual help (e.g., role playing, cognitive strategies, and relaxation) to give him the skills needed to change entrenched problematic behavior. At the same time that the behavior is being dealt with directly in this way, the unconscious concerns that made the symptom necessary are also addressed. The types of interventions described in Chapter 7 are used to help the child own denied aspects of herself and resolve the unconscious conflicts that may be contributing to her difficulties. Third, the systemic issues surrounding the child's difficulties are also addressed. Work on marital conflict, hidden alliances, projection of aspects of self onto a child, and rigidly defined roles in the family are all a crucial part of the work.

It is important to note that although interventions can be thought of as deriving from a particular perspective, in fact there is a good deal of overlap between categories. Interventions of any sort, including those whose conceptual basis is behavioral or psychodynamic, for example, inevitably alter the family system as well. In general, the set of interventions is best understood not only as complementary but synergistic as well (Schacht, 1984). Fauber and Kendall (1992) have pointed out that when child-focused and family-focused interventions are used together, each is likely to enhance the effectiveness of the other. So too do interventions derived from different theoretical perspectives; one is not simply adding together behavioral and psychodynamic considerations but enhancing the power of each through an integrative approach (P. Wachtel, 1977).

Thus, for example, in the case of Jenny, the Play Baby technique not only addressed her particular psychodynamic conflicts but also enhanced the effectiveness of systemic interventions aimed at helping her give up the "parentified" role. Similarly, in this case as in many others, negative responses to unwelcome behavior on the part of the child had much more impact when the parent began to meet some of the child's unexpressed needs. In turn, the Play Baby method gained effectiveness because it was offered in the context of behavioral and systemic interventions as well.

In the case of Mathew, disengaging him from his role as parentified child enhanced the effectiveness of interventions aimed at addressing his unconscious conflicts around being "bad." Similarly, strengthening the relationship between his parents made it safer for him to become more comfortable with his own sexuality.

At the heart of this integration is a cyclical understanding of psychodynamic formulations that makes them compatible with systemic and behavioral perspectives (P. Wachtel, 1987, 1993). Unconscious conflicts, defenses, and fantasies are seen as both causing and caused by the child's interactions with others. It is the aim of generating synergistically interacting interventions that is the hallmark of the integrative work described in this volume.

JENNY: A DEPRESSED CHILD

Jenny, age 10, was having difficulty with her school work. A psychoeducational evaluation which had been done prior to seeking therapy indicated that although she had some mild learning disabilities, these were not sufficient to account for the problems she was having. Rather, her learning difficulties seemed to be primarily due to constrictedness and anxiety when confronted with challenging material. She was reported to have been cautious and inhibited in her response to the tester's questions. In addition Mrs. Mitchell, Jenny's mother, was quite concerned about the very negative statements Jenny had been making for quite some time. It was not uncommon for Jenny to say such things as, "I shouldn't have been born," "Life is too hard," "I have no energy to try it." She often got upset when getting dressed and cried about how ugly she was. An energetic career woman, Jenny's mother was worried about her daughter's mood and also found the youngster's low energy level and lack of enthusiasm for things quite hard to deal with.

The following case report demonstrates a relatively short-term (16 sessions over 6 months) integrative approach to the difficulties described above. The work consisted of four individual sessions with Jenny, four individual sessions with Mrs. Mitchell, two individual sessions with Mr. Mitchell, and six sessions that Jenny and one or both of her parents attended together.

Family Background

Mrs. Mitchell and her husband had been separated for 6 years (from the time Jenny was 4) but they had still not actually gotten a legal divorce. Although Mr. Mitchell's primary residence was in Europe, he would come to New York three or four times a year and reside with his father, who lived in an apartment next door to the one in which Jenny and her mother lived. At the time of the initial consultation, Jenny's father was expected to return permanently to New York within the next few months. He was described by Mrs. Mitchell as a brilliant man who had a position of some prominence in the foreign service but whose career and personal life continued to be seriously hampered by alcoholism. Mr. Mitchell had been involved in a serious relationship for a number of years, and Jenny would occasionally visit with her father and the woman with whom he lived. Recently that relationship had ended and Mrs. Mitchell was concerned that in returning to New York, Mr. Mitchell had hopes of renewing their failed marriage.

Mrs. Mitchell is a hard-working, highly responsible single parent who in addition to her job is active in church affairs and school functions. In the past year she had also assumed primary responsibility for the care of Mr. Mitchell's father, who had become increasingly senile.

In describing Jenny's early childhood, Mrs. Mitchell reported that she was an easy baby who could easily be comforted. The only "peculiarity" she had was that she would cry whenever a man other than her father came into the room. By the time she was in nursery school she had outgrown this fear and adjusted well to the male assistant teacher. Mrs. Mitchell related this early fear of men to the violent temper Jenny's father exhibited when he was drunk. Though he never hit, he did throw and break objects when arguments got very heated. Mrs. Mitchell said she doubted that Jenny had any memory of these arguments since they had occurred when she was around 3 years old and she had been in another room. By the time Jenny was 4, Mrs. Mitchell and her husband had separated, and even though she continues to have a good deal of contact with him, she now knows how to sidestep his hostility and avoids these kinds of explosions.

Meetings Alone with the Child

In my first meeting alone with Jenny, it was clear that she had a great desire to please me. She was cooperative to excess, and only with great encouragement would she voice a preference for one activity over another. As we talked, drew, and played projective games (over several sessions), a number of issues began to emerge. She expressed a good deal of concern about her grandfather, who she looked after some days after school. She recounted on several occasions a time when her grandfather was trapped in a locked apartment and Jenny could not get in to help him. Although it was clear that Jenny was a child who felt burdened by being responsible, it was not until further sessions with both her parents that I realized that Jenny's concern for her grandfather also reflected an identification with his helplessness and the "burden" he seemed to be to Jenny's mother. In a session held with Jenny and her mother, the youngster speculated about philosophical issues of morality; for example, whom should you save if in danger, the one you love the most or the one who has the greatest need for you. She wondered whether one was "good" if one took care of another person but did not love them and related this issue to her mother's care of her grandfather.

Jenny had a great need to be adored. She stated that she wished she had known her paternal uncle and grandmother (both deceased) since "they would have adored me." When talking about her father, she primarily emphasized how much he valued good grades and worried that he would not be happy with how she was doing in school. She also expressed concern that he drinks too much and that although he was going to be living next door, she probably would not get to see him as much as she wished.

Although Jenny could express criticism of her mother, it was quite difficult for her to say anything negative about her father. On one occasion, for instance, when Mr. Mitchell forgot to pick Jenny up from school and come with her to therapy, Jenny blamed herself for not calling him during the day to remind him.

Formulating a Multidimensional Hypothesis

Psychodynamic Issues

Jenny's constrictedness and depressed affect seemed to be related to a serious inhibition against the expression of aggression. When asked to draw the scariest thing she could think of, she drew a store stocked with kegs of some chemical which she labeled in the drawing "explosives" and a man with a gun holding up the storekeeper and threatening to shoot the kegs. She defended against her angry feelings by working hard to be "good to others" but nonetheless felt "bad." The worry that she was in fact bad was expressed in her negative self-image and in her seemingly intellectual interest in discussions of morality.

It also seemed that Jenny, who appeared to be a very mature and responsible youngster, had a strong wish to be babied. She would get "cranky" at night and when she got very upset about how she looked or the difficulty of her school work, she would sob to her mother and was soothed by being rocked on her mother's lap. Jenny worried a good deal about her senile grandfather, whom she described once as "like a baby."

It was also hypothesized that Jenny had repressed some traumatic memories of violence and that in order to maintain this repression she needed to ward off current perceptions of hostility and expressions of anger. Thus, for instance, when shown the Divorce Story Cards, Jenny interpreted a scene in which a couple was clearly arguing as one in which they were putting on a play.

Systemic Contributions to Difficulties

Jenny's difficulty with anger was a direct reflection of her mother's issues around the same topic. Mrs. Mitchell felt guilty about having "pushed out her husband." She felt that he was "sick" and that in some sense she had abandoned him. Though Mrs. Mitchell had some perspective on this, and joked that she had always wanted to be a "saint," her guilt was reflected in her commitment to personally devote herself to the care of her father-in-law (with almost no assistance from her ex-husband). She also worked hard to preserve Jenny's relationship with her father and would encourage Jenny to be understanding when she had been disappointed by her father's failure to live up to significant promises like attending her birthday party. Although Mrs. Mitchell could see that much of Mr. Mitchell's irresponsible behavior occurred even when he had not been drinking, she explained to Jenny that her father had a difficult childhood and was under great stress.

Setting boundaries was very difficult for Mrs. Mitchell. When her ex-husband was in New York for only brief periods of time she allowed him to come to her apartment whenever he liked and tiptoed around him to avoid provoking outbursts. Now that he had returned permanently, Mrs. Mitchell felt some pressure to come up with new rules since she did not want the intrusion on her privacy to go on indefinitely.

Mr. Mitchell also contributed to Jenny's inability to express anger. Though he was concerned about how unassertive the youngster was with her peers, and felt that she "let people walk all over her" and was "always too kind," he had little tolerance for assertiveness directed toward him. He complained that she had become "a little fresh lately." In talking about Jenny's childhood, he said he felt badly about the fights that he had had with Jenny's mother and that he sees that Jenny is overly concerned whenever he and her mother have the slightest disagreement. He minimized the seriousness of his problem with alcohol and refused to consider getting any help. On several occasions he came to a meeting at my office with a strong smell of liquor on his breath.

The Behavioral and Cognitive Dimensions

Jenny had received a lot of positive reinforcement for being a highly responsible youngster. In school and Sunday school she was often given responsibilities that she carried out assiduously. Teachers recognized that she needed this as a boost to her self-esteem, but being "good" and "mature" in this way inadvertently reinforced the very constrictedness which in large part was responsible for her academic and social difficulties. Both parents are proud—perhaps too proud—of how Jenny can be relied on.

When Jenny expresses criticism, she gets a strong negative response, which is aversive to her. For instance, when Jenny complained in a session about the need to go to her mother's office after school or the need to go supermarket shopping on the way home, Mrs. Mitchell responded with a reminder to the youngster of just how overworked and stretched to the limits *she* was feeling. And when Jenny criticized her father, she was more likely than not to get an angry response in return.

Jenny experienced all anger as potentially devastating. One could say that she had overgeneralized from early traumatic experiences with anger. Thus her fear of assertiveness was not simply based on the negative reactions she got from her parents when anger was expressed but also reflected excessive sensitivity to people being angry at her.

The other cognitive dimension of this child's difficulties was her overvaluation of academic achievement, which was linked in her mind to paternal approval. Jenny was quite creative. She wrote wonderful stories, loved music, and was a good dancer. None of these qualities, however, figured in her assessment of her self-worth, which was narrowly based on academic performance alone.

The Child's Contribution

It is always important to understand a child not just as a victim of a family system but as someone who in turn also contributes to the interactions. Therapists must try to ascertain the child's role in problematic interactions. When a clear sense of this is obtained it is often possible to use individual sessions with the youngster to playfully coach him in ways to surprise adults with unexpected behavior. Having a well-articulated sense of how the child participates in and even evokes dysfunctional systemic interactions also enables the therapist to coach parents in resisting the child's bait.

There were several ways in which Jenny actively, albeit unwittingly, participated in perpetuating a system that led to difficulties. First, it was noted that Jenny often volunteered to take on responsibilities even when they had not been asked of her. It was difficult for her overburdened mother to resist Jenny's offer of help for the care of her grandfather even when it seemed to be excessive.

Another way that Jenny contributed to the system was in the pleasure she took in being "good." She irritated her mother by having even higher moral standards than the mother herself had.

Perhaps the most important way that Jenny's actions played a part in establishing a family system that left the youngster feeling bad about herself was that she had learned to express some of her anger in indirect ways. Thus, instead of directly voicing criticism of her mother she punished her by moping around and whining. Criticism expressed in this way was dismissed or was responded to angrily. By whining and moping rather than confronting directly, Jenny contributed to interactions that made her feel that she was not being heard.

Interventions and Tasks

It has been my experience that approaching parents in as "collegial" a manner as possible results in the greatest cooperation and flexibility on their part. Explaining in detail one's understanding of the child's difficulties is particularly helpful in most cases. Thus it was explained to Mrs. Mitchell (and later to Jenny's father when he became involved in the treatment) that many of Jenny's difficulties stemmed from an excessive fear of anger and an attempt to ward off disturbing memories. Similarly, the youngster's conflicts around being "adult" and "responsible" were described. An explanation of the treatment strategies that follow from such an analysis helps parents accept "coaching" on how they each can be therapeutic to the child.

Interventions with Mother

The initial intervention involved Mrs. Mitchell's side of the interaction with her daughter. In order to make angry feelings more acceptable to Jenny, Mrs. Mitchell was given the task of noticing and telling Jenny about her own annoyed reactions to daily events that might otherwise go unnoticed. Some time was spent giving examples of the types of daily events that one might normally ignore but which now would be helpful to notice and mention. For instance, she might mention to Jenny something like, "I'm annoyed at my friend Sandra. She was supposed to call me back today but she didn't." She was also asked to express aloud some of her anger at Jenny's father so that she was no longer exclusively modeling "acceptance," "understanding," and "forgiveness."

Mrs. Mitchell was also asked to think of times in the past when she had negative feelings about someone she was *supposed* to love or like and felt guilty about it. She was asked to weave into her conversations with Jenny any memories of that type.

These interventions can be thought of in two ways; in addition to modeling the acceptability of negative feelings, it also made it more difficult for Jenny to defend against her own warded-off feelings because she was being confronted with the topic. Furthermore, doing this exercise "for Jenny" exposed Mrs. Mitchell to *her own* disowned negative feelings. In order to accept these feelings in Jenny, she had to become more comfortable with them in herself; being given permission and encouragement to feel these negative emotions was in fact therapeutic to them *both*.

An important aspect of the work entailed helping Mrs. Mitchell find a way to be sympathetic to Jenny when she was upset without simultaneously reinforcing the child's "falling apart." Prior to our discussions, Mrs. Mitchell would rock and comfort Jenny when Jenny would say very self-critical things about herself. The first step in changing this interaction was to convey to Jenny that her "little girl" self could be "babied" sometimes without having to fall apart. After explaining the Play Baby technique, the therapist asked Mrs. Mitchell to adapt this method to Jenny. Perhaps she could tell anecdotes about Jenny as a little girl or take out some of the youngster's cherished baby toys for them to look at together. Statements such as, "You're getting to be big, but in a way you'll always be my baby," are very reassuring to youngsters who are conflicted about their dependency needs. Mrs. Mitchell was encouraged to find ways to work similar statements into her conversations with Jenny.

The importance of *not* babying or "jollying" Jenny out of her crying jags was emphasized. Instead, the Play Baby method should be used when it would not be experienced as a response to emotional upset but rather as something that occurred even when she was her most mature and emotionally composed self. Breaking the cycle of reinforcement for self-loathing statements also involved encouraging Mrs. Mitchell to respond to Jenny's self-criticism with a statement on the order of, "I don't like when you talk that way. Please stop it!" Two weeks after these interventions were suggested, Mrs. Mitchell reported that Jenny seemed to be responding very well. She had calmed down considerably and even seemed to welcome being told to stop it. Often, being firm with a child in this way reinforces the child's own wish to gain self-control, and the external support helps buttress the youngster's own coping mechanisms.

Another important intervention with Mrs. Mitchell involved alerting her to how easily tempted she was to give Jenny more responsibility than Jenny could actually handle. She was encouraged to resist some of Jenny's requests for responsibility and was urged to find ways to relieve the youngster of some of the responsibilities she had assumed in regard to the care of her grandfather.

One session was spent alone with Mrs. Mitchell helping her become clearer about setting appropriate boundaries on Mr. Mitchell's visits. This was important because it modeled for Jenny the ability to sometimes say "no."

Interventions with Jenny

Though the primary goal of the meetings I had with Jenny was simply to get to know her better, some direct interventions were offered in these sessions as well. Latency-age children usually love to make lists, and Jenny was no exception. She was asked to make a list (which I would write down) of three things that she liked about each parent. Then she was asked to list three things that annoyed her about each of them. The aim of this was to legitimize that she could feel both positively and negatively simultaneously. Since negative feelings had been minimized between all members of the family as well, she was also asked to list three things that annoyed her father about her mother and vice versa.

Jenny was quite worried about the reaction she might get if she expressed displeasure at her parents, particularly her father. In sessions held with each parent and Jenny, the youngster was supported in expressing some of her feelings directly and was encouraged to discuss her fear of the reaction she would get.

Jenny needed help in being more assertive with peers as well. In an individual session, the therapist and Jenny role played being direct with a friend who had hurt her feelings.

We also discussed how Jenny volunteered to take on responsibilities and wondered together whether she might prefer to have less responsibility.

Interventions with Father

Though Mr. Mitchell refused to consider getting help for his drinking problem, he was eager to do what he could to assist in helping his daughter. He was concerned more about her timidity and lack of assertiveness than he was about her academic success. It was explained to him that Jenny might try out being more assertive *with him,* and that it would be helpful if he could respond to her beginning attempts at assertiveness with as much acceptance and lack of defensiveness as possible. In order to assist him in doing this, I predicted the difficulty that I thought might occur; many of Jenny's assertions would seem like unjust "complaints" to him, and it might be difficult to listen to them without getting angry in return. Although he felt he did not really need it, he did cooperate in doing role playing in which I played Jenny being "unreasonably" assertive and he practiced responding nondefensively and calmly.

Negative Reminiscing

It was explained to both parents that Jenny's constrictedness probably had its roots in her need to ward off memories of frightening events. Each parent was shown the picture Jenny had drawn (described earlier) of explosives. Both parents had dealt with the past in the same way—by not talking about it. They were each asked if they would be willing to have a session alone with Jenny in which they would help her recollect some of the scary events she had witnessed. Both were willing to do this, and we talked prior to the meeting about some of the events they would be describing. In the actual Negative Reminiscing session, Jenny was asked to recall in each parent's presence some of the fights she had witnessed. She had very sketchy memories in which the fighting was minimized. In each session Jenny's parents were encouraged to fill in some details of the events Jenny was describing. They also were encouraged to discuss some disturbing scenes Jenny had witnessed about which she seemed to have no conscious memory. In the session with her father, Jenny talked about remembering lying in bed with her hands over her ears to block out the noise. She remembered thinking that the house was shaking and being afraid that if they killed each other there would be no one to take care of her. Both Jenny and her father cried when these events were recounted.

In addition to helping Jenny recall some frightening events, the discussion reinforced for each parent the need to prevent these kind of occurrences from happening again. Although Mr. Mitchell continued to refuse to acknowledge his alcoholism (even when he would come to an early-afternoon appointment smelling of liquor) he did follow through on the plans and agreements made in sessions and more willingly accepted the new boundaries that Mrs. Mitchell had established.

Follow-Up

At the point that I stopped working with the family, Jenny's school work was improving and she seemed considerably less lethargic. She was beginning to spend more time with friends and had a regular once-a-week play date. She had not had a sobbing episode in months and rarely made self-critical statements. The school reported a noticeable change in her mood and felt that she was participating much more actively in class. discussions.

Mrs. Mitchell came in to see me 4 years later, when Jenny was 14 years old. She reported that until the past few months Jenny had been doing fine. Her academic work was good and she enjoyed a number of extracurricular activities. Mrs. Mitchell had remarried and Jenny got along well with her stepfather. Although Jenny continued to worry about her father (whose alcoholism had made normal functioning impossible), she seemed to have come to terms with it and knew that there was nothing she could do to help.

Mrs. Mitchell had consulted me because Jenny seemed to be having a hard time adjusting to high school. She had been used to a small supportive environment and was now in a rather large school in which she had to make new friends and get in on ongoing activities. Given Jenny's history of having been overly mature while wishing to be babied, I thought it would be useful for Mrs. Mitchell to actively intervene rather than letting Jenny work it out herself. I suggested that Mrs. Mitchell (with Jenny's knowledge) let the school psychologist and the teachers know that Jenny was feeling isolated and lonely. If they could invite her to join some activities this might ease the transition. Mrs. Mitchell called back a few weeks later to say that everything was going better and that she agreed with me that it was not necessary to work with Jenny. Giving Jenny a little assistance rather than accepting her initial protestations that she could handle things herself had a big impact and soon Jenny was once again able to handle things herself.

Conclusion

In working with Jenny and her parents it was important to devise strategies that would not only alter dysfunctional family patterns but would also address the child's fear of her angry feelings and dependency needs. Two interventions seemed particularly crucial. Playing Baby with Jenny and at the same time responding negatively rather than positively to her self-critical outbursts had an immediate impact, and within 2 weeks Jenny seemed much calmer. The other turning point in this brief therapy occurred in the 10th and 11th sessions (out of a total of 16) when Jenny engaged in Negative Reminiscing with each parent. These sessions interfered with her rigid defense against anger, and she was able after that to work on being more assertive.

MATHEW: A CHILD WHO HATED SCHOOL

Mathew, a mature, cooperative, and "good" 10-year-old (as his parents described him) had recently become "impossible to handle." Apparently, 3 weeks into the new school year he had become desperately unhappy about school. Although he had been going by bus for the past 2 years, he now refused to do so. Once in school, he would periodically start to cry quietly and whimper that he missed his mother and wanted to go home. Even visits to his younger sister's classroom or calls home could not console him. The situation was getting worse and worse, and Dr. and Mrs. Jones were being called to take their son home almost every day. By the time they came to see me, the Joneses were feeling hopeless. They had let Mathew stay home from school for the past week, and now Mathew would not leave his mother's side. He wanted no visitors and would not even visit the close friend who lived nearby for fear of missing his mother.

Family Background

Laura and William Jones had been married 10½ years. They had dated for several years but had not lived together before they were married because William could not decide whether he wanted to make a commitment to marry Laura. When Laura became pregnant with Mathew, William felt he had no choice but to propose. Both Laura and William came from rather strict Catholic families, and although at that time they regarded themselves as "secular" Catholics, they both felt strongly that it would be wrong for Laura to have an abortion. Laura stated that although she had not purposely become pregnant, it was probably a good thing because "William would probably never have been able to make up his mind." William grudgingly agreed with this statement, saying that he too was glad it had happened but he resented how "Laura always pushes me so that she gets just what she wants."

Three years later, the Joneses had another child, Claudia, now age 7. Claudia was described as being a bit wild and much more difficult than Mathew had been at that age. The children were very close, and Mathew was "a wonderful big brother" who really looked after his little sister.

When the Joneses met, William had finished medical school and was in the middle of a residency. He decided afterwards not to go into private practice but rather to work at a Veterans Administration (VA) hospital where he would be able to have reasonable hours and some time for research. Laura had been a nursery school teacher prior to their marriage but had not worked since Mathew was born. Much of her time was spent doing volunteer work for various church and community organizations. She had received a good deal of recognition for her ability to organize and mobilize people and both described their home as a hub of activity.

A Systemic Understanding of Mathew's Difficulties

In the first meeting with the whole family, it became clear that Mathew's behavior was mature beyond his years, and that he was perceived that way by his parents as well. He took a parental role with his sister, urging her, for instance, to "be quiet and listen" and saying to his mother in reference to his sister's whininess "I don't think she got enough sleep." The degree to which Mathew was encouraged to participate in major family decisions was dramatic. It was hard at first to register that the Joneses were not placating him but were in fact absolutely sincere when they stated that his opinion would be decisive on such major questions as whether Mr. Jones should take a job in another city or whether they should buy a new car. Since Laura and William often disagreed—William was far more conservative and preferred to leave things as they were rather than to make changes—Mathew was in a difficult spot.

There was a great deal of tension between William and Laura. William was quite overt in his complaints that his wife was like a bulldozer against whom he had no power. Although William admired his wife's exuberance and forcefulness, and admitted that he often ended up enjoying the family activities she had set in motion, he often felt that he was incapable of influencing, much less stopping, any plan she had set her mind to do. Feeling helpless and resentful, he would reluctantly submit to what he felt was a much too packed schedule and resented the constant presence of neighbors and guests.

Mrs. Jones in turn felt that her husband always said "no" to the slightest variation in his routine. She felt that he stayed at his job at the VA hospital not because it was really what he wanted to do but because he was fearful, anxious, and rigid. She felt resentful that he did not earn the kind of money that doctors normally earn and that they always had to scrimp and save. "Instead of appreciating how hard it is to do the things we do on his income he's always sullen and resentful and thinks I'm pushing him."

Mrs. Jones was also hurt by the fact that William almost never exhibited any affection to her, and she admitted with some embarrassment that she was jealous of the affection he lavished on their two children. Laura kept trying to win her husband's respect and affection by planning wonderful activities for the family, which she felt he would finally appreciate. Sadly, as is so often the case, her attempts to get what she wanted had the ironic consequence of alienating him still further.

In family meetings, it became clear that Dr. Jones tried to enlist Mathew in his battle against his wife's persistent pushing. He would cue Mathew to join him in laughing at and "tattling" to me about how intrusive and controlling Laura could be. There was a "we boys have to stick together" tone to much of what was said. Mathew seemed to be very much enmeshed in a relationship with his parents in contrast to his sister, who played off to the side and was not expected by either parent to participate in the discussion. She seemed to need very little attention and happily became quite absorbed in fantasy play as the three "adults" in the family talked.

From a systemic point of view, Mathew's current difficulties could be understood as both a rejection of the parentified child role—he was now acting like a little boy instead of a boy who was making the decisions that his father should be making—and, simultaneously, a way of doing battle for his father. Furthermore, his trouble with school had thrust his father into a more involved role in the family. Mathew would only go to school if brought there by his father and would stay only if his father actually brought him into the classroom and chatted with the teacher for a few minutes before leaving. Mathew was much more "stubborn" with his mother and she felt totally thwarted in her attempts to handle the school problem. It was as if the child and father were saying in unison, "for once *you* can't control everything."

The Behavioral Perspective

From a behavioral perspective each parent could be seen as rewarding and thereby encouraging Mathew's symptoms. William clearly took pride in his strong-willed son's absolute refusal to do what he did not want to do and communicated this pride to the child. Though agreeing that children had to go to school, William saw nothing wrong with his son's preferring to be at home than out visiting friends. Acting out of his own concerns about being pushed—and perhaps his own wish to be left alone—William took a strong stand regarding the importance of not pushing Mathew to do anything he did not want to do except attend school.

Laura also reinforced Mathew's withdrawal. She hated seeing him play alone after school (his sister was often on play dates at other children's homes) and to cheer him up she spent much more time than usual playing with him.

The Individual Perspective

Meetings alone with Mathew were used to gain an understanding of his school difficulties in individual as well as systemic terms. The aim was to discover what might be going on at school that made him uncomfortable. Knowledge of the systemic dynamics at home provided an initial focal point for exploration. Given the power struggles in the family and his role as a parentified child, it was important to get some detail about his relationships with his peers. It was also important to elicit his feelings about being regarded by both parents and school as unusually mature and responsible—he was a year ahead in school and many of the children in his class were considerably older than he.

Through drawings, stories, projective board games, and just straightforward talking, an understanding of what Mathew was upset and conflicted about was gained. In school, it seemed that Mathew experienced himself as being pushed too hard to be mature. He longed to be in the lower grade where not as much would be expected of him intellectually. This wish to be with younger children was also fed by Mathew's discomfort with the preadolescent behavior of some of his classmates. As some of the children in his class were as much as 2 years his senior, there was a lot of talk about sex with which he was very uncomfortable. Cursing, sexual innuendos, and simply "bad" behavior such as pushing ahead in line on the part of classmates upset him tremendously.

Mathew spoke about these occurrences in a highly moralistic manner. This moralistic stance was understood at least in part as a defense against his own aggressive urges. He very much thought of himself as and wanted to be a "good boy." Although his discomfort with sexuality was not atypical for his age, it did seem excessive, and one wondered how the family dynamics were contributing to this reaction.

Since the crisis, even when playing with children his own age, Mathew would feel waves of homesickness and wanted to be with his mother. When the visit was taking place in his own home, he became eager for the visit to end. As we discussed what exactly he was feeling in those situations, it became clear that Mathew often felt angry and powerless with friends who did not want to play the games he suggested. By doing some role plays with Matthew, it became evident that he tended to invite and create power struggles, which he then felt helpless to win. Mathew spoke of being "bored" with other children because they seemed to want only to hang around and watch television rather than actively play. It seems that Mathew was recapitulating with other children the power struggles that he was witnessing, and had become a party to, at home. He had learned poor social skills in regard to enlisting cooperation and resolving conflict.

It also became clear from the projective material that Mathew did not always feel as kindly and nurturant toward his little sister as his parents believed. He envied her "wildness" and what he regarded as her license to act babyishly.

Interventions

On the systemic level, the first intervention was to get Mathew's father to make clear to Mathew that from now on he would not seek him as an ally in his conflict with Mathew's mother. Making the conflicts between the parents more explicit and helping them keep this between themselves is of course standard family therapy procedure. This was accomplished by meeting with the couple alone after the family meeting in which this dynamic became apparent and discussing with them privately the ways in which Mathew was enlisted to be his father's support.

The benefit of first talking about this with the parents alone rather than in a family session was twofold. First, it avoided the risk of embarrassing the father in front of his children—to a man sensitive to power issues, to be "uncovered" as an instigator of Mathew's resistance to his mother's power could easily feel humiliating. Second, it provided an opportunity to discuss and explore in depth the various ways, often subtle, that Mathew was enlisted as an ally. A detailed understanding of just how this is done is important in order to ensure that any resolve to no longer do it will really be effective and will not just shift to more subtle forms of engaging Mathew in their conflict. For instance, in that session Laura complained that she felt like she had three children rather than two. She gave as an example the typical scenario when she called them all down to a meal. Claudia would generally come soon after called. William and Mathew however would continue playing a game together until at least 10 minutes after she had put the meal on the table. They both recognized that this was an instance of communicating to Mathew that he should not be too submissive to his mother.

Mathew's refusal to go to school or to socialize could be thought of, in part, as a "sit-down strike" in support of his father. And except for school, his father supported him in his wish not to have to do the activities that his mother was pushing on him. Although resolving their marital difficulties would take some time, they could get Mathew out of the middle of their conflict almost immediately.

Because Dr. Jones, although he clearly wanted help for Mathew, was very sensitive to being told what to do, it was quite important to leave it entirely up to him to figure out how he was going to communicate to Mathew that his support was no longer needed. He accomplished this rapidly (apparently by simply talking directly to Mathew about what had been happening) and the difference was apparent in the next family meeting.

The same approach was taken in regard to the way both parents encouraged Mathew to be an overly responsible parentified child and engaged him in decisions that gave him too great a sense of responsibility. It was explained that the sessions alone with Mathew had disclosed his longing to be just a little boy and that the conflict around his wish to be a baby and the sense that he was regarded and expected to be mature and responsible was contributing to his distress at school. We discussed the specific ways in which Matthew was thrust into an overly responsible role at home. Since this was so habitual it was important to give Dr. and Mrs. Jones many concrete examples of ways in which they could communicate to Mathew that *they*, not *he*, were responsible for important decisions and that they would take charge of Claudia when it was necessary.

Both parents recognized in this discussion that Claudia was quite peripheral in the family. Mrs. Jones had been looking to Mathew as a substitute "husband" and Dr. Jones had looked to him as an ally in guerrilla warfare. Meanwhile Claudia was cast into the role of the "difficult" one who did not seem to need either parent's involvement. Dr. Jones in particular felt that he did not have much of a relationship with his daughter and we talked about ways he could become closer to her.

Once Dr. Jones made it clear both that he did not need Mathew's help in doing battle with Mother and that he wanted the child to go to school without a fuss, Mathew was quite willing to take gradual steps toward overcoming the anxiety. This family had little experience in negotiating effectively, and the initial sessions were spent helping them plan the gradual steps Mathew would take toward tolerating the bus and school. For example, Dr. Jones agreed to take the boy to school for 1 week only, after which time Mathew agreed that he would once again take the bus.

Although there was clearly some systemic meaning to Mathew's withdrawal from school, it was also clear that he was feeling extremely anxious in the school environment. Thus, the initial interventions with Mathew involved giving him some ways to feel less anxious when he was overcome by a strong desire to go home. He liked the idea of carrying a picture of his family, which he could look at whenever he felt homesick. We also practiced some deep-breathing and relaxation techniques which he thought would be useful to do on the bus.

An intervention was designed that would reinforce his efforts at overcoming his anxiety and would at the same time address his unconscious longing to regress. If he got through the day in the classroom, he would be rewarded at the end of the day with some "young" play with his mother. Mathew was initially embarrassed by the suggestion that it would be good for him to play with something that he generally regarded as babyish (teddy bears, finger paints). It was clear from his response, however, that this prescription was tapping into unspoken desires and he, in fact, was enthusiastic about the prospect of these kinds of activities at the end of the day.

Feeling at a loss to know how to help this child, the school was quite receptive to advice and guidance. The administration agreed to let Mathew join the younger children in another classroom 1 hour a day for woodworking. The teacher also agreed to temporarily give Mathew alternative assignments rather than encouraging him to do the challenging work that he was, in fact, capable of doing. Along these same lines a suggestion was made that she say to him several times a day, "You're a little young for this so let me give you something more for your age." These interventions were aimed at Mathew's unspoken longing to be younger and less responsible.

Mathew's difficulties with other children were worked on in individual sessions with the therapist in which role playing was used to teach alternatives to power struggles. As the children he played with had already gotten into a set with Mathew in which they would, in fact, reject his suggestions, we talked about his initially joining in with what they suggested so as to change his part in the interpersonal system. After his joining with others, they would be more likely to be receptive to his wishes. We rehearsed some possible scenarios, including what he could do if his attempts at cooperation nonetheless failed.

Individual sessions were also used to help Mathew feel more comfortable with being "bad." He was asked to tell me curse words, and together we planned some "not nice" behavior he could do at home and in school. The parents and teacher were alerted to this and were asked to be supportive in this loosening up of Mathew's inhibitions.

The parents' assistance was elicited in helping Mathew be more comfortable with sexuality. They had always been very restrained in front of the children and were now encouraged to talk more openly about things being "sexy." We talked about whether they might be comfortable using some mildly "offensive" language in his presence and even to tell some off-color jokes if possible. Of course, as discussed in Chapter 7, this type of intervention often involves the parents talking about issues they are having trouble dealing with themselves. This suggestion, along with their understanding that the conflicts in their marriage were directly affecting their son, led the Joneses to decide that they really wanted to work on problems in their relationship. It was hard for them to show physical affection to one another in front of Mathew or to talk about things being sexy when they felt that there was so little affection, intimacy, and sex in their marriage.

Conclusion

Mathew was seen over the course of 4 months for a total of eight individual sessions interspersed between sessions with the whole family and sessions with just his parents. Within a few weeks of beginning therapy Mathew was taking the school bus and attending school for the whole day. This change can be attributed both to the fact that he was getting a clear message from his father that he was no longer needed in the marital battle and that both parents stopped reinforcing his withdrawal from the anxiety-producing situations at school. By working on social skills as well as Mathew's discomfort with being regarded as mature beyond his years, he gradually began to be more comfortable with children. His teacher reported that he seemed quite engaged and relaxed most of the time.

After Mathew's difficulties were largely resolved, William and Laura continued in couples therapy for an additional 10 months. During that time Laura decided to go back to work so that the money she would earn could be used for the "luxuries" William's salary could not provide. William overcame some of his resistance to change and even seemed "almost" excited about the prospect of moving to the suburbs. Laura slowed down the pace of the activities she still planned for the family and William sometimes seemed appreciative rather than resentful of her energy. They both felt that they were closer and sexual intimacy was now possible.

In a "checkup" visit 8 months later, they reported that Claudia had gradually become less difficult and was blossoming in school. Mathew continued to like school, had overnight visits with friends, and was now far from the "perfect" child he had been. William and Laura still struggled over many issues but they felt that their disagreements were resolved much more quickly.

JOHNNY: AN ENCOPRETIC 10-YEAR-OLD

Johnny, slightly built and extremely short for his age, made up in "toughness" and a "macho" demeanor what he lacked in stature. Although he generally liked school and was a conscientious student, he had always been mildly challenging of authority and engaged (in his parent's words) in "minor delinquent" acts. In the last few months, however, Johnny had developed a real hatred for his teacher. He believed that she was picking on him and treating him harshly for doing things that "everybody did." After weeks of saying to his parents such things as "you never believe me" or "you always take the adult side," he succeeded in getting them to pressure the school to transfer him to a new class. Now, in a new class, the complaints had begun again. The Sloans were concerned about how terribly upset Johnny got when he was questioned about his complaint that once again, he was being treated unfairly.

Recently, hidden in closets and cabinets, they had begun to find Johnny's underwear soiled with feces. Confronted with this, Johnny stated that he did not want to go to the bathroom in school. He confessed that he sometimes could not hold it in and defecated in his pants just as he reached home. His promises to stop doing this were to no avail and the Sloans came to therapy when they continued to find soiled underwear hidden throughout the house.

Family Background

The Sloan family currently consisted of Charles, age 50, Rita, age 40, Johnny, age 10, and Rich, Mr. Sloan's son from his first marriage, age 17. Rich had always spent a good deal of time with the Sloans but it was not until 2 years ago, when he was 15, that he and his sister Shelly, then age 21, moved in with them full time. At that time Rich and Shelly's mother had moved to California after getting a divorce from her second husband, and the two children decided they preferred to stay in New York. Shelly lived with the Sloans for 6 months until she completed college and then moved to California to be with her mother. The Sloans reported that those 6 months were very difficult largely because their living space was small. Having Rich with them, however, was not a problem since Johnny "adored" him and they were used to sharing a room during holidays.

Rich was described by the Sloans in our first meeting as "intense, introspective, and a loner." He had transferred into his current school at the age of 15 when he moved in with his father and stepmother and had only made one real friend who unfortunately had moved away this year. He participated in a number of after-school activities (orchestra, newspaper) but spent the remainder of his free time listening to music in his room or playing with Johnny.

Rich had seen his mother two or three times since she had moved to California 2 years ago. His relationship with his mother had always been difficult, and he seemed to have little interest in contact with her. He did, however, have a good deal of contact with his ex-stepfather, whom he liked a lot. Sometimes the Sloans and Rich's ex-stepfather would go out to dinner together. Although they were not friends, the relationship between the two families had been good, and the Sloans were upset when that marriage broke up. They fostered the continuing relationship between Rich and his ex-stepfather.

Mrs. Sloan worried a good deal about Rich and tried hard to get close to him. At times he did open up to her, and she felt that it was unfortunate that he would be going away to college just when he was beginning to bond with her.

Shelly was described as an outgoing young woman who was much closer to her mother than Rich was. Mrs. Sloan liked her, but they had never become close. She was relieved when Shelly moved to California.

Mr. and Mrs. Sloan had been married for 15 years. They reported that there had been a lot of tension between them until a few years ago when, through couples counseling, they had learned to be "more rational with one another." Mrs. Sloan recognized that one effect of their not very close relationship was that she and Johnny had "a lot of intense time together." She hated winters in New York, and Mr. Sloan, although he ran his own business, never could or wanted to take the breaks from his work that his business partners routinely took. Her solution was to take long winter vacations alone with Johnny, often keeping him out of school for a week or two beyond the official school vacation. She reported that they were incredibly close and that even now Johnny was much closer to her than he was to his father.

A lot had changed 2 years ago when Johnny entered the third grade. His half siblings Rich and Shelly had moved in and Rich's stay was permanent. Mrs. Sloan started working part time in her husband's business. And Mr. Sloan, perhaps because he and his wife had begun to get along better, was able to take some time off in the winter and the couple began to go away on long vacations while Johnny and Rich were looked after by their paternal grandmother, who would move in with them whenever the couple went away.

Recently, Mr. Sloan had encountered significant business difficulties. He had decided to let his partner buy him out and he was currently out of work and worried about long-term finances and what to do next.

A Psychodynamic Understanding of Johnny's Difficulties

In two individual meetings with Johnny, it became clear that he was worried about being a "wimp." Woven throughout the projective material he produced was the theme of "dorks," who having been victimized by bullies eventually get their revenge. Characters in his stories "clobbered" their enemies, "punched in the nose" tough guys, and built their muscles up so that they could take care of those who had harmed them. Throughout the conversation, Johnny made comments about the "sexiness" of girls. These remarks felt tacked on and inauthentic — intended primarily to prove to himself and others that he was more like a teenager than a mere young boy.

Using a pretend car speedometer as a gauge of feelings (see Chapter 4), Johnny positioned himself as feeling very unhappy most of the time. He stated that he was happiest when he got sick and was waited on. It seemed that Johnny was feeling powerless and unprotected. Asked to draw something frightening, he drew a boy being pushed off the top of the world trade center by a bully and a teacher on the ground who would not catch him because she disliked the soon to be "squashed" youngster.

A number of psychodynamic hypotheses emerged from the above data. When, as a result of couples counseling, Mr. and Mrs. Sloan became closer, Johnny may have felt dethroned. He was no longer his mother's little man and travel companion. Nor was he a "baby" who could easily miss school to accompany his mother on her trips. Johnny's wish for the "babying" he used to have could be seen in his statement that "being sick is the best time. You don't have to go to school and you get everything you want."

The transition to "little boy" status was made more difficult by the fact that Johnny's older half siblings moved in with the family just around the same time that Mr. and Mrs. Sloan began to travel together. Johnny had to cope with having an older brother who would tease and "outsmart" him as well as with the fact that his mother was giving a lot of attention to Rich in order to help Rich express "pent-up feelings."

Johnny's soiling his underpants could be understood in a number of different ways. It was both an expression of a wish to be a baby as well as an angry statement regarding his feelings about what was going on at home. The hidden feces could also be understood as a statement that there was a lot of hidden nastiness in the home (see later section on family system dynamics).

Battles with Johnny's teacher were understood as displaced confrontations with his mother, whom he felt was expecting too much of him and who was no longer his protector.

Johnny's need to be "macho" could be understood as a way he was trying to renounce his strong dependency needs. His concerns about being a wimp were understood as related both to his relationship with his older brother and to his father's gnawing worry that he had caved in to his partner's demands and had consequently gotten a bad deal.

The Systemic Perspective

In the initial family meeting that included just Johnny and his parents (Rich was away visiting his maternal grandmother), Johnny directed his parents in a role play of a scene at home. He played the part of the absent Rich, making a sarcastic and insulting comment toward Johnny (played by a large stuffed doll) as he entered the room. In the scene, Dad was asleep and Mom, though sitting in the room, barely looked up as Rich hurled insults at Johnny.

The role play became clearer when Johnny, rolling up a sheet of paper into a long cylinder, placed the "joint" in his mother's hand. With much embarrassment, the Sloans explained that Rita was often very tense and sometimes smoked marijuana to calm herself down.

With this scenario, Johnny made it clear that he believed neither parent noticed the level of hostility Rich was directing toward him. Further family meetings that included Rich revealed that other problematic interactions went unnoticed as well. Thus, for example, when the hostile bantering between Mr. Sloan and both boys was commented on, they all reported that this was much the way they always were together. "Put-downs" and "comebacks" were so much part of the modus operandi of the males in the family that the hostility involved in it was scarcely noticed. It seemed that Johnny was not the only one in the family concerned about acting "tough." The ability to withstand insults and to give them back seemed to be a way that all the males in the family demonstrated that they could "take it."

The systemic changes that occurred when Rich moved in 2 years earlier, and when Rita stopped relating to Johnny as her partner and turned instead to her husband, did not account for the immediate dramatic symptoms that Johnny was exhibiting. Thus, it was important to look for more recent changes in what was going on in the family. Family meetings revealed that Johnny had noticed that "Dad sleeps all the time." It seems that Charles was feeling rather depressed about his job situation, and both boys had observed that he just did not seem to care as much about their homework or even their fighting. Mrs. Sloan seemed to the boys to be more tense than usual, and she acknowledged that she had been smoking marijuana more frequently and would start earlier in the evening than she had done in years.

The atmosphere in Johnny's home was also being affected by the fact that Rich, who was in the process of applying to colleges, was also more tense. He felt he had not done so well on his Scholastic Aptitude Tests and was feeling enormous pressure to do better on his second trial. Rich was also in conflict about whether to apply to schools in areas nearer to where his mother had moved. As a result of these tensions, Rich had become increasingly difficult with Johnny and mocked him incessantly.

Johnny's symptoms had sounded an alarm. Like his barely hidden soiled underpants, depression, anxiety, and hostility occupied every corner of their home. Concern about Johnny had not only brought this all out in the open but also to some extent pushed Charles to refocus his attention on his sons.

The Behavioral Perspective

Although Johnny's difficulties with his teacher clearly had psychodynamic meaning, as expressed for example in his drawing of the teacher who would not save him, the problem was being furthered by the fact that it was in this situation that Johnny's mother once again gave him the support and protection he craved. By convincing the school to transfer him to a new class, Rita demonstrated her loyalty to her son and inadvertently made having difficulties in school a rewarding experience.

So too with Johnny's encopresis. Although it was best understood as a "statement," some problematic bowel habits had developed that had gained some measure of secondary autonomy from their original meaning. Johnny usually "let it out" after days of being constipated, and he now found sitting on the toilet frustrating and moving his bowels painful. Thus, even after the meaning of the encopresis had become apparent and was being worked on in family sessions, Johnny had difficulty establishing regular bowel habits and much to his chagrin, still would "explode" sometimes.

Interventions

As discussed earlier, Johnny revealed in the very first family meeting that both his parents were too "out of it" to notice that Rich was giving him a very hard time. Since one of the reasons for Johnny's symptoms was that upsets in the family were acted out (father slept a lot, mother smoked marijuana) rather than talked about, the aim of the initial family meetings was to help family members feel more comfortable talking about what bothered them. Thus, the first session focused on both the discomfort each felt in overtly talking about problems and, to a lesser extent, the actual content of what was worrying and bothering each person. It became clear to all of them that talking openly about one's worries did not feel safe because the family style was to tease and be teased, and this was hard to take when one was really feeling vulnerable. Almost immediately after the first meeting, Johnny's complaints about "not being listened to" by his teacher and parents subsided. Rich, who was very guarded in the session, began to talk a little more openly at home, particularly to Rita.

With some prodding, subsequent family meetings focused not on Johnny's presenting problems but rather on more general emotional issues such as fear of failure (a topic of particular relevance to Charles and to Rich who was applying to college) or on how each of the males coped with the fact that he was slightly built and far shorter than average, or on how Rita felt about the responsibilities of parenting. The boys were each encouraged to talk about how they felt when "insulted" by the other and about the pros and cons of their competitiveness. Some new rules regarding "nastiness" and teasing between the two boys were agreed on which would be enforced by the parents by not allowing the boys to spend time together if they heard them being nasty. Enforcement turned out to be quite unnecessary since the level of hostility in the family markedly decreased after just a few family sessions.

Two sessions were held with just Mr. and Mrs. Sloan. Rita expressed her resentment that Charles had withdrawn so much and that this had left her feeling like a single parent. He, in turn, felt that Rita was not dealing with the seriousness of his career problem and was not supportive. Two agreements arose out of these meetings. Mr. Sloan would take over the role of working with Johnny on his homework and Mrs. Sloan would seriously consider and talk over with her husband a move to the West Coast.

It was hypothesized that the recent tension between the couple had reawakened in Johnny the unconscious wish to be his mother's partner. Both his wish to be close to her and his need to separate were demonstrated in the arguments they would have over his homework. It was felt that Mr. Sloan's taking over of the homework would be helpful because it would remove Johnny from an overly dependent relationship with his mother. It was also suggested that being more openly demonstrative with one another in front of Johnny could be reassuring to Johnny in that it would help put to rest any fantasies he still had about taking his father's place.

Johnny's dependency yearnings, which he renounced by being "tough," were addressed in several ways. A part of one family meeting (the same meeting in which mocking had been discussed) was devoted to reminiscing about each boy as a baby and young child. The family was also asked to discuss just how each of them currently liked to be babied. The aim was to normalize and make more acceptable dependency needs for both Rich and Johnny. Rich was encouraged to talk about some of the things he remembered doing with his mother as well as with his father. Johnny's renunciation of dependency needs was exacerbated by the fact that Rich acted very "cool" about not seeing his mother and conveyed a sense that only "dweebs" cried and needed "Mommy."

In one of the separate meetings with the parents, they were advised to continue this normalizing of dependency needs at home. They decided, in this spirit, that this might be a good time to organize the family photos. Charles, at Rita's suggestion, agreed to contact his ex-wife so that he could obtain more photos of Rich as a young child. They were also encouraged to recount instances in their own life when they felt embarrassed about being dependent and afraid and perhaps covered such feelings up with a cool or "tough" facade.

An individual meeting with Rich focused on his relationship with his mother and whether he might choose a college near to where she lived. It became clear in our discussion that Rich regarded his leaving for college as a rather final leaving of his father's home and believed that he would then be "on his own." Rich was extremely guarded about discussing anything else but did acknowledge that he had been feeling tense and angry. He was more communicative in family meetings than he was in individual sessions and this brought home all the more clearly how difficult "being on his own" might be for him. A subsequent family session clarified everybody's expectations. Rich was concerned about whether he would be considered a "guest," as he had been before he moved in 2 years ago, or whether he would actually still be part of the family even though his main home would be at his college. Assurances were offered that wherever they lived he would be part of their family.

An individual session was held with Johnny to which he brought the new puppy the family had recently acquired. As he talked about the things that the puppy was still afraid of and how much the little dog needed to be held and petted, a soft tender side of Johnny emerged. We talked about whether, and how, he, like the puppy, could make it clearer when he too needed a little comforting.

In another individual session, Johnny indicated that he "wouldn't mind" getting some help with his problem about going to the bathroom. Although he had stopped soiling his underpants almost immediately after our family sessions began, he was having trouble getting back to regular bowel habits. He was very constipated and hated going to the bathroom. When he did have a bowel movement it was painful and increased his aversion to sitting on the toilet. He still would never go to the bathroom in school.

Johnny did not want to discuss this difficulty in a family meeting. Instead, Johnny and I planned a simple behavioral strategy to help him overcome his anxiety and then informed his parents of how they could participate. Like many boys his age, Johnny enjoyed charts and reward systems. After discussing with him what foods he could eat to increase his fiber intake, Johnny came up with a plan in which he would get a check if he sat on the toilet for 10 minutes after each meal and a star if he actually had a bowel movement. The most striking aspect of this intervention was that Johnny clearly enjoyed figuring out a solution. There was a feeling of mastery and competence in how he tackled the problem, much like the way he was training his puppy. Bowel difficulties were no longer being used as a way to express his need to be babied.

Termination

Therapy with the Sloans lasted for 4 months. During that time there were five family meetings, three meetings with the parents, four individual meetings with Johnny and one with Rich. Charles had been offered a new job in California, which he was interested in taking, and Rita agreed that she, Johnny, and Rich would move out there at the end of the school year, which was 3 months away. Johnny's teacher reported that he had made a good adjustment to the new class, and both parents felt it would not be fair to Johnny or to Rich to ask them to move at this point in the school year. Rich had made a decision to go to college in California, where he would be near his mother as well as his father.

Everybody in the family seemed to feel that there was less tension at home. Nonetheless, sarcastic repartee remained the dominant mode of communication and Johnny continued to assume a "macho" attitude when interacting with his friends or with Rich. Rita and Charles reported that their relationship was on the mend but by no means "perfect." Rita had given up smoking marijuana entirely. Charles no longer seemed depressed. The boys continued to fight, but the fighting seemed much less mean spirited. The whole family adored the new puppy and spent a lot of time together playing with her.

SARA: A CHILD WHO HATED HERSELF

Sara, a 4½-year-old, sturdy, poised, and outgoing little girl, was referred by her pediatrician because her mother, Mrs. Ryan, was greatly distressed by Sara's sudden outbursts of rage. For several weeks, this normally pleasant youngster (at least at home) had exhibited extremely erratic behavior. Suddenly, she would scream, "I don't need my mother!" and scowl, kick, and say "dirty" bathroom words. Sara's mother could not figure out what was triggering these episodes. They appeared to be unrelated to anything that had transpired between them. Mrs. Ryan was particularly disturbed by the mean things Sara would say (in her presence) to other children.

Background information provided by Sara's mother revealed that Sara had not spoken to her father for almost 2 months. The parents had separated 9 months earlier and in the fall, Sara's father had moved far away. Although he spoke occasionally with Mrs. Ryan, he never asked to speak with his daughter and Mrs. Ryan did not ask Sara to come to the telephone.

This absence of communication must have been particularly difficult for Sara, because, until the time of the separation, father and daughter had been unusually close. Despite her very negative feelings regarding her ex-husband, Sara's mother felt that he had been extremely attentive, albeit somewhat unpredictable. A charismatic character, Sara's father used to swoop in and out of the house, involving Sara in a swirl of exciting activity. Later sessions with the babysitter confirmed that Sara had seemed to be extremely attached to her father prior to the separation.

Both Sara's mother and her babysitter reported an event at age 2½ that they regarded as very significant in Sara's life. From the time Sara was 2 months old, when Mrs. Ryan resumed working full time, Mrs. Blake, the babysitter, took care of the baby all day and was regarded by the whole family as a much needed surrogate mother. For a variety of reasons, the most conscious one being financial, a decision was made when Sara was 2½ years old to send Sara to a playschool day-care program. Terribly distressed by the separation from her beloved babysitter, Sara cried inconsolably at night and in the morning. Continued contact with Mrs. Blake seemed not to help and finally a decision was made to sever all ties so that Sara could adjust to the change. After about 6 weeks, the crying stopped and Sara seemed to make a good adjustment to the day-care arrangement. She no longer talked about Mrs. Blake.

When Sara started nursery school, Mrs. Ryan was able to rehire Mrs. Blake. When I first started working with the family Mrs. Blake had been back in Sara's life for several months. She picked her up every day after school and stayed with her until Mrs. Ryan came home from work. They seemed to get along very well and there were no noticeable scars from the seemingly traumatic separation.

Initial Interventions

Mrs. Ryan was asked to describe how she handled the fact that Sara's father never called or visited. Both because she did not want to remind the youngster of her loss and because she wanted to protect the child from the intensity of her own negative feelings toward her ex-husband, Mrs. Ryan tried to avoid the subject of her ex-husband as much as possible. Neither Sara nor her mother brought up the subject of how it felt not to have Daddy involved in her life. Very concerned with not burdening Sara with her own problems, Mrs. Ryan also studiously avoided talking negatively about any aspect of her life. When upset about something she tried to keep her feelings to herself.

The combination of sympathy for the child and discomfort with negative feelings was also reflected in Mrs. Ryan's way of handling Sara on the occasions when she inexplicably exploded. She would engage in lengthy attempts to reason with Sara and found it extremely frustrating that despite Sara's verbal precocity, she could not influence the child with reason. Finally, when totally exasperated, she would walk away and the incident would stop.

As described in Chapter 2, the work almost always begins by my sharing with parents some tentative thoughts I have about the problems which have been described. With Mrs. Ryan I discussed the idea that Sara's outbursts of anger were probably connected to feelings she had about her father but did not feel able to express or even acknowledge to herself. In addition, she might be testing out whether she can be a "bad" girl and still retain her mother's love. In trying not to remind Sara of her loss by not talking about her ex-husband, Mrs. Ryan was inadvertently giving the child the message that it was wrong to talk about her father and any negative feelings she might have about him.

We also talked about the interpersonal consequences of Mrs. Ryan's attempts to be understanding, rather than firmly setting limits when Sara misbehaved. Her frustration and emotional withdrawal from Sara in a sense confirmed the child's worst fears (i.e., "If I'm not good, my mother will leave me.").

To deal with these issues, three specific suggestions were made.

1. Mrs. Ryan was to find ways to casually mention her ex-husband so that he was no longer a taboo subject. She was not to ask the child directly how she was feeling but simply to provide an opportunity for the little girl to talk about her father if she wanted to. Something as simple as, "Your Daddy used to have that kind of car," would do.

2. In order to reassure Sara that her negative feelings were acceptable and understandable, Mrs. Ryan was asked to tell the child stories from her own childhood in which she was jealous, angry, or misbehaving.

3. It was suggested, too, that Mrs. Ryan be firmer with Sara, making clear to her what behavior would not be accepted. Even though the child's outbursts were the result of emotional pain it was important to set clear limits. We discussed changing her tone of voice when telling Sara

that the way she was acting was not permissible. Time Out could also be used if necessary.

When Mrs. Ryan returned 2 weeks later, she reported that her relationship with Sara had greatly improved and Sara was no longer having inexplicable tantrums at home. As was hoped, Sara had begun to speak a little bit about her father and asked some questions about the breakup of the marriage. Relating stories from her childhood had been more difficult for Mrs. Ryan than she expected, and she did not follow through on that suggestion. She had, however, set limits, to which Sara responded well, and there were far fewer times that Mrs. Ryan became frustrated and withdrawn.

Although Sara was no longer difficult at home, either with her mother or her babysitter, school was still very much of a problem. The next intervention was to work with the teacher. With Mrs. Ryan's permission, I explained the probable source of the hostility Sara was displacing onto her classmates. Having felt frustrated and exasperated, the teacher had begun to feel hostile toward Sara and had had a difficult time avoiding power struggles. Explaining the problem to the teacher, asking for her observations, and enlisting her help through specific tasks helped to give the teacher the distance she needed to resist Sara's provocations.

The teacher was asked to give the child as much attention as possible when she was cooperating. She was told that pats on the head or a smile or kind word whenever Sara was doing what was expected of her, even for intervals as short as 5 minutes, would be helpful. It became apparent that in her own way the teacher too had been trying to hide her angry feelings about Sara's misbehavior. She was encouraged to be more open with Sara about feeling annoyed with her, just as she would be more open about the more positive feelings.

A Psychodynamic Understanding of Sara's Concerns and Conflicts

For the sake of conciseness, information obtained over several months and from three different people (mother, sitter, and teacher) will be condensed into one composite description of this child. With a child as young as Sara, it is important to use what one learns about the child from the reports of her statements and behaviors to formulate hypotheses regarding unconscious conflicts. Thus, I will begin by describing some of the information obtained that led to the psychodynamic formulations to be discussed shortly.

In addition to the sudden rages and nastiness Sara displayed to classmates, all three adults reported that Sara would be absolutely insistent that she was 10 or 12 years old rather than age 4. This was said with no humor or acknowledgement that it was a wish rather than a reality. If questioned about this, Sara would become angry and adamant.

After seeing the Walt Disney movie *Pollyanna,* Sara insisted that her name was Pollyanna and she would not respond to the name Sara. Contrary to my association to "pollyannish behavior," Sara clearly identified with the character of Pollyanna having hurt herself in a fall from a tree. Thus, at home, Sara would frequently play act that she had been in an accident and would improvise bandages, casts, and crutches. She insisted on her mother and sitter responding to her as if she really had been hurt.

Sara was so adamant about her name being Pollyanna that, to avoid a tantrum, the teacher finally started to call her Pollyanna and even listed her name that way on the board.

All three adults reported that Sara would, on occasion, say such things as, "I want to break my fingers all up" or, "I hate my body." These statements sometimes seemed to follow some frustrating experience (e.g., her attempt and inability to write in script), but often seemed to the adults in Sara's life to be "totally out of the blue."

When Sara's father began to call her almost daily, much of the time Sara would only speak gibberish and babytalk. Sometimes, she denied that it was her father who had called. After one conversation with her father, she lay down on the floor and screamed, "I don't want to live, I want to die! Can I eat poison to make myself die? Jesus died and he came back to life." After another conversation with her father, Sara angrily accused her mother of not being nice to him and making him leave.

Mrs. Ryan reported that Sara said, "I love you" to her a million times a day. On one occasion, she expressed concern for her mother's safety and wondered, "What if a bad stranger gets her?".

The babysitter said that on several occasions Sara expressed the opinion that a beetle had gotten inside her and that was what was making her "bad."

Daily, when Mrs. Ryan returned from work, Sara would demand to know whether a present had been brought for her and would get angry if she in fact did not receive anything.

Sara repeatedly stated that she hated school, even when the teacher reported that she seemed to be having a fine time.

For a number of weeks (toward the end of treatment) Sara shouted, quite randomly, "Dirty, dirty, dirty . . . " "Poo-poo," "Pissy," and so on.

Based on the events and conversations described above, the following hypotheses were formulated regarding the issues that Sara seemed to be struggling with.

1. Sara seemed to be very uncomfortable with the dependency inherent in being a small child. Her protestations that she was really 10 or 12 could be seen as her way of expressing her strong desire to be more in control of her life. Extreme frustration at her inability to do certain things that were well beyond her developmental capabilities and her insistence that she *could* do these things reflected the intensity of her discomfort at simply being a little girl and her wish to be powerful and in control.

2. Much of Sara's behavior seemed to indicate deep feelings of deprivation. Her rejection of dependency needs prevented her from asking directly for the reassurance and attention that she so sorely needed. By play-acting injuries, she could get (as did Pollyanna in the movie) the longed-for display of deep love. Similarly, her desire for a gift from mother as she returned from work was an indirect way of asking for some reassurance regarding her mother's love.

3. Angry feelings toward her father or mother were very frightening to Sara. Splitting of the "bad" and "good" Sara was apparent in her belief that a beetle had gotten inside her and was making her bad. Her wish to die after speaking to her father and her expression of hatred for her body can be seen as expressions of self-hatred when she has unacceptable feelings. Compulsive expressions of love for her mother and the concomitant concern that a bad stranger might hurt her are further indications of conflict over aggression that has been resolved by reaction formation.

4. "Will I still be loved if they (mother, father, and babysitter) know about my dark side?" Looking for an answer to this question seemed to be behind Sara's need to shout "dirty" and to use whatever expletives she could come up with in her still limited vocabulary.

Many of these hypotheses were explicitly confirmed in the individual sessions with Sara. For instance, in response to a story in which the therapist described being jealous, as a child, of her best friend's family, particularly her father, Sara asked:

SARA: Why didn't he play with you?
THERAPIST: I don't know. What do you think?
SARA: Maybe he didn't love you.

Then, in a tone of voice that seemed to the therapist like a pathetic attempt to grasp at straws, she said of her father, whom she had just heard from after 2 months of no contact, "My father loves me *so much* he's going to make me a tape and send it to me."

In many sessions Sara demonstrated both her tremendous desire to be a baby and her strong discomfort with that idea. For instance in one session Sara had dolls "poop" in their pants. She went on to claim that she too had just "pooped" in her pants but then stated that she was just joking and instead went to the bathroom.

Interventions and Tasks That Address the Child's Concerns

A number of Sara's concerns were addressed by interventions designed to influence specific intrapsychic conflicts.

Fear of Dependency and Need to Be in Control. The first intervention was to help Mrs. Ryan, *for Sara's sake,* be more accepting of her own dependency needs. She was encouraged to ask her parents for help despite her feeling that "I would rather die than ask for anything."

All the adults in Sara's life were asked to give this little girl as many choices as possible. Having had the experience of highly significant events just happening to her (e.g., the loss of her babysitter at age 2 and the loss of contact with her father), Sara, even more than most 4-year-olds, needed to feel that she had a say in things that affected her.

The Play Baby technique (see Chapter 7) was suggested as a way to address Sara's conflicts around her dependency wishes. As described in Chapter 7, it was important to make sure that Play Baby was used only at times that Sara was acting appropriately so that the gratification of the game would not inadvertently reinforce problematic behavior. In Sara's case it was particularly important not to Play Baby with her when she was pretending to be the injured Pollyanna, as this would reinforce disturbed behavior.

Feelings of Jealousy and Deprivation. Both Sara's mother and her babysitter were asked to tell Sara stories about being jealous or envious of friends and coming to terms with the feelings (see the Story-Telling technique in Chapter 7). It was suggested that these stories be about both past and current experiences. Thus, Mrs. Ryan might say about a friend, "I wish I could dance as well as she can, but I guess there are a lot of other things I can do well." This intervention was aimed at addressing Sara's concerns through the way her mother talked about herself.

Whenever Sara pretended to be the physically injured Pollyanna, everyone was instructed not to play this game with her. They were to say instead that they did not want to play this game because it was not fun even to pretend that Sara was hurt. Sara always responded well to this and dropped the game. Shortly after these events a game of Play Baby was initiated but with enough distance in time so, as described earlier, Sara would not be getting reinforcement for pretending to be hurt.

Demands for daily gifts were seen as a self-defeating attempt at asking for reassurance regarding her mother's concern for her when she was away at work. Because Mrs. Ryan found this very annoying, she was instructed to make clear to Sara that this was unacceptable behavior and to use Time Out if Sara persisted in the whining demand for presents. It was important, however, to combine this approach to Sara's behavior with comments that would address the child's underlying concern. It was suggested that soon after arriving home Mrs. Ryan should mention that she was thinking during the day about something Sara had said or done and had been eager to come home to see her. It was also suggested that the mother buy Sara a locket to take to school in which she would put a picture of her mother.

The Splitting Off of Angry Feelings and the Fear That She Will Not Be Loved if Her Dark Side Is Known. Both mother and babysitter were asked to tell stories about very angry feelings they had toward people that they also loved. They were to show their dark side as much as possible without "prettying it up" for public consumption. It was important that current "bad" feelings be expressed as well as experiences in the past. Sara was fascinated by stories about her mother's anger at her parents during adolescence. She also seemed very interested in hearing about times that the babysitter was irritated with her fiance.

When Sara obsessively repeated, "I love you, I love you," to her mother, Mrs. Ryan was not to say, "I love you, too." Instead, she was to say, "I know you love me but that doesn't mean you don't get angry at me sometimes."

In response to Sara's saying that she hated her body or wished to break her fingers, all the adults were to reply with the seeming nonsequitur "I know you feel very angry sometimes."

All the adults found it very annoying when Sara shouted and laughed, "Dirty," "Poo-poo," and so on. She was truly "offensive" in that when she was engaged in this behavior she kept everyone at a distance. It was impossible to talk to her because she was totally ignoring what was said and instead continued to talk in unpleasant gibberish. In response to this behavior, everyone was instructed to firmly let her know that they found it very annoying and that if she persisted she would be given a Time Out. They were also to say that they understood she was angry and that they were willing to hear about it in words but this form of expression was not permissible.

Conclusion

Though the work described here focused primarily on the identified patient, many noticeable and significant changes occurred in the system during the 6 months (23 sessions) of treatment.

Perhaps the most important change was that Mr. Ryan started to call every day at an agreed-upon time. This change can be attributed to both Sara's growing comfort with the expression of need (she requested the call) and Mrs. Ryan's encouragement of this contact.

When therapy first started, Mrs. Ryan expressed feeling burdened and resentful at having to raise Sara on her own. In sessions toward the end of treatment, she said instead that she felt lucky to have a child and felt sorry for her single friends who did not have children in their lives. This change probably reflected Mrs. Ryan's greater comfort in asking for help, as well as her growing ability to set limits without feeling guilty.

The teacher became very supportive of both the mother and the child. In feeling praised and supported by the therapist, the teacher was able to disengage from power struggles with Sara.

Sara became much more comfortable expressing her feelings. She was able to tell her mother that she wanted her Daddy back. Mrs. Ryan was able to tolerate hearing about these feelings. In general, Sara seemed more relaxed and happy.

Perhaps the greatest evidence of how Sara changed comes from the teacher's end-of-the-year report:

> Sara . . . has worked hard to come to terms with things this year. At circle time she is now a good listener and a ready participant. She has made so many happy steps: we believe she is pleased with herself, and thus calmer and more accepting of other classmates. We, too, are greatly pleased with her efforts. . . . Sara's intellect and loving nature have made her an endearing student. She has worked hard this year, gained confidence and made peace with herself. She is ready for the increased academic challenges in Kindergarten next fall and will be an interesting and lively student!

MICKEY: A BOY WITH A DANGEROUS TEMPER

Mickey, 7 years old, made his teachers and parents very anxious. Though a sweet and cooperative child a good deal of the time, he had a volcanic temper that transformed this slightly built youngster into a terrifying and truly dangerous force. It was hard to predict when his temper would erupt: When it did, he would strike back at those he felt had hurt him with all the power and lack of concern for consequences that out-of-control rage can produce. Prior to coming to therapy, Mickey, screaming and cursing, had pulled a bookcase over on a classmate, poked a child in the eye, bent another child's finger back so severely that a doctor needed to be consulted, and terrorized a group of older neighborhood children by wielding a bat until he cornered them.

Sometimes instead of lashing out, Mickey would simply withdraw when he was angry. According to his teacher, "a wall descends and he's simply not reachable" at those times. For as long as it lasted, Mickey would answer no questions and accept no physical comforting. Then, after about an hour or so, he would usually calm down and voluntarily rejoin his classmates.

Although Mickey did play with some of his classmates after school, his teacher reported that a number of parents were becoming increasingly apprehensive about the risks involved in inviting him over for play dates.

Academically, Mickey was having a good deal of difficulty. One year earlier he had been evaluated for learning disabilities and was found to have some significant problems with sequencing and retrieval of words. Mickey had been receiving twice a week tutoring with the hope that this extra help would enable him to remain in a regular class. He had made little progress, however and his reading and math levels remained considerably below those of his classmates. The tutor working with Mickey felt that his relative lack of improvement reflected a very resistant approach to learning. She described him as extremely averse to risk taking and reported that he simply would not try academic tasks that he believed he could not do.

Mickey was described by his parents, teacher, and tutor as having extreme responses to failure. If he tried to do something but did not succeed, he might rip up the sheet of paper he had been working on, break his pencil, or throw a book on the floor. Athletic accomplishment came easily to Mickey. He was advanced for his age at a number of sports. Yet even in this area he was extremely upset by failure. For instance, he might react to a fall when skating by cursing at himself and leaving the rink.

Mickey and his family were seen weekly over a 4-month period. When they stopped for the summer, Mickey had not had one rage reaction for the past 3 months, seemed much more relaxed, and not only read but had begun to really enjoy it. A follow-up report from the school in the fall indicated that he had begun to catch up considerably and was no longer a problem in the classroom. This case report will try to account for the dramatic improvement.

Family Background

Roger and Sally Walker, both age 50, had been teenage sweethearts who at the time they consulted me had been married for 28 years. They had tried for many years to have children and finally, after surgery, Sally became pregnant and gave birth to their first child when she was 39 years old. After 3 more years of trying and numerous medical interventions, Mickey was born. The difference in temperament between the two boys was obvious from the start. Kevin, physically much bigger and bulkier in stature than his slightly built younger brother, was described as friendly, relaxed, social, and open. Mickey, on the other hand, was cranky and difficult from the time he was a toddler. The difference in verbal ability between the two boys was great. Kevin spoke early and his speech was extremely clear and articulate by the time he was 3 years old. Mickey, on the other hand, said almost nothing until he was 2, and did not really speak in paragraphs until he was almost 4. Even now, at the age of 7½, Mickey had a good deal of difficulty expressing himself verbally. The boys differed too on how readily they expressed affection. Having had a snuggly first child, the Walkers were surprised and disturbed by how seldom Mickey seemed to want to be hugged or comforted. They could tell, however, that he was very attached to them because he had a hard time when they left him with a babysitter. In fact, when they were away overnight he would not speak to them on the telephone for fear that he would start to cry and be unable to "hold himself in."

The two brothers had what the parents called a "love–hate" relationship. They enjoyed roughhousing quite a bit, but often this would end in tears and violence. Overpowered by his much bigger and stronger older sibling, Mickey would resort to unfair tactics like biting and "hitting below the belt." However, although the fighting was intense, they never stayed mad at each other very long and Kevin seemed to admire what a "monster" his little brother could be.

The Walkers had grown up in the Midwest and lived there until a few years before Kevin was born. Roger was the youngest of four brothers who "fought all the time." Sally had two younger brothers who "were always kind to each other," and she was much more dismayed than her husband by the intensity of the fighting that occurred between her sons.

The couple moved to New York when Roger decided to go to law school, and at the time of the consultation he had become a rather successful criminal lawyer. Sally, who had been a nurse, had begun working part time when Mickey entered first grade.

The Walkers described their marriage as a very good one. As the work progressed it was clear that there were some tensions between them regarding the hours Roger worked and Sally's feeling that she carried too much responsibility and had become the family's drill sergeant. They described being each other's "best friend" but seldom spent any private time together since the children had been born.

Understanding the Systemic Context of Mickey's Difficulty with Anger

Both the family meetings and the sessions alone with Mickey's parents shed considerable light on important systemic aspects of Mickey's difficulties. It was clear that both Roger and Sally were very sympathetic to Mickey when he had outbursts. He had a way of being angry that made his parents and even his teachers aware that he was in fact suffering. Although both parents regarded Mickey as highly vulnerable, Roger particularly identified with his youngest son. He often felt angry at how Kevin and his friends "picked on little Mickey." Roger was quite concerned about the severity of Mickey's temper outside the home since he himself had seriously injured a classmate when he was growing up. He believed, however, that the way Mickey fought with his brother was "pretty typical" and though violent, was not nearly as rough as the fighting that he and his three older brothers engaged in when he was growing up. Sally acquiesced to her husband's judgment regarding the "normalcy" of the boys' fighting, stating that she did not feel qualified to judge since in her family *no* fighting was permissible.

Roger Walker described himself as someone who once had a terrible temper but who no longer loses control. He stated that he never forgot an injury and found some way, even if years later, to get back at those whom he felt had wronged him. He viewed himself as aggressive and highly competitive, but not at home. He had great sympathy for underdogs and would often take a case free of charge if he felt that an injustice was being done. Aware that he regarded Mickey as "weaker" than his brother, not only because he was younger but because he was more slightly built and not nearly as verbally adept, Roger struggled with the inclination to take the younger boy's side in disputes. He felt a good deal of pride in Mickey's ability to hold his own against his brother and other older children without much help from adults.

In various ways it became clear that Roger was experienced as "outside" the core family, which consisted of the two boys and their mother. He worked long hours during the week, and on weekends the family "understood" that when they were not visiting other families or having guests over, Dad needed time for himself. When the boys' fighting became intense he would be awakened by Sally to assist in settling them down. He would also be drawn in when the boys "tormented" their mother until she was in tears—a not infrequent occurrence.

The fighting between the boys was in contrast to the extremely amicable relationship between their parents. Despite the fact that Roger tended to be quite aggressive in his dealings with the rest of the world, both parents agreed that they seldom argued or got into power struggles.

It seemed possible that the boys were expressing in their fighting not only their desire to have more contact with their father but also the mother's unspoken unhappiness with the traditional roles that had evolved. Roger also seemed to be using the boys to express some hostility toward his wife. He chuckled at how impossible it was for Sally to control the boys and only when she collapsed in tears did he see their misbehavior and relentless teasing as being excessive.

Another quite common systemic dynamic was at work in this family. Older, "good" children often get great pleasure at the wildness of the younger more difficult sibling. At the same time that they are annoyed by how much the family revolves around the demands of a difficult younger child, they may also get vicarious pleasure in the uncontrollable child's provocations and confrontations. In this case, Kevin, like his father, laughed appreciatively at how Mickey had terrorized the neighborhood when wielding a bat. There was pride and admiration in what a "monster" Mickey could be, and Kevin enjoyed pushing the buttons that could get Mickey going.

Psychodynamic Considerations

My first contact with Mickey was in a family session that included both parents and Kevin. Mickey, in contrast to his parents and older brother, seemed extremely tense. In a barely audible voice, he would, answer questions in one or two words and then only when prodded by his mother. When I asked Mickey to tell me more about something he had said, Kevin would jump in with information long before Mickey could utter a word. Mickey did not seem to mind that Kevin would take over for him. In fact, he seemed quite relieved by it.

Even when there was "activity" in the family session instead of talking, Mickey was quite content to let Kevin take the lead. Asked to decide on a skit that would show a scene that happens at home, Kevin eagerly picked a scene and told everyone what they should be doing. Mickey seemed to enjoy the activity but said very little. Only when Kevin started "tackling" him did he really relax.

Not surprisingly, when I next met with him in an individual session he seemed even more tense and constricted than he had been previously. He complied with what I asked of him but clearly looked frightened and pained by being asked to talk. He answered questions in a guarded manner and the picture he drew of his family doing something was striking in how hard it was to actually see; he had chosen a piece of yellow paper and a yellow marker of almost the exact hue to draw with.

Similarly, his stories and Squiggle drawings were very simple and unelaborate. With encouragement he would tell a story that was an almost an exact duplicate, with only the slightest variations, of one that I had just told. His parroting of my stories seemed to be more a reflection of an assumption that he could not make up a story that would be any good than one of guardedness.

As the session progressed and Mickey was praised for his efforts, his body visibly relaxed. He spontaneously picked up an orange marker and added to his theretofore virtually invisible picture.

Detail obtained from talking with Mickey's teacher about his eruptions in school led me to conclude that his extreme aggression was in response to what he perceived as intentional attacks. He seemed to misread other children's behavior and frequently saw as an attack something that had clearly been accidental. The severity of Mickey's distortions were such that some time was spent in an individual meeting with him assessing his ability to distinguish reality from fantasy. It appeared that on reflection Mickey did realize that he had misperceived something. He could clearly distinguish his thoughts from external realities, and there were no indications of delusions or hallucinations.

Mickey's feelings of vulnerability were related to very low feelings of self-worth. A request to help me list some of the things that he was "pretty good" at was met with silence. When I mentioned things that I knew he did well, he assented with a quiet "I guess." The first picture Mickey drew (the yellow on yellow one) showed a boy entering his house having just found a $100 bill. He seemed to feel that being who he was just was not good enough.

The Behavioral Perspective

Mickey had been receiving a good deal of reinforcement both for his fierce temper and for his misinterpretation of slights and injuries. Both his mother and his father responded with sympathy to his upset rather than negatively to his outbursts. For instance, Roger reported on an incident that had happened when they were visiting another family with three children. Mickey exploded and withdrew from a game of Monkey in the Middle when a knotted up sock hit him in the face. He was in a rage that the other children, all of whom were older, were teasing him and would not let him catch the sock. As we have seen, Roger was very aware of injuries and identified with Mickey as an underdog. Thus, when he intervened it was to comfort his son and to offer assurances that he would deal with the older children who had behaved "meanly" to Mickey. This response not only communicated an acceptance of Mickey's dealing with upset through rage but further reinforced the youngster's perception that something *very* bad had actually been done to him.

Sally too inadvertently reinforced Mickey's overreactions. When Mickey acted out in fury she responded to the tears and obvious emotional pain of the youngster rather than to his anger. She would hug and stroke him until he calmed down and would only very mildly rebuke him for his out-of-control behavior.

Kevin's reaction was also reinforcing. When he had succeeded in provoking a rage reaction in his younger brother, Kevin would not strike back but would instead laugh with admiration at the fury of the "monster."

Even in school, where there was a good deal of concern about whether he could be worked with in a regular classroom, the immediate consequence of Mickey's outbursts was the attention of caring and worried adults. These responses were very understandable since it seemed inappropriate to be angry at a youngster who seemed liked he just could not help what he had done and whose emotional distress was palpable.

Interventions

Working with the Parents

In the second meeting alone with Mr. and Mrs. Walker I discussed my observations regarding Mickey's low self-esteem and feelings of vulnerability. In the course of "brainstorming" with the parents about the roots of these feelings (e.g., Mickey's learning disability and comparing himself to his older brother), it felt natural and nonaccusatory to discuss the ways in which each parent inadvertently reinforced Mickey's feelings of vulnerability by responding so much to his obvious hurt. It was also easy in this context to discuss how Roger, in particular, was reinforcing Mickey's excessive sensitivity to feeling "wronged."

A fundamental tenet of this work is that one does not simply ask parents to stop doing something without carefully planning with them alternative responses. Thus, we reviewed various situations that had already occurred and the types of situations that were likely to arise in the future, and together we formulated plans for responding in new ways. As we talked, Roger got in touch with his own wish at times to be more mellow and to let things roll off his back more easily. By focusing on instances in his own life when he had been able to be more "philosophical" and "nonreactive," Roger came up with some statements he could make in response to Mickey's complaints that might help Mickey shrug off "insults" a little better. For instance, instead of saying, "I'm going to yell at them for how they teased you," he could say something such as, "Don't let it bother you, they were only playing."

A statement like this would only be effective, of course, if Roger himself really could see the behavior of the other children as not so terrible or that an injury inflicted was in fact only an accident. This shift in perspective was possible because Roger's negative views derived largely from a protective feeling toward his son. Once he realized that angry statements at others was not helpful, Roger was able to get in touch with the other side of how he saw things, namely that aggressive play is "normal" and that "accidents happen."

It was explained that Mickey also needed to learn some cognitive strategies like "self-talk" to control his anger. Although this was something Mickey and I would work on in some individual sessions, the parents were asked to help in several ways. First, they needed to let their son know that "loss of temper," at others as well as at himself, would no longer be permitted. We discussed together exactly what was meant by loss of temper. I felt that it was important, for the time being, to include in loss of temper some things that might, at a later date when Mickey had more consistent control over his anger, not be considered unacceptable. It was explained that it was important to try to make Mickey's attempts at developing impulse control successful and if he was allowed to go too close to the line of loss of temper, he was likely to lose control. For example, behavior such as storming off in anger when he lost a game or mild cursing and punching his brother when they were play fighting might not normally be considered much of a problem. But to allow this behavior in Mickey while he was struggling with his temper might result in his throwing the bat *at* someone or punching his brother *too* hard. Both parents could easily relate to the idea that the more one lets go of one's temper, the harder it is to regain control. Together, Roger and Sally decided what they would allow and what they would consider unacceptable.

When Mickey did something in the category of loss of control, some negative consequence had to follow. This could be anything from not being allowed to play with his brother for the rest of the afternoon to not being allowed to watch television to having to immediately leave a play situation he was enjoying.

Another important behavioral intervention was to have the parents reward Mickey for maintaining self-control at moments when that was not easy for him to do. Before going to bed, Mickey and one of his parents would review the day and make a list of instances when the youngster had in fact controlled his temper. The parents would contribute to the list events that they had observed, and Mickey would add to it moments of the same sort at school. As Mickey accumulated points for self-control, he could redeem them for rewards.

Such an exercise serves many functions. It further emphasizes the seriousness of the parents wish for development of self-control. It rewards Mickey for his efforts. And finally, by labeling somewhat ambiguous situations as instances of self-control, Mickey is helped to change his self-image and to think of himself as a person who can handle difficult situations without losing his temper.

While Mickey was working on developing self-control, it was suggested that as much as possible his parents keep him away from situations that were difficult for him to handle calmly. Participation in Little

League, visits with families with older children, long play dates, or overnight visits with classmates should all be deferred until Mickey seemed better able to handle these potentially stressful situations. They were encouraged to resist Mickey's requests and assurances in regard to these activities. It was important to make absolutely clear to Mickey that the intent was not to punish him but rather to help him be successful at his attempts to gain self-control. Mickey was reassured that after a few weeks of practice, these activities would be gradually reintroduced.

Restrictions of these sorts not only enabled Mickey to have more of a sense of success but also increased his motivation to try hard to learn methods of self-control. If he in fact failed to control himself when these experiences were reintroduced, they would temporarily be deferred again. It must be emphasized that although this may seem harsh, it is occurring in the context of a great deal of attention to and rewards for self-control. The deprivation of temporarily not being able to engage in desired activities is mitigated by the youngster's pride in his success, and the comfort he feels by learning to be more mellow and less angry.

As is the case with most parents, the Walkers were willing to institute these behavioral methods because they understood that the deeper issues would be addressed too. They were concerned about Mickey's poor sense of self and the vulnerability that lay behind his overly aggressive responses. Simply training Mickey to control these feelings better would not suffice. Better behavior, though important to them, was not nearly as crucial as Mickey's really feeling better about himself.

It was explained that the first step toward this end would be to help Mickey understand that feelings of vulnerability were acceptable and even "normal," and thus they did not have to be defended against by being guarded, withdrawing from activities, or converting them into anger. The Story-Telling technique (see Chapter 7) as a way to address these issues was described to the Walkers, and a good part of a session was spent working with the Walkers on the types of stories it would be most useful for them to tell.

Roger recalled many instances when one of his older brothers would say something that made him feel foolish and babyish and in response he would attack back physically, like a "wild dog." Although this story had been told before, Roger had always previously put the emphasis on his *fierceness* rather than on how humiliated and stupid he felt in relation to his older brothers.

Sally talked about feeling very foolish and embarrassed by her poor athletic ability. She recalled some childhood events in which teachers took a lot of class time to get her to learn some basic physical skills (e.g., rope climbing and somersaults) that others had learned easily. She had felt great shame about the attention she needed and for years avoided learning the sports she now enjoyed. She also recalled feeling not quite as intelligent as one particular older brother and to this day tending to confine conversation with him to "light, superficial subjects" rather than feel overwhelmed by the breadth of his knowledge in comparison to her own. By talking about current feelings of embarrassment and vulnerability of this sort, Mickey's parents would be communicating that these feelings are something everybody has sometimes and that they are not "childish" and therefore necessary to disavow as an adult.

In order to sensitize the Walkers to even very minor feelings of vulnerability that they could discuss, it was helpful to review the types of situations that could evoke even brief moments of embarrassment. For instance, perhaps Sally felt a bit foolish about having to ask a salesperson something that she thought she should know (e.g., converting European sizes into American sizes). Or perhaps Roger felt foolish when, after asking directions, he was told that he was driving in the wrong direction. Or perhaps they felt shame for having ordered something from television that they "should have known" would be junk, or misspelling a word on a business memo and having a colleague circle and correct it, or going bowling for the first time in years and having many balls go down the gutter.

Whenever possible they were encouraged to include in the story something about their own defensive reaction when feelings of shame occurred, be it withdrawal or anger. Roger's story about becoming a wild dog when teased was a good example of linking feelings of vulnerability to reactions that ward off those feelings. Whereas Roger tended to fight when he felt shame, Sally was much more apt to withdraw. Mickey did both, and stories about these reactions could sensitize the youngster to his own defensive posture without making "interpretations."

Perfectionism

A family meeting was planned in which Roger and Sally would be asked to talk about times when each of them was upset about failing to live up to some self-imposed mental standard regarding the level of performance required for a particular task. A session alone with them was used to help them think through their feelings about standards and ways they coped with not being able to do everything really well. It was particularly important for them to become aware of the cognitive strategies they used so that doing something in a less than perfect way did not lead to intense self-criticism and private verbal abuse of themselves.

In the course of this discussion, Sally recognized how in recent years she had overcome inhibitions about participating in sports simply by telling herself that "it was just for fun" and she did not have to be very good in order to enjoy using her body and participating in family outings that involved athletics. Her wish to do things as a family had motivated her to overcome some perfectionistic tendencies.

Roger, on the other hand, did not have any cognitive strategies of this sort. In our discussion he recognized that he just did not do things unless he could do them really well. The process of becoming good at something often was "no fun at all," but he felt it was important to stick with things until he mastered them. Thus, Roger did have things he said to himself that enabled him to persist at things that he was not initially good at. He would say to himself for instance, "I've been through this before, and I know gradually I'll get better." When he was certain, in advance that he would "never be much good at this," he just did not bother to try. Thus, for example, he never would do anything involving arts and crafts. Nor would he watch on television or read anything about science since he was sure he would "be lost."

In a family meeting, the various facets of each parent's reactions to his own performance difficulties was opened up. Both Kevin and Mickey were encouraged to give their views on how Mom and Dad differed in how they handled not being very good at something. A discussion of each boy's way of dealing with that circumstance readily followed. The fact that some things that came easily to Kevin were difficult for Mickey was explicitly dealt with. Together the family decided that both parents' attitudes were useful. Some activities could be done "just for fun" without working too hard to become good at them. Other tasks required Dad's stick-to-itiveness, which was only possible if one could accept the inevitable feelings of frustration one encountered in the process of developing mastery.

The ideas developed in this family meeting were used to develop a task that would playfully "detoxify" the issue of perfectionism. Each family member agreed to try doing something that he or she believed they would definitely not do well. The aim was to help them all be more comfortable "making fools of themselves." An animated discussion ensued regarding what each person would have to try. Roger playfully groaned when the children decided that they wanted him to learn to cook. Mom, on the other hand, was required to learn to play some video games. Kevin, who "couldn't even carry a tune," would try learning to play the harmonica. And Mickey, who would never join in games that involved "a lot of words," agreed to try Kevin's word puzzle books and, with some modification of the rules, Junior Scrabble. It was up to each of them to decide what kind of cognitive strategy to use so as not to get frustrated. They could either label the activity as something they were doing, to use Mom's words, "just for fun," or could use Dad's approach, which was to remind oneself that "if I keep at it I'll get better."

The purpose of this exercise was both to put into practice what had been spoken about and also to help Mickey verbalize rather than act out some of his feelings. The problem of handling perfectionistic expectations, rather than being something that only Mickey had difficulty with, became a family project.

Working with Mickey to Develop Impulse Control

Individual sessions were used primarily to help Mickey develop methods of staying calm in situations in which he was apt to lose his temper. Mickey was quite highly motivated to work with me on this problem. He was clearly in a good deal of emotional pain when he had an outburst, and was as eager as his parents to prevent these occurrences. Furthermore, the interventions discussed earlier (e.g., rewarding him for self-control and removing him from high-stress situations) increased his motivation to solve this problem. We started simply by making a list of some of the things that happen that led to his losing his temper. The list included specific events that had already happened as well as types of situations that could occur in the future. By suggesting various situations that could be a problem for him, we were, together, able to come up with a fairly broad range of situations. The very act of making the list had some therapeutic value, as it alerted and somewhat desensitized Mickey to problem situations. Each time I asked Mickey to think about a situation that might be included on the list (e.g., "What if somebody calls you a jerk?" "What if one of Kevin's friends laughs at you for 'not getting it'?" "What if someone gives you a good hard push on purpose?" "What if you trip over someone's foot and you are not sure it's an accident?"), Mickey was having the experience of staying calm while imagining something he normally experienced as provocative.

Mickey was then taught Kendall's Stop and Think method (1992) in which the child is trained to define problems, think about various solutions, evaluate the probable consequences of each choice, and finally either to reward himself with a congratulatory self statement (e.g., "I did it right!") or, if he chose incorrectly, to use a coping statement (e.g., "On the next problem I'll slow down and concentrate."). Together we made a bright orange sign and wrote "Stop and Think" boldly on the front of it. Then Mickey was asked to think about what he could say to himself so that he would not explode. "I don't care what he thinks" seemed to work best in a number of situations. If actually hit by another child, he thought it would be best to say "you idiot," and tell the teacher. An important part of the Stop and Think method is teaching the child to praise himself for handling things well. Mickey and I talked about his saying something to himself like, "I did it! I stayed calm! I have to remember to put this on my list tonight!" If he did not stay calm it was important for him not to be demoralized by it but instead to say, "Next time I'll try harder."

Once strategies of this sort were developed, we began to practice them by my taking the part of the annoying or aggressive kids with whom he had to interact. As described in the previous chapter, role playing generally evokes quite vivid and real feelings despite the fact that at one level the child knows we are only pretending. After role playing a few of the situations on his list, we then did some *in vivo* practice. Having explained at the outset of our next activity (hitting a balloon back and forth to one another) that I was going to do something annoying to him, I intentionally stepped (not very hard) on Mickey's foot. Even though he had been prepared for this "assault," Mickey instinctively began to step on my foot but then stopped himself and said, "It's only a game and she didn't really hurt me."

In the next session, Kevin was included in Mickey's impulse control practice. Again, with advance notice, Mickey was going to try to stay calm even when Kevin and I behaved provocatively toward him. This time he was told that Kevin and I would hit a balloon back and forth and either not let him get it or hit it at him in an annoying way. In response to this Mickey sat down on the floor with a bag of miniature cars and proceeded to amuse himself and, interestingly, entice Kevin away from his game with me. To further strengthen Mickey's ability to be nonreactive, I asked Kevin to try to take away some of Mickey's model cars. As Kevin grabbed them, Mickey grabbed them back, but only with a minimum of force. As Kevin persisted, Mickey loudly said, "Stop it" but did not hit.

At this point, I stopped the play and enthusiastically congratulated Mickey on how well he had done. Again, it was important for him to think of himself as someone who could stay calm when he wanted to do so. Sally was invited in so that Mickey could show her how well he could do. Once again, Kevin was asked to behave provocatively. This time he hit Mickey in the face with a balloon and again Mickey handled the situation assertively but calmly—he loudly said, "Stop," and grabbed the balloon when Kevin kept doing it.

Systemic Interventions

Attempts to explore conflict between Roger and Sally proved to be futile. Even with gentle prodding, both insisted that they got along really well and did not accept that there might be a link between the boys' fighting and their own conflicts. Nor did they make much of the fact that Roger clearly thought that "up to a point" it was funny that the boys "tortured" their mother by being disobedient. Although Sally expressed some wish that her husband would not work as late as he did and would participate more with the boys, the dissatisfaction she expressed was of the mildest sort.

What the Walkers were more able to accept was that the relationship between the two boys, although very close, was also contributing to Mickey's rage and low self-esteem. In my sessions alone with Mickey, it became clear that he really experienced Kevin as not liking him. It was important for the parents to be less tolerant of the barbs and "playful" insults that Kevin directed at Mickey, as they appeared to be more wounding to Mickey than had been realized. The Walkers made it clear to both boys that squabbling and fighting so much would not be accepted. They carried through on a plan to not allow the boys to play together for some significant amount of time if they started fighting. Again, in order to help Mickey strengthen his ability to control his temper, the parents were encouraged to be rather strict about this prohibition. Given this clear message, Kevin's behavior toward Mickey changed dramatically, and it became clearer to both boys how much they wanted to be able to play together.

The Walkers were quite aware that Kevin overpowered Mickey with his far superior verbal ability. They had not, until receiving feedback on the family session, really registered just how much Kevin tended to answer for Mickey and how this contributed to the younger boy's feeling that he could not express himself. Kevin, of course, was not to blame for this. Mickey contributed to the interaction both by inviting Kevin to talk for him and by not protesting even when Kevin was in fact interrupting. Just as a reward system had been set up for Mickey regarding impulse control, Kevin would be rewarded for allowing Mickey to collect his thoughts and express his ideas. Each parent would try to notice during family conversations the times that Kevin waited patiently while Mickey made his own contribution to the discussion and these would be recorded on a reward chart.

An inadvertent systemic change took place as part of the plan to temporarily keep Mickey away from situations that might be overstimulating to him while he was in the process of developing impulse control. Both parents found that they enjoyed the somewhat quieter and less hectic weekends that resulted from this change. They were doing less visiting, had fewer guests, and were not on as tight a schedule because Mickey's organized sports had been temporarily eliminated from the family's agenda. Although they were all eager to get Mickey back into sports, they did discuss planning some more time that they would just have low-key time.

Summary

The Walkers were see for a total of 14 sessions which were divided as follows: Four were with the parents alone, three were with Mickey alone, one was with Kevin alone, four were with the whole family, one was with Mickey and Kevin, and one was with Sally alone.

Within 3 weeks of the Walkers' first visit, Mickey's mood and behavior began to change markedly. From that point on, the school reported no incidents of loss of control. Sally noticed that Mickey was easier to awaken in the morning and seemed much more relaxed getting ready for school. As competitive and stimulating activities were reintroduced, Mickey, having rehearsed and prepared in advance for potentially provocative situations, handled himself appropriately. At the time therapy was concluded the coach of Mickey's soccer team noted that Mickey "fussed now like any other kid." His teacher also noticed that Mickey was much more comfortable writing in his journal and did not seem nearly as pained when asked to participate in classroom discussions.

When Roger and Sally returned for a follow-up visit a few months later, they reported that both boys had had a good summer. Both parents felt that Mickey was generally much more self-confident. For instance, he would now sometimes sit with them when they had friends over and would participate in the conversation. He was doing his homework fairly independently and they could not think of a time when he had stormed off in frustration. During the summer, he had developed a number of new skills in day camp and did not withdraw from activities that did not come easily. The boys were spending less time together because Mickey had made a number of new friends and had begun to have overnight play dates.

Generally the atmosphere at home was calmer but the roles each parent played in the family remained fundamentally unchanged. The boys continued to be "difficult" with Sally and she continued to accept this as just the way boys are. On occasion, Roger would intervene and tell them to stop giving their Mom such a hard time, but neither parent regarded this scenario as much of a problem.

Although the cognitive-behavioral aspect of the interventions with Mickey and his family were certainly central, it is my belief that the parents' understanding of the psychodynamic issues underlying Mickey's behavior was a crucial piece of the work. The willingness of Roger and Sally to follow through on rather radical changes in what they rewarded and punished was based on their understanding of the interaction between the psychodynamic and the behavioral. Recognizing that Roger's "pride" in Mickey's fierceness or Sally's sensitivity to Mickey's vulnerability reinforced the beliefs and behaviors that contributed to Mickey's low self-esteem and high anxiety enabled the Walkers to feel much more comfortable with being "harder on him."

Roger and Sally made it clear that they were not interested in changing anything about their own relationship, but their willingness to work on doing things differently with the children was strong enough that it was highly effective without ever really addressing problematic issues in their relationship.

CONCLUSION

What enabled these rather dramatic changes to occur in the cases described here? Clearly it must be acknowledged that to some degree the cases were selected to illustrate how the process goes when it is working well. No therapist can guarantee that in every case everyone lives happily ever after. Nonetheless, I think that these case examples are reasonably illustrative of what happens when one works in the way that I am describing. The specifics of the cases differed, but in each I believe it was the synergistic effect of combining systemic, individual, and behavioral perspectives that enabled such significant changes to be achieved in a relatively brief time.

There is clearly a good deal that still remains to be developed in the child-in-family approach described here. I hope, however, that the reader has come away with a better sense of how viewing individual and systemic perspectives as complementary rather than antagonistic provides the therapist with new possibilities for helping children and their families.

Notes

CHAPTER ONE

1. Korner and Brown's (1990) study of 173 family therapists' beliefs and practices in regard to the inclusion of children in family sessions found that the tendency to exclude children and to work only with the adults was directly related to the amount of specific training with children therapists had received.

2. This phenomenon is not limited to parent–child interactions. Many theorists have written about the collusive defensive system that exists between marital partners in which they each carry psychic functions for the other (Bowen, 1978; Framo, 1981; Sager, 1978). For present purposes, however, I am focusing only on this process in regard to children.

3. Gurman and Kniskern (1981) do include a chapter on behavioral parent training in the *Handbook of Family Therapy* but comment as follows:

> Behavioral parent training (BPT) certainly has not evolved in the mainstream of family therapy and indeed, we think there are a number of family therapists who do not consider BPT to be a method of family therapy at all. Our view is that such a position derives both from a very narrow definition of what constitutes family therapy and from a good deal of ignorance about the premises and practices of BPT. Moreover, it is our experience that large numbers of family therapists, while owing primary allegiance to some other approach to treatment, selectively include parent training interventions in their work. (p. 517)

CHAPTER TWO

1. Kessler (1966), a child therapist, has pointed out that "parents are impressed by what 'you got' out of their child. . . . Intellectual abstractions are much less impressive than your ability to illuminate even some small aspect of their child's behavior" (p. 442).

2. Although it is important for the therapist to have detailed information about the child's symptoms, behaviors, and history, one must be careful that the child and his difficulties are not the main topic of the family sessions. Too much focus on the parents' concern about the symptomatic child can be humiliating to the youngster and can lead to pathologizing and scapegoating of the child by other family members.

CHAPTER THREE

1. The Talking, Feeling, and Doing Game was created by Richard Gardner (1973) and is available from Creative Therapeutics, Cresskill, New Jersey. It combines challenging and provocative questions with silly ones and is consistently a favorite among children and adults.

Scruples is a commercially available game in which moral and ethical dilemmas are posed. I combine the child and adult version and create simplified rules in which the parent and child are scored on their ability to guess correctly the answer the other will give.

My Two Homes is available through the Center for Applied Psychology, P.O. Box 1586, King of Prussia, Pennsylvania 19406. It has proven to be extremely useful in facilitating discussion of concerns and problems relating to divorce and separation.

Feeling Checkers (also available through Center for Applied Psychology) is just like regular checkers except that in order to take the captured checker one must say something about the feeling listed on the underside of the checker.

The Ungame (commercially available), like the Talking, Feeling, and Doing Game, provides an opportunity for talking about feelings and answering some questions that are more straightforward. It has the benefit of choosing cards that are geared to a specific age group but, as it is a commercially available game, its questions are somewhat less psychologically challenging.

Family Happenings, as well as My Ups and Downs, can also be obtained through the Center for Applied Psychology.

2. It is important to inquire whether the tolerance observed is representative of the way parents actually act at home. Sometimes the parent's acceptance of such behavior is an artifact of the therapy situation: The parent may be embarrassed to get angry at the child in front of the therapist because she thinks that the therapist believes parents should be permissive.

3. When there is suspicion of child abuse the therapist not experienced in such evaluations should have the youngster seen by a well-trained colleague.

4. Some parents have a strong need to pathologize a child. They dismiss observations about strengths as superficial and can feel angry at the therapist for not seeing the seriousness of the problem. This reaction is highly informative and is, of course, one of the things that must be worked on in the therapy.

CHAPTER FOUR

1. Violet Oaklander (1988), working from a Gestalt model, has numerous highly creative suggestions for how clay can be used to help constricted children become more comfortable with their body as well as for helping them release and talk about unexpressed anger.

2. It is interesting to note that writing for child analysts, Anna Freud cautions against underestimating the powerful influence of the environment on the child's symbolic play. Freud (1965) points out that in play

> [the child] communicates not only his internal fantasies; simultaneously it is his manner of communicating current family events, such as nightly intercourse between the parents, their marital quarrels and upsets, their frustrating and anxiety-arousing actions, their abnormalities and pathological expressions. The child analyst who interprets exclusively in terms of the inner world is in danger of missing out on his patient's reporting activity concerning his—at the time equally important—environmental circumstances. (p. 51)

CHAPTER FIVE

1. The notion of latency in young children is a questionable one. In psychoanalytic theory it refers to a period of assumed quiescence in which sexual drives are repressed. Clinical experience, however, points to more continuous psychosocial and sexual development and, perhaps because of greater exposure to sexual stimuli, there does not seem to be a developmental switch that turns off such impulses until adolescence. Thus, I use the term *latency* only to denote the ages between 6 and adolescence.

CHAPTER SIX

1. The reader interested in a comprehensive overview of the various schools of psychoanalytic thought and the implications for psychotherapy of these theoretical differences should consult the excellent chapter by Eagle and Wolitzky in the *History of Psychotherapy* (1992).

2. Fathers often do not seem to realize how important they are to their children. One wonders whether they are simply using denial or whether they have in a sense given the child to the parent who they are leaving as a substitute for themselves. And, of course, family dynamics may be such that the importance of the father has been minimized by the mother as well as the father. Whatever complex reasons exist, it is unfortunately true that many children have vastly changed contact with their fathers when a separation takes place.

3. See P. Wachtel (1993) for further discussion of the ways in which our diagnostic terms can be demeaning and counterproductive rather than helpful guides to conceptual clarity.

CHAPTER SEVEN

1. Violet Oaklander in her workshops on Gestalt methods with young children has made the same observations.

CHAPTER EIGHT

1. Although Haley (1976) explicitly distinguished his approach from a step-by-step deconditioning process and believes that "If family relationships are changed, the boy will be over the problem" (p. 227), his suggestion that the family adopt a puppy does, in fact, introduce an opportunity for highly effective *in vivo* desensitization.

2. Similarly, therapists can bring out more positive behavior in *parents* by noticing and affirming their steps in the right direction. Minuchin and Fishman (1981), in a session in which Minuchin asks a mother to take control in getting her two young daughters to play quietly in a corner of the room, keeps prodding the mother to "make it happen." After many delays and disruptions the girls play quietly for a few moments. Minuchin then comments, "You have been successful at this point" (p. 89). Minuchin states:

> The enactment of this situation finished with the mother being effective. Of course, this outcome is an artifact of punctuation. The therapist selects a moment at which the mother has been able, with his help, to organize the behavior of the two girls, and at this particular moment he declares the end of the enactment. The purpose of this strategy is to help the mother to experience herself as competent. . . . (p. 89)

3. There are a number of books written for parents which I frequently recommend. These include the following: *SOS! Help for Parents* (Clark, 1985); *How to Help Children with Common Problems* (Schaefer & Millman, 1988); *Toilet Training without Tears* (Schaefer & DiGeronimo, 1989); *When Your Child Is Afraid* (Schaefer & McCauley, 1988); *The Fears of Childhood* (Serafino, 1986); *The Difficult Child* (Turecki, 1985).

4. A good description of how to get a child to focus on the physiological aspects of feelings can be found in the chapter by Kendall et al. titled "Treating Anxiety Disorders in Children and Adolescents" in Kendall (1991).

5. The reader is again reminded that the behavioral work with Suzanne and her parents was only one aspect of a multifaceted approach that included attention to psychodynamic and systemic issues as well.

References

Ackerman, N. (1966). *Treating the troubled family*. New York: Basic Books.

Ackerman, N. (1970). Child participation in family therapy. *Family Process, 9*, 403–410.

Ainsworth, M. D. S., Blehar, M., Waters, E., & Wall, S. (1978). *Patterns of attachment*. Hillsdale, NJ: Erlbaum.

American Psychiatric Association. (1987). *Diagnostic and statistical manual of mental disorders* (3rd ed., rev.) (DSM-III-R). Washington, DC: Author.

Anderson, C., & Stewart, S. (1983). *Mastering resistance: A practical guide to family therapy*. New York: Guilford Press.

Barton, C., & Alexander, J. F. (1981). Functional family therapy. In A. Gurman & D. Kniskern (Eds.), *Handbook of family therapy* (pp. 403–443). New York: Brunner/Mazel.

Bell, R. Q. (1974). Contribution of human infants to caregiving and social interaction. In M. Lewis & L. A. Rosenblum (Eds.), *The effect of the infant on its caregiver* (pp. 1–19). New York: Wiley.

Benson, M. J., Schindler-Zimmerman, T., & Martin, D. (1991). Accessing children's perceptions of their family: Circular questioning revisited. *Journal of Marital and Family Therapy, 17*, 363–373.

Bergman, J. S. (1985). *Fishing for barracuda*. New York: Norton.

Bloch, D. A. (1976). Including the children in family therapy. In P. J. Guerin (Ed.), *Family therapy* (pp. 168–181). New York: Gardner Press.

Bloch, D. A., & LaPerriere, K. (1973). Techniques of family therapy: A conceptual frame. In D. A. Bloch (Ed.), *Techniques of family psychotherapy* (pp. 1–20). New York: Grune & Stratton.

Bogard, M. (1986). A feminist examination of family systems models of violence against women in the family. In J. C. Hansen & M. Ault-Riche (Eds.), *The family therapy collections: Women and family therapy* (pp. 34–50). Rockville, MD: Aspen.

Bogdan, J. (1986, July–August). Do families really need problems: Why I am not a functionalist. *Family Therapy Networker*, p. 30.

Boggiano, A. K., & Ruble, D. N. (1985). Children's responses to evaluative feedback. In R. Schwarzer (Ed.), *Self-related cognition in anxiety and motivation*. Hillsdale, NJ: Erlbaum.

Boszormenyi-Nagy, I., & Ulrich, D. (1981). Contextual family therapy. In A. Gurman & D. Kniskern (Eds.), *Handbook of family therapy* (pp. 159–186). New York: Brunner/Mazel.

Bowen, M. (1978). *Family therapy in clinical practice*. Northvale, NJ: Jason Aronson.

Bowlby, J. (1982). *Attachment*. New York: Basic Books. (Original work published 1969)

Braswell, L., & Kendall, P. C. (1987). Treating impulsive children via cognitive-behavioral therapy. In N. S. Jacobson (Ed.), *Psychotherapists in clinical practice: Cognitive and behavioral perspectives* (pp. 153–189). New York: Guilford Press.

Brett, D. (1986). *Annie stories*. New York: Workman.

Brody, S. (1964). Aims and methods in child psychotherapy. *Journal of the Academy of Child Psychiatry, 3,* 385–412.

Carter, C. A. (1987). Some indications for combining individual and family therapy. *American Journal of Family Therapy, 15,* 99–110.

Cassidy, J. (1988). Child–mother attachment and the self in six-year-olds. *Child Development, 59,* 121–134.

Chasin, R., & White, T. (1989). The child in family therapy: Guidelines for active engagement across the age span. In L. Combrinck-Graham (Ed.), *Children in family contexts: Perspectives on treatment* (pp. 5–24). New York: Guilford Press.

Chess, S., & Thomas, A. (1986). *Temperament in clinical practice*. New York: Guilford Press.

Chethik, M. (1979). The borderline child. In J. Noshpitz (Ed.), *Basic handbook of child psychiatry* (pp. 305–321). New York: Basic Books.

Chethik, M. (1989). *Techniques of child therapy: Psychodynamic strategies*. New York: Guilford Press.

Clark, L. (1985). *SOS! Help for parents*. Bowling Green, KY: Parents Press.

Combrinck-Graham, L. (1986). Preface. In L. Combrinck-Graham (Ed.), *Treating young children in family therapy* (pp. ix–x). Rockville, MD: Aspen.

Combrinck-Graham, L. (1989). Family models of childhood psychopathology. In L. Combrinck-Graham (Ed.), *Children in family contexts: Perspectives on treatment* (pp. 67–90). New York: Guilford Press.

Combrinck-Graham, L. (1991). On techniques with children in family therapy: How calculated should it be? *Journal of Marital and Family Therapy, 17,* 373–379.

Cottone, R. E., & Greenwell, R. J. (1992). Beyond linearity and circularity: Deconstructing social systems theory. *Journal of Marital and Family Therapy, 18,* 167–177.

Deci, E. I., & Ryan, R. M. (1985). *Intrinsic motivation and self-determination in human behavior*. New York: Plenum Press.

Dell, P. F. (1982). Beyond homeostasis: Toward a concept of coherence. *Family Process, 21,* 27–42.

Dell, P. F. (1986). In defense of lineal causality. *Family Process, 25,* 513–522.

deShazer, S. (1985). *Keys to solutions in brief therapy.* New York: Norton.

Diller, L. (1991, July–August). Not seen and not heard. *Family Therapy Networker,* p. 18.

Duhl, B., & Duhl, F. (1981). Integrative family therapy. In A. Gurman & D. Kniskern (Eds.), *Handbook of family therapy* (pp. 483–513). New York: Brunner/Mazel.

Duncan, B. L., & Parks, M. B. (1988). Integrating individual and systems approaches: Strategic–behavioral therapy. *Journal of Marital and Family Therapy 14,* 151–162.

Dunn, J., & Plomin, R. (1991). Why are siblings so different? The significance of differences in sibling experiences within the family. *Family Process, 30,* 271–284.

Eagle, M. N., & Wolitzky, D. L. (1992). Psychoanalytic theories of psychotherapy. In D. K. Freedheim, H. J. Freudenberger, J. W. Kessler, S. B. Messer, D. R. Peterson, H. H. Strupp, & P. L. Wachtel (Eds.), *History of psychotherapy* (pp. 109–158). Washington, DC: American Psychological Association.

Fairbairn, W. R. D. (1952). *Psychoanalytic studies of the personality.* London: Tavistock and Routledge & Kegan Paul.

Fauber, R. L., & Kendall, P. C. (1992). Children and families: Integrating the focus of interventions. *Journal of Psychotherapy Integration, 2,* 107–124.

Feldman, L. B. (1985). Integrative multi-level therapy: A comprehensive interpersonal and intrapsychic approach. *Journal of Marital and Family Therapy, 11,* 357–372.

Feldman, L. B. (1988). Integrating individual and family therapy in the treatment of symptomatic children and adolescents. *American Journal of Psychotherapy, 42,* 272–279.

Feldman, L. B. (1992). *Integrating individual and family therapy.* New York: Brunner/Mazel.

Ferreira, A. J. (1963). Family myth and homeostasis. *Archives of General Psychiatry, 9,* 457–473.

Fish, V. (1990). Introducing causality and power into family therapy theory: A correction to the systemic paradigm. *Journal of Marital and Family Therapy, 16,* 21–37.

Frame, C. L., Johnstone, B., & Giblin, M. S. (1988). Dysthymia. In M. Hersen & C. G. Last (Eds), *Child behavior therapy casebook* (pp. 71–83). New York: Plenum Press.

Framo, J. (1980). Foreword. In J. K. Pearce & L. J. Friedman (Eds.), *Family therapy: Combining psychodynamic and family systems approaches* (pp. vii–xi). New York: Grune & Stratton.

Framo, J. (1981). The integration of marital therapy with sessions with family of origin. In A. Gurman & D. Kniskern (Eds.), *Handbook of family therapy* (pp. 133–158). New York: Brunner/Mazel.

Friedman, L. J. (1978). Integrating psychoanalytic object-relations understanding with family systems intervention in couples therapy. In J. K. Pearce & L. J. Friedman (Eds.), *Family therapy: Combining psychodynamic and family systems approaches* (pp. 63–80). New York: Grune & Stratton.

Freud, A. (1946). *The ego and the mechanisms of defense.* New York: International Universities Press.

Freud, A. (1964). *The psychoanalytical treatment of children.* New York: Schocken.

Freud, A. (1965). *Normality and pathology in childhood.* New York: International Universities Press.

Freud, S. (1937). Analysis terminable and interminable. *Standard Edition, 23,* 216–253. London: Hogarth Press, 1964.

Gardner, R. A. (1971). *Therapeutic communication with children: The mutual storytelling technique.* Northvale, NJ: Jason Aronson.

Gardner, R. A. (1973). *The Talking, Feeling, and Doing Game.* Cresskill, NJ: Creative Therapeutics.

Gardner, R. A. (1985). *Separation anxiety disorder: Psychodynamics and psychotherapy.* Cresskill, NJ: Creative Therapeutics.

Gold, J. (1988). An integrative psychotherapeutic approach to psychological crisis of children and families. *Journal of Integrative and Ecletic Psychotherapy, 7,* 135–152.

Goldner, V. (1985). Feminism and family therapy. *Family Process, 24,* 31–47.

Goldner, V., Penn, P., Sheinberg, M., & Walker, G. (1990). Love and violence: Gender paradoxes in volatile attachments. *Family Process, 29,* 343–364.

Goodman, J. D., & Sours, J. A. (1967). *The Child Mental Status Examination.* New York: Basic Books.

Goolishian, H. A., & Anderson, H. (1992). Strategy and intervention versus nonintervention: A matter of theory. *Journal of Marital and Family Therapy, 18,* 5–15.

Gordon, S. B., & Davidson, N. (1981). Behavioral parent training in. In A. Gurman & D. Kniskern (Eds.), *Handbook of family therapy* (pp. 517–555). New York: Brunner/Mazel.

Guerin, P. J., Jr., & Gordon, E. M. (1986). Trees, triangles and temperament in the child-centered family. In H. C. Fishman & B. L. Rosman (Eds.), *Evolving models for family change: A volume in honor of Salvador Minuchin* (pp. 158–182). New York: Guilford Press.

Gurman, A. (1981). Integrative marital therapy: Toward the development of an interpersonal approach. In S. Budman (Ed.), *Forms of brief therapy.* New York: Guilford Press.

Gurman, A., & Kniskern, D. (Eds.). (1981). *Handbook of family therapy.* New York: Brunner/Mazel.

Haley, J. (1976). *Problem solving therapy.* San Francisco: Jossey-Bass.

Haley, J. (1979). *Leaving home: Therapy with disturbed young people.* New York: McGraw Hill.

Haley, J. (1986). Behavior modification and a family view of children. In H. C. Fishman & B. L. Rosman (Eds.), *Evolving models for family change: A volume in honor of Salvador Minuchin* (pp. 44–61). New York: Guilford Press.

Haley, J. (1987, March–April). Interview. *Family Therapy Networker,* p. 39.

Harter, S. (1983a). Cognitive–developmental considerations in the conduct of play therapy. In C. E. Schaefer & K. J. O'Connor (Eds.), *Handbook of play therapy* (pp. 89–127). New York: Wiley.

Harter, S. (1983b). Children's understanding of multiple emotions: A cognitive–developmental approach. In W. F. Overton (Ed.), *The relationship between social and cognitive development* (pp. 147–194). Hillsdale, NJ: Erlbaum.

Harter, S. (1986). Cognitive–developmental processes in the integration of concepts about emotions and the self. *Social Cognition, 4,* 119–151.

Hoffman, L. (1981). *Foundations of family therapy.* New York: Basic Books.

Hoffman, L. (1988, September–October). An interview with Lynn Hoffman. *Family Therapy Networker,* p. 56.

Hoffman, L. (1990). Constructing realities: An art of lenses. *Family Process, 29,* 1–12.

Hoffman, L. (1991). A reflexive stance for family therapy. *Journal of Strategic and Systemic Therapies, 10,* 30–38.

Holder, A., & Holder, E. (1978). *Bulletin of the Hamstead Clinic, 1,* 111–114.

Horney, K. (1945). *Our inner conflicts.* New York: Norton.

Imber-Black, E. (1986). Maybe "lineal causality" needs another defense lawyer: A feminist response to Dell. *Family Process, 25,* 523–527.

Irwin, E. C. (1983). The diagnostic and therapeutic use of pretend play. In C. E. Schaefer, & K. J. O'Connor (Eds.), *Handbook of play therapy* (pp. 148–173). New York: Wiley.

Isaacs, M. B., Monatalvo, B., & Abelsohn, D. (1986). *The difficult divorce: Therapy for children and families.* New York: Basic Books.

James, B. (1989). *Treating traumatized children: New insights and creative interventions.* Lexington, MA: Lexington Books.

Kagan, J. (1984). *The nature of the child.* New York: Basic Books.

Kaslow, N. J., & Racusin, G. R. (1990). Family therapy or child therapy: An open or shut case. *Journal of Family Psychology, 3,* 273–289.

Keith, D. V. (1986). Are children necessary in family therapy. In L. Combrinck-Graham (Ed.), *Treating young children in family therapy* (pp. 1–10). Rockville, MD: Aspen.

Keith, D. V., & Whitaker, C. A. (1981). Play therapy: A paradigm for work with families. *Journal of Marital and Family Therapy,* 243–254.

Kendall, P. C. (Ed.). (1991). *Child and adolescent therapy: Cognitive-behavioral procedures.* New York: Guilford Press.

Kendall, P. C. (1992). *Cognitive-behavior therapy for impulsive children: The manual* (2nd ed.). Philadelphia: Temple University Press.

Kernberg, O. (1975). *Borderline conditions and pathological narcissism.* Northvale, NJ: Jason Aronson.

Kernberg, P. (1983). Issues in the psychotherapy of borderline conditions in children. In S. K. Robson (Ed.), *The borderline child: Approaches to etiology, diagnosis and treatment.* New York: McGraw-Hill.

Kessler, J. W. (1966). *Psychopathology of childhood.* Englewood Cliffs, NJ: Prentice Hall.

Kestenbaum, C. J. (1983). The borderline child at risk for major psychiatric disorder in adult life. In S. K. Robson (Ed.), *The borderline child: Approaches to etiology, diagnosis and treatment.* New York: McGraw-Hill.

Kirschner, D. A., & Kirschner, S. (1986). *Comprehensive family therapy.* New York: Brunner/Mazel.

Korner, S. (1988). Family therapists and children: A case of neglect. *Psychotherapy in Private Practice, 6,* 101–113.

Korner, S., & Brown, G. (1990). Exclusion of children from family psychotherapy: Family therapists' beliefs and practices. *Journal of Family Psychology, 4,* 420–430.

Kramer, C. (1980). *Becoming a family therapist.* New York: Human Sciences Press.

Laing, R. D. (1965). Mystification, confusion and conflict. In I. Boszormenyi-Nagy & J. Framo (Eds.), *Intensive family therapy* (pp. 343–364). New York: Harper & Row.

Lebow, J. L. (1984). On the value of integrating approaches to family therapy. *Journal of Marital and Family Therapy, 10,* 127–138.

Lebow, J. L. (1987). Integrative family therapy: An overview. *Psychotherapy, 24,* 584–594.

Levy, D. M. (1955). Oppositional syndromes and opppositional behavior. In P. Hoch & J. Zubin (Eds.), *Psychopathology of childhood.* New York: International Universities Press.

Lewis, M., Feiring, C., McGuffog, C., & Jasher, J. (1984). Prediction of psychopathology in six-year-olds from early social relation. *Child Development, 55,* 123–126.

Lindblad-Goldberg, M. (1986). Elective mutism in families. In L. Combrinck-Graham (Ed.), *Treating young children in family therapy* (pp. 31–41). Rockville, MD: Aspen.

Lochman, J. E., White, K. J., & Wayland, K. K. (1991). Cognitive-behavioral assessment and treatment with aggressive children. In P. C. Kendall (Ed.), *Child and adolescent therapy: Cognitive-behavioral procedures* (pp. 25–65). New York: Guilford Press.

Luepnitz, D. A. (1988). *The family interpreted: Feminist theory in clinical practice* New York: Basic Books.

Madanes, C. (1980). Protection, paradox, and pretending. *Family Process, 19,* 73–85.

Madanes, C. (1984). *Behind the one-way mirror.* San Francisco: Jossey-Bass.

Madanes, C. (1986). Integrating ideas in family therapy with children. In H. C. Fishman & B. L. Rosman (Eds.), *Evolving models for family change: A volume in honor of Salvador Minuchin* (pp. 183–203). New York: Guilford Press.

Mahler, M., Pine, F., & Bergman, A. (1975). *The psychological birth of the human infant.* New York: Basic Books.

Main, M., Kaplan, N., & Cassidy, J. (1985). Security of attachment in infancy, childhood, and adulthood. In I. Bretherton & E. Waters (Eds.), Growing points in attachment theory and research. *SRCD Monographs, 49* (6, Serial No. 209).

Marks, I. M. (1969). *Fears and phobias.* New York: Academic Press.

McDermott, J. F., & Char, W. F. (1974). The undeclared war between child and family therapy. *Journal of the American Academy of Child Psychiatry, 13,* 422–426.

Meichenbaum, D. H., & Goodman, J. (1971). Training impulsive children to talk to themselves: A means of developing self-control. *Journal of Abnormal Psychology, 77,* 115–126.

Michelson, L., Sugai, D. P., Wood, R. P., & Kazdin, A. E. (1983). *Social skills assessment and training with children.* New York: Plenum Press.

Mills, J. C., & Crowley, R. J. (1986). *Therapeutic metaphors for the children and the child within.* New York: Brunner/Mazel.

Minuchin, P. (1985). Families and individual development: Provocations from the field of family therapy. *Child Development, 56,* 389–302.

Minuchin, P. (1988). Relationships within the family: A systems perspective on development. In R. A. Hinde & J. Stevenson-Hinde (Eds.), *Relationships within families: Mutual influences.* Oxford: Oxford University Press.

Minuchin, S. (1974). *Families and family therapy.* Cambridge, MA: Harvard University Press.

Minuchin, S., & Fishman, C. (1981). *Family therapy techniques.* Cambridge, MA: Harvard University Press.

Minuchin, S., Rosman, B., & Baker, L. (1978). *Psychosomatic families* Cambridge, MA: Harvard University Press.

Montalvo, B., & Haley, J. (1973). In defense of child therapy. *Family Process, 12,* 227–244.

Moultrup, D. (1981). Toward an integrated model of family therapy. *Clinical Social Work Journal, 9,* 111–125.

Moultrup, D. (1986). Integration: Coming of age. *Contemporary Family Therapy, 8,* 157–167.

Napier, A. Y., & Whitaker, C. A. (1978). *The family crucible.* New York: Harper & Row.

Nichols, M. (1987, March–April). The individual in the system. *Family Therapy Networker,* pp. 32–39.

Oaklander, V. (1986). *Helping children and adolescents to become self-nurturing* (Audiotape). Seattle, WA: Max Sound Tape Co.

Oaklander, V. (1988). *Windows to our children.* Highland, NY: Center for Gestalt Development.

Ollendick, T. H., & Cerny, J. A. (1981). *Clinical behavior therapy with children.* New York: Plenum Press.

Palazzoli, S., Cecchin, M., Prata, G., & Boscolo, L. (1978). *Paradox and counterparadox.* Northvale, NJ: Jason Aronson.

Papp, P. (1986). Letter to Salvador Minunchin. In H. C. Fishman & B. L. Rosman (Eds.), *Evolving models for family change: A volume in honor of Salvador Minuchin* (pp. 204–213). New York: Guilford Press.

Patterson, G. R. (1975). *Families: Application of social learning to family life.* Eugene, OR: Castalia.

Penn, P. (1982). Circular questioning. *Family Process, 21,* 267–281.

Penn, P. (1985). Feed-forward: Future questions, future maps. *Family Process, 24,* 299–310.

Penn, P., & Sheinberg, M. (1992). Stories and conversations. *Journal of Strategic and Systemic Therapies, 10,* 30–38.

Piaget, J. (1962a). *Play, dreams and imitation in childhood.* New York: Norton.

Piaget, J. (1962b). *The moral judgment of the child.* London: Kegan Paul.

Pine, F. (1974). On the concept "borderline" in children. *Psychoanalytic Study of the Child, 29,* 342–368.

Pine, F. (1985). *Developmental theory and clinical process.* New Haven, CT: Yale University Press.

Pinsof, W. M. (1981). Symptom/patient defocussing in family therapy. In A. S. Gurman (Ed.), *Questions and answers in the practice of family therapy.* New York: Brunner/Mazel.

Pinsof, W. M. (1983). Integrative problem-centered therapy: Toward the synthesis of family and individual psychotherapies. *Journal of Marital and Family Therapy, 9,* 19–36.

Redl, F. (1976). The oppositional child and the confronting adult: A mind to mind encounter. In J. E. Anthony & D. C. Gilpin (Eds.), *Three clinical faces of childhood* (pp. 41–50). New York: Spectrum.

Rehm, L. P., Gordon-Leventon, B., Ivens, C. (1987). Depression. In C. L. Frame & J. L. Matson (Eds.), *Handbook of assessment in childhood psychopathology: Applied issues in differential diagnosis and treatment evaluation.* New York: Plenum Press.

Reynolds, W. M. (1988). Major Depression. In M. Hersen & C. G. Last (Eds.), *Child behavior therapy casebook* (pp. 85–100). New York: Plenum Press.

Rosman, B. L. (1986). Developmental perspectives in family therapy. In H. C. Fishman & B. L. Rosman (Eds.), *Evolving models for family change: A volume in honor of Salvador Minuchin* (pp. 227–233). New York: Guilford Press.

Rutter, M. (1988). Depressive disorders. In M. Rutter, A. H. Tuma, & S. I. Lann (Eds.), *Assessment and diagnosis in child psychopathology* (pp. 347–376). New York Guilford Press.

Sager, C. (1978). *Marriage contracts and couples therapy.* New York: Harper & Row.

Sander, F. M. (1979). *Individual and family therapy: Towards an integration.* Northvale, NJ: Jason Aronson.

Sarnoff, C. A. (1976). *Latency.* Northvale, NJ: Jason Aronson.

Sarnoff, C. A. (1987). *Psychotherapeutic strategies in the latency years.* Northvale, NJ: Jason Aronson.

Satir, V. (1964). *Conjoint family therapy.* Palo Alto: Science & Behavior Books.

Schacht, T. E. (1984). The varieties of integrative experience. In H. Arkowitz & S. B. Messer (Eds.), *Psychoanalytic therapy and behavior therapy: Is integration possible?* (pp. 107–131). New York: Plenum Press.

Schachter, R., & MaCauley, C. S. (1988). *When your child is afraid.* New York: Simon & Schuster.

Schaefer, C. E., & DiGeronimo, T. F. (1989). *Toilet training without tears.* New York: Signet.

Schaefer, C. E., & Millman, H. L. (1988). *How to help children with common problems.* New York: Signet.

Scharff, D., & Scharff, J. (1987). *Object relations family therapy.* Northvale, NJ: Jason Aronson.

Scheflen, A. E. (1978). Susan smiled: On explanation in family therapy. *Family Process, 17,* 59–68.

Schwartz, R. (1987, March–April). Our multiple selves. *Family Therapy Networker,* p. 24.

Serafino, E. P. (1986). *The fears of childhood.* New York: Human Sciences Press.

Shapiro, L. E., & Thiobdeau, M. (1987). *The Divorce Story Cards.* Philadelphia, PA: Center for Applied Psychology.

Shapiro, T. (1983). The borderline syndrome in children. In S. K. Robson (Ed.), *The borderline child: Approaches to etiology, diagnosis and treatment.* New York: McGraw-Hill.

Sheinberg, M. (1992). Navigating treatment impasses at the disclosure of incest: Combining ideas from feminism and social constructivism. *Family Process, 31,* 201–216.

Shelov, S., & Kelly, J. (1991). *Raising your Type A child.* New York: Pocket Books.

Sider, R. C. (1984, March). The ethics of therapeutic modality choice. *American Journal of Psychiatry, 141,* 390–394.

Simmons, J. E. (1987). *Psychiatric examination of children.* Philadelphia: Lea & Febiger.

Singer, J. (1975). *The inner world of daydreaming.* New York: Harper & Row.

Skynner, R. (1981). An open-systems, group analytic approach to family therapy. In A. Gurman & D. Kniskern (Eds.), *Handbook of family therapy* (pp. 39–84). New York: Brunner/Mazel.

Slipp, S. (1984). *Object relations: A dynamic bridge between individual and family treatment.* Northvale, NJ: Jason Aronson.

Sroufe, L. A. (1988). The role of infant–caregiver attachment in development. In J. Belsky & T. Nesworski (Eds.), *Clinical aspects of attachment.* Hillsdale, NJ: Erlbaum.

Stern, D. N. (1985). *The interpersonal world of the infant.* New York: Basic Books.

Stierlin, H. (1977). *Psychoanalysis and family therapy.* Northvale, NJ: Jason Aronson.

Sullivan, H. S. (1953). *The interpersonal theory of psychiatry.* New York: Norton.

Tomm, K. (1987). Interventive interviewing: Part I. Strategizing as a fourth guideline for the therapist. *Family Process, 26,* 3–13.

Tomm, K. (1987). Interventive interviewing: Part II. Reflexive questioning as a means to enable self-healing. *Family Process, 26,* 167–183.

Tomm, K. (1988). Interventive interviewing: Part III. Intending to ask circular, strategic or reflexive questions? *Family Process, 26,* 3–15.

Turecki, S. (1985). *The difficult child.* New York: Bantam.

Vela, M. R., Gottlieb, E. H., Gottlieb, H. P. (1983). Borderline syndromes in childhood: A critical review. In S. K. Robson (Ed.), *The borderline child: Approaches to etiology, diagnosis and treatment.* New York: McGraw-Hill.

Wachtel, E. F. (1979). Learning family therapy: The dilemmas of an individual therapist. *Journal of Contemporary Psychotherapy, 10,* 122–135.

Wachtel, E. F. (1987). Family systems and the individual child. *Journal of Marital and Family Therapy, 13,* 15–25.

Wachtel, E. F. (1990). The child as an individual: A resource for systemic change. *Journal of Strategic and Systemic Therapies, 9,* 50–59.

Wachtel, E. F. (1992). An integrative approach to working with troubled children and their families. *Journal of Psychotherapy Integration, 2,* 207–224.

Wachtel, E. F. (1993). Postscript: Therapeutic communication with couples. In P. Wachtel, *Therapeutic communication: Principles and effective practice* (pp. 273–293). New York: Guilford Press.

Wachtel, E. F., & Wachtel, P. L. (1986). *Family dynamics in individual psychotherapy: A guide to clinical strategies.* New York: Guilford Press.

Wachtel, P. L. (1977). *Psychoanalysis and behavior therapy: Toward an integration.* New York: Basic Books.

Wachtel, P. L. (1987). *Action and insight.* New York: Guilford Press.

Wachtel, P. L. (1989). *The poverty of affluence.* Philadelphia: New Society Publishers.

Wachtel, P. L. (1993). *Therapeutic communication: Principles and effective practice.* New York: Guilford Press.

Waters, D., & Lawrence, E. C. (1993). *Competence, courage and change.* New York: Norton.

Wynne, L. C. (1986). Structure and lineality in family therapy. In H. C. Fishman & B. L. Rosman (Eds.), *Evolving models for family change: A volume in honor of Salvador Minuchin* (pp. 251–260). New York: Guilford Press.

Willock, B. (1983). Play therapy with the aggressive, acting out child. In C. E. Schaefer & K. J. O'Connor (Eds.), *Handbook of play therapy* (pp. 387–412). New York: Wiley.

Wilson, G. T., & Davison, G. C. (1971). Processes of fear reduction in systematic desensitization: Animal studies. *Psychological Bulletin, 76,* 1–14.

Winnicott, D. W. (1965). *The maturational process and the facilitating environment.* New York: International Universities Press.

Winnicott, D. W. (1971). *Therapeutic consultation in child psychiatry.* New York: Basic Books.

Zeanah, C. H., Anders, T. F., Seifer, R., & Stern, D. N. (1989). Implications of research on infant development for psychodynamic theory and practice. *Journal of the American Academy of Child and Adolescent Psychiatry, 28,* 657–668.

Zilbach, J. J. (1986). *Young children in family therapy.* New York: Brunner/Mazel.

Index

n indicates that entry will be found in a footnote